ESSENTIAL MEDICINE

This book is to be returned on or before
the last date stamped below.

For Churchill Livingstone:

Publisher: Laurence Hunter
Project Editor: Barbara Simmons
Copy-Editor: Ruth Swan
Project Controller: Nancy Arnott
Design Direction: Erik Bigland

For information on Churchill Livingstone titles, or to place
an order, call:

UK: Freephone 0500 566 242
Europe: +44 131 535 1021
USA/Canada: +1 201 319 9800
Australia/New Zealand: +61 3 9699 5400

ESSENTIAL MEDICINE

Edited by

John Vann Jones PhD FRCP
Professor, Department of Cardiology, Bristol Royal Infirmary

Charles R.V. Tomson MA DM (Oxon) FRCP
Consultant Nephrologist, Southmead Hospital, Bristol

SECOND EDITION

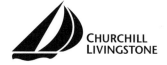

CHURCHILL
LIVINGSTONE

EDINBURGH LONDON MARID MELBOURNE NEW YORK
SAN FRANCISCO AND TOKYO 1998

CHURCHILL LIVINGSTONE
Medical Division of Pearson Professional Limited

Distributed in the United States of America by Churchill
Livingstone Inc., 650 Avenue of the Americas, New York,
N.Y. 10011, and by associated companies, branches and
representatives throughout the world.

First edition edited by A. E. Read and J. Vann Jones 1993
Second edition 1998

Standard edition ISBN 0443 058113

International Student Edition ISBN 0443 058105

British Library of Cataloguing in Publication Data
A catalogue record for this book is available from the British
Library.

Library of Congress Cataloging in Publication Data
A catalog record for this book is available from the Library
of Congress.

Produced by Longman Singapore Publishers (Pte) Ltd
Printed in Singapore

PREFACE

The purpose of this book is to provide a concise account of modern medicine in a format that is easy to read and to revise from. For younger medical students it provides the core, or essential, information about all the common medical conditions, while for more senior students it is designed to be compact but comprehensive. The layout is intended to be easy on the eye, avoiding long uninterrupted pages of text and using colour to highlight important points.

The chapters have all been written by consultants from the Bristol Hospitals. All contributors regularly teach medical students both at the bedside and in more formal surroundings. They have, as a result, an understanding of what the student needs to be competent in medicine and to be able to pass final examinations. Wherever possible, younger consultants were chosen for their enthusiasm and freshness of approach to teaching and writing.

In the brief period since the publication of the first edition, one of the editors of that edition, Professor A. E. Read, has died, as has, prematurely, Professor A. E. Raine, who wrote the renal chapter. Charles Tomson has stepped in to fulfil both roles, but our former colleagues are sadly missed by us all. The new edition, while obviously being brought up to date has, most unusually for a second edition, been reduced in size to make it even more concise and readable. The editors and publishers were very keen that the size and weight of this book should enable it to be taken in a pocket to the bedside or outpatient clinic and for it to be easy to refer to whenever appropriate. Numerous suggestions from readers and course organisers have also been incorporated to bring the text more in line with integrated undergraduate courses.

Present-day medicine has to take into account demographic changes. Care of the elderly is an increasingly complex and respected specialty and we have included a brief separate chapter on this. Air travel has brought tropical and infectious diseases to our hospitals that we may not have seen a few years ago.

It is also commonplace for medical students to spend elective periods abroad, often in exotic places where the pattern of disease is different. We would hope that this book would travel conveniently with them and prove useful.

Genetics is a subject that is increasingly important and the treatment of many diseases in the future may depend on a good knowledge of this subject. Deliberate self-harm is increasing and it has been given extensive coverage in Chapter 17, together with a comprehensive chapter on the psychiatric aspects of disease. All the conventional subjects such as neurology, cardiology, gastroenterology, respiratory medicine, etc, have been covered in considerable detail but concentrating on the basic, or essential, facts.

In this day of increasing demands on student time – even to the extent of some subjects being dropped from the medical curriculum in some medical schools – we feel there is a place for a compact, comprehensive, readable account of general medicine as practised today. We hope we have achieved this with Essential Medicine.

J.V.J.   Bristol
C.R.V.T.   1998

ACKNOWLEDGEMENTS

Plate 11 is reproduced with the kind permission of Professor Neil McIntosh. Plates 13 and 14 are reproduced from Infectious Diseases by A P Ball and J A Gray, Churchill Livingstone, 1992, by kind permission of the authors.

CONTRIBUTORS

Clive B. Archer BSc MD PhD FRCP (London, Edinburgh) Consultant Dermatologist, Bristol Royal Infirmary

Caroline Bell MB MRC Psych
Research Fellow, Bristol Royal Infirmary

Ralph E. Barry BSc MD FRCP
Clinical Dean, Bristol Royal Infirmary

James R. Catterall BSc MD FRCP FRCP (Edinburgh)
Consultant Physician, Bristol Royal Infirmary

David Coates MB BS LRCP MRCS FRCA
Consultant in Anaesthesia and Intensive Care, Bristol Royal Infirmary

Roger J.M. Corrall BSc MD FRCP FRCE
Consultant Physician, Bristol Royal Infirmary

Iain T. Ferguson MD FRCP
Consulant Neurologist, Southmead and Frenchay Hospitals, Bristol

Stuart C. Glover MB ChB (Hons) FRCP FRCPE
Consultant Physician, Southmead Hospital, Bristol

Kenneth W. Heaton MA MD FRCP
Reader in Medicine, Bristol Royal Infirmary

Peter Hollingworth FRCP
Consultant Rheumatologist, Southmead Hospital, Bristol

Richard F. Harvey MD FRCP
Consultant Physician, Frenchay Hospital, Bristol

John R. Kirwan BSc MD FRCP (UK)
Reader in Rheumatology, Bristol Royal Infirmary

Gabriel Laszlo MA MD FRCP
Consultant Physician, Bristol Royal Infirmary

Peter W. Lunt MA MSc FRCP
Consultant Clinical Geneticist, Institute of Child Health, Bristol Children's Hospital

David Nutt DM MRCP FRC Psych
Professor of Psychopharmacology, Bristol Royal Infirmary

Clive J.C. Roberts MD FRCP
Senior Lecturer in Clinical Pharmacology, Bristol Royal Infirmary

A. Jane Scott MB BS
Consultant in Genitourinary Medicine, Bristol Royal Infirmary

Geoffrey L. Scott MD FRCP
Consultant Haematologist, Bristol Royal Infirmary and Weston General Hospital

David Stansbie BSc PhD FRCPath
Consultant in Chemical Pathology, Bristol Royal Infirmary

Patrick K. Taylor FRCOG
Consultant in Genitourinary Medicine, Bristol Royal Infirmary

Charles R.V. Tomson MA DM (Oxon) FRCP
Consultant Nephrologist, Southmead Hospital, Bristol

John Vann Jones PhD FRCP
Professor, Department of Cardiology, Bristol Royal Infirmary

Gordon K. Wilcock BSc DM (Oxon) FRCP
Professor of Care of the Elderly, Frenchay Hospital, Bristol

CONTENTS

1

DISEASES OF THE HEART AND CIRCULATION

John Vann Jones

Diseases of the heart are common the world over. In Western countries ischaemic heart disease predominates while in the Third World rheumatic heart disease remains a major problem. Heart disease often strikes in the prime of life; it is the most common cause of death in males aged 34–65 in industrialised countries. Its treatment and, ultimately, its prevention remain a major health priority in all communities.

ISCHAEMIC HEART DISEASE

Ischaemic heart disease (IHD) is the most common cause of death in the Western World. In males of working age it causes about 40% of all deaths. In underdeveloped countries it remains relatively uncommon but is increasing whereas it has started to decline in the industrialised nations. In the form of heart failure or angina, IHD also greatly contributes to morbidity.

Atheroma (fatty tissue) is deposited in the walls of blood vessels, and the coronary arteries seem particularly susceptible. Atherosclerosis develops and is a complex mixture of fatty deposits, fibrous tissue, smooth muscle proliferation and some blood constituents. Several predisposing, or risk, factors have been identified for IHD.

Risk factors

Irreversible

Age. IHD increases with age. Not only is it more prevalent but it tends to be more devastating with fewer elderly people surviving their first heart attack.

Sex. Females have much lower rates of IHD before the menopause. Later the prevalence increases rapidly until females in their seventies have the same high risks for developing IHD as do males of equivalent age. The role of hormone replacement therapy (HRT) in delaying the onset of IHD remains to be determined.

Family history. There are undoubtedly families with a strong history of IHD in whom none of the other risk factors can be identified. The offspring of such parents are at risk but it is common to find that the parents were heavy smokers or had hypertension and allowance must be made for this when ascribing a genetic influence to the likelihood of IHD.

Premature baldness, premature grey hair and the presence of an arcus senilis (thin line of fatty tissue at the outer edge of the cornea of the eye) before the age of 40 are said to carry some increased risk of IHD.

Reversible

High blood pressure. Hypertension seems to accelerate the atheromatous process and is the major potentially reversible risk factor for IHD.

Smoking. Heavy smokers are at roughly three times the risk of their non-smoking counterparts. All smokers are at substantially less risk if they do not inhale. Usually this means pipe or cigar smoking.

Hyperlipidaemia (elevated blood fat, or lipid, levels). An elevated blood cholesterol level seems to carry an increased risk of premature atherosclerosis which is linearly related over the range of cholesterols found in the population. Unless substantially elevated, triglycerides do not carry a risk of IHD but when both cholesterol and triglyceride levels are elevated the triglycerides appear to contribute additionally to the risk. Increased high density lipoprotein (HDL) cholesterol levels may be protective.

Diet. Low-fat eaters do seem to live longer. The relationship of this to IHD prevention in people with normal lipid levels has not been clearly established. Coffee excess and soft water drinking have also been linked with an increased risk of IHD.

Exercise. Regular exercise lowers both cholesterol levels and blood pressure and such people seem to live longer and have healthier lives.

Stress. The haemodynamic upset of stress can precipitate ischaemic chest pain in those with pre-existing atheroma, e.g. the racing heart and raised blood pressure following an argument. It is doubtful whether stress actually causes atheroma deposition although chronic stress can persistently raise the blood pressure in some people and may therefore have an indirect effect.

Obesity. Obese people have high blood pressure and often hypercholesterol-aemia, latent diabetes or glucose intolerance. When these are not present obesity does not carry a separate risk for IHD but if atheroma is already present these people will be more likely to get chest pain because of the physical exertion involved in getting themselves around.

Race. Racial influences are probably environmental, e.g. Japanese Americans have the same incidence of IHD as do white Americans whereas the Japanese in Japan have a low incidence of IHD. Similarly, as African people become urbanised there is evidence of increasing IHD, which is virtually unknown in rural African communities.

Table 1.1. Symptoms of heart disease

Dyspnoea (breathlessness)
   Classified by the New York Heart Association as
      Grade 1 Uncompromised
      Grade 2 Slightly compromised
      Grade 3 Moderately compromised
      Grade 4 Severely compromised
Orthopnoea—dyspnoea occurring when the patient lies flat
Paroxysmal nocturnal dyspnoea (PND)—dyspnoea often acute and severe occurring during sleep. The patient awakens acutely breathless
Chest pain
Syncope
Palpitations
Fatigue and lethargy

Associated diseases

There are some specific medical conditions predisposing to IHD. The most noteworthy are diabetes hypothyroidism and transplantation. These conditions will be considered in the relevant sections.

Symptoms and signs (Table 1.1)

Angina pectoris

This is a descriptive term for a certain pattern and type of chest pain arising from the ischaemic heart. Retrosternal chest discomfort or pain comes on with exertion and settles within a few minutes with rest or easing back. It may also come on with emotion (which increases the work of the heart) or excitement. Cold weather makes it worse and it may be more obvious shortly after meals. Often the patient is a little breathless (dyspnoeic) and at times the dyspnoeic aspect seems to be dominant.

The pain or discomfort may radiate to either or both arms but more usually to the left, to the jaw or teeth and more unusually through to the back. It is the relationship to exertion or exercise that largely makes the diagnosis but it is important not to confuse movement with exertion: a strained intercostal muscle can give a history that sounds like angina but it is movement rather than exercise that is causing the problem. Similarly, the site of pain or discomfort arising from the heart is never tender to the touch. Indigestion or gastro-oesophageal pain can be confused with angina and unsuspecting patients often initially think they have indigestion, especially as it may present following a meal. The patient with angina pectoris usually has no abnormal physical signs.

Investigations (Table 1.2)

Resting electrocardiogram (ECG) (Fig. 1.1). This is normal in up to 80%

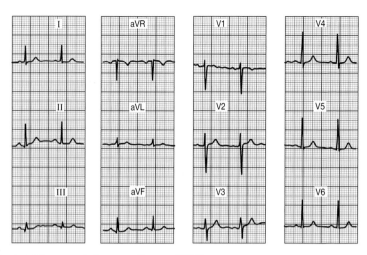

Fig. 1.1 The normal electrocardiogram (ECG).

Table 1.2. Techniques used in the investigation of heart disease

Chest X-ray	
Postero-anterior (PA) to assess	Heart size
	Heart shape
	Specific chamber enlargement, e.g. left atrial size
	Lung fields
	Presence of calcification
Antero-posterior (AP) Left lateral Penetrated PA	Used in selected patients
Electrocardiogram (ECG)	Specific patterns, e.g. infarction
	Rhythm
	Cardiac axis
	Electrical conduction
Exercise electrocardiography	Ischaemic heart disease
Echocardiography	Cardiac anatomy
	Left ventricular function
	Pericardial effusion
	Valve function

of people with angina. When it is abnormal, T wave changes predominate, e.g. inversion or flattening when they should be upright.

Exercise ECG (Fig. 1.2). Between 90 and 95% of people with angina will show changes on an exercise ECG, usually ST segment depression. Exercise

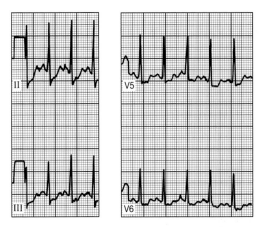

Fig. 1.2 Positive exercise test. ST segment depression has developed with the increased cardiac work of exercise, seen here as a tachycardia.

tests are normally conducted in a standardised way using either a treadmill or a bicycle ergometer. It is possible to obtain false negative and, in females particularly, false positive results.

Not only is the ECG observed during an exercise stress test but so too are the patient and their symptoms. People with false negative exercise tests often give a good description of angina even when the ECG does not change.

Blood pressure should be measured at intervals during an exercise test. A drop in blood pressure usually reflects important myocardial ischaemia but people who are nervous or not used to exercise can develop near faints and this, too, will decrease the blood pressure. Exercise-induced arrhythmias or conduction abnormalities also generally reflect underlying ischaemia while those arrhythmias which disappear with exercise are usually benign.

Radioisotope studies. These can be used to diagnose ischaemia when combined with an exercise test and will further increase the diagnostic rate.

Coronary arteriography. X-ray studies of the coronary arteries are sometimes needed to finally establish a diagnosis. More usually, they are performed where the diagnosis has already been established by exercise ECG testing in order to obtain information prior to consideration for coronary artery surgery or balloon dilatation.

Treatment

Patients told they have angina naturally become anxious. Correct management, therefore, includes:

1. *A full explanation.* Often when patients understand their angina they are better able to cope with it.
2. *Sensible limitation of activity.* The patient should avoid strenuous exertion, e.g. rushing up stairs.

3. *Addressing risk factors*, e.g. smoking, high blood pressure, lipids.
4. *Reducing weight and getting fitter.*
5. *Prescribing glyceryl trinitrate (GTN).* This drug is taken sublingually either as a small tablet or a spray with a metered dose. GTN dilates the coronary arteries and reduces cardiac work by dilating the peripheral arteries and, especially, the veins. It is very potent in relieving angina and works extremely rapidly. The effect of each dose lasts 20–30 minutes.

Often, patients use GTN before situations that might precipitate their angina, e.g. before a winter's walk, after Sunday lunch. At this stage, many patients also start regular aspirin treatment for its antiplatelet effect. Narrowed coronary arteries are often finally blocked off by clotting and aspirin may help to prevent this.

Sustained anti-anginal therapy

If the above simple measures do not control the patient's symptoms then drugs are used. These include long-acting nitrates, beta-adrenergic blocking drugs and the calcium channel blocking agents. They may be used singly or in combination. Patients with severe angina often take all three.

1. Long-acting nitrates. These are chemically related to GTN and may be unpredictable in their response partly because tolerance develops and partly because they are extensively metabolised by the liver. The mononitrates are best. Like GTN they dilate coronary arteries and also, by dilating arteries and veins, they reduce cardiac work and lessen angina. Their principal side-effect is headache, which often settles in a few days. GTN may itself be given percutaneously by means of patches applied to the skin.

2. Beta-adrenergic blocking agents (beta-blockers). These drugs modify the heart's response to exercise so that it works less hard, i.e. the heart rate response is lessened as is the rise in blood pressure. In this way the patient's angina threshold is raised and activity is increased before discomfort begins. Beta-blockers can cause people to feel 'washed out' and lethargic because of a drop in cardiac output. They may also complain of cold limbs. These drugs are contraindicated in heart failure and asthma and relatively contraindicated in peripheral vascular disease, chronic obstructive airways disease and diabetes.

3. Calcium channel blockers. This heterogeneous group of drugs prevents the normal movement of calcium in myocardial cells. They thus reduce energy requirement and oxygen utilisation and are effective in treating angina. Some of the drugs resemble beta-blockers in their actions on the heart, e.g. verapamil and diltiazem, whereas others appear to stimulate the heart, e.g. nifedipine. Flushing, headaches and fluid retention are the major side-effects.

Coronary angioplasty (percutaneous transluminal coronary angioplasty, PTCA)

Patients who fail to respond to medical therapy may be considered for surgery but first a coronary arteriogram is needed. This sometimes shows relatively localised discrete lesions and in some cases these can be dilated using small inflatable balloons.

Coronary artery bypass grafting (CABG)

If the coronary arteriogram shows extensive disease, the patient is referred for surgery where grafts bypassing the coronary lesions will be constructed.

There are three factors that might potentially benefit from surgery.

1. Angina. The operation is very successful in relieving angina with up to 95% of such patients substantially improved or free of pain.

2. Life expectancy. There is increasing evidence that surgery prolongs life. This is established where the proximal left coronary artery is diseased (left mainstem stenosis) and also when all three major branches are affected.

3. Cardiac function. Bypass grafting improves cardiac function in some patients but may reduce it in others. There is no consistent overall benefit.

Prognosis of angina pectoris

The mortality of these patients is 4% per year. The more extensive the disease, the worse the prognosis. It is also worse if the patient's blood pressure drops on exercise, the exercise test is strongly positive, the angina has developed following a myocardial infarct, or if there is heart failure. The prognosis is better if the patient is a non-smoker, has not had heart failure, the resting ECG is normal and there is no history of previous heart damage.

Unstable angina

A few people will follow an accelerated course and may need urgent surgery despite full medical treatment. They are said to have unstable or pre-infarction angina.

Prinzmetal's angina (coronary artery spasm)

In some people the coronary arteries can go into spasm. It is very rare and the ECG usually shows gross ischaemic changes during an attack. Treatment is with nitrates and calcium channel blockers.

MYOCARDIAL INFARCTION

Most myocardial infarctions (MI) occur in relation to an occluded coronary artery. At post-mortem 90% of patients will be found to have a clot blocking their artery where it is already narrowed by atheroma. In some, the vessel is still patent but the flow down it is so poor that the muscle downstream infarcts. In others haemorrhage into the atheromatous plaque occurs.

Symptoms and signs

Chest pain behind the sternum is the most common presentation. It ranges from mild to agonising in its severity but some MIs are silent and not associated with significant pain (especially in the elderly and in those with diabetes).

The pain is usually crushing and may radiate to either arm but especially to the left and to the jaw and neck. The patient is often nauseated, may even vomit, is usually sweaty, and may be breathless particularly if the infarct has resulted in a degree of heart failure.

In an uncomplicated infarct, signs are remarkably few. The heart sounds may be soft and there may be an added third heart sound but often there is remarkably little to find unless a complication has set in. The complications giving rise to physical signs are:

Left ventricular failure. The patient is breathless, usually has a tachycardia and there are crepitations in the lung fields. Third or fourth heart sounds may be heard and give rise to a particular cadence when the heart is listened to which sounds like a horse galloping in the distance (gallop rhythm).

Cardiogenic shock. This occurs when the left ventricular damage is great. The patient is shocked with thready pulses, low blood pressure and tachycardia, usually looks pale owing to constriction of the skin blood vessels (vasoconstriction) and is clammy and sweaty. Prognosis is poor.

Arrhythmias. Most patients have some form of heart rhythm disorder (arrhythmia). Treatment depends on the type of arrhythmia, its consequences (e.g. drop in blood pressure) and its duration.

Inflammation of the pericardium (pericarditis). Pericarditis is one of the causes of continuing pain after MI and there is an associated pericardial rub. This is a superficial scratching sound caused by the surfaces of the inflamed pericardium rubbing together in time to the heartbeat. There is often a respiratory variation as well. It usually passes off within 1–2 days and the rub, in particular, can be very transient.

Mitral valve incompetence. Because the papillary muscles are often involved in the infarction, the mitral valve cusps then become out of alignment and allow degrees of mitral incompetence. In some cases the papillary muscles rupture and so allow free reflux through the damaged valve. A pansystolic murmur of varying intensity is heard over the mitral area. It is usually very loud and obvious if the papillary muscle has ruptured.

Ventricular septal defect (VSD). Occasionally the interventricular septum ruptures and allows a VSD to form. There is a pansystolic murmur at the left sternal edge.

Emboli. These may occur either to the systemic side of the circulation and lead, for example, to strokes or to the pulmonary side giving rise to pulmonary emboli. They are especially common in relation to large infarcts on the anterior surface of the heart.

Investigations

ECG. This shows a characteristic pattern in MI. The dead muscle is no longer electrically active and so the recording leads 'look through' the infarcted area. This generally means that the electrical activity being recorded is moving away from the electrode and is therefore negative. This negative wave is called a Q wave. In the early stages there are usually ST segment changes (Fig. 1.3) as well as various T wave abnormalities, e.g. T wave inversion. Changes occur in leads II, III and aVF for inferior infarcts (Fig. 1.4) and V1–V4 for anterior infarcts (Fig. 1.5). Partial thickness infarcts also give their own ECG appearances (Fig. 1.6).

Enzymes. The dead myocardial cells release enzymes into the blood. Some of those measured, lactate dehydrogenase (LDH) and aspartate transferase

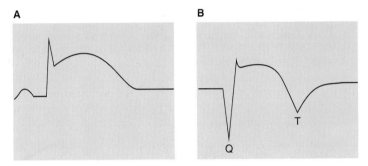

Fig. 1.3 The evolving ECG in myocardial infarction. (A) Acute stage shows ST segment elevation; (B) later stage shows less ST segment elevation together with appearance of Q waves. The T waves are also usually inverted.

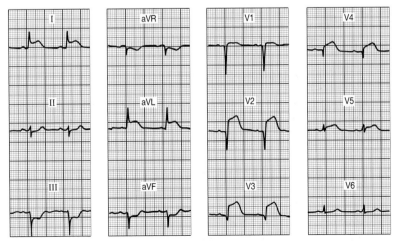

Fig. 1.4 Acute anteroseptal myocardial infarction showing Q waves and ST segment elevation in leads V1–V4. Reciprocal ST segment depression is seen in the inferior leads II, III and aVF.

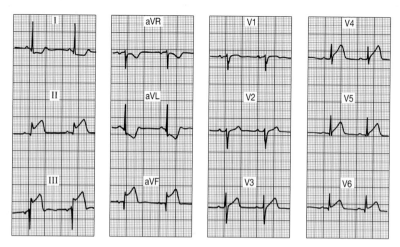

Fig. 1.5 Acute inferior myocardial infarction showing ST segment elevation in the inferior leads II, III and a VF. Q waves have not yet developed. There is reciprocal ST segment depression in I and aVL.

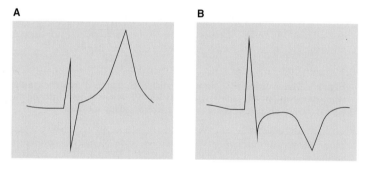

Fig. 1.6 The ECG in partial thickness (non Q-wave) myocardial infarction. (A) Tall peaked symmetrical T waves; and (B) sharp T wave inversion. This type of infarction is sometimes called subendocardial. Tall T waves may also be seen in ischaemia.

(AST), are not specific to the heart and may be released by other tissues, e.g. lung and liver. Creatinine phosphokinase (CPK) is released by damaged muscle and is generally more useful in diagnosis but intramuscular injections, such as might be given for pain relief, can cause an elevation. Only the cardiac isoenzyme is specific for myocardial infarction. The time course of the release of the enzymes differs (Fig. 1.7).

Temperature. This often rises for a few days.

Blood. The white cell count may be raised. The erythrocyte sedimentation rate (ESR) or viscosity may increase as in any major stressful illness. Similarly the blood glucose level may rise, often to quite high values.

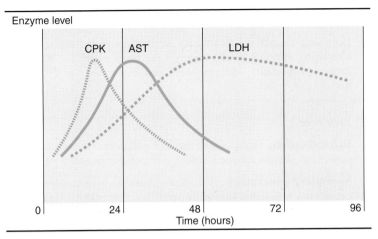

Fig. 1.7 Time course of the release of 'cardiac' enzymes in myocardial infarction.

Treatment

The four broad aims are pain relief, treatment of complications, salvage of the myocardium, and restoration of patency of the coronary arteries. The risk of dying from a heart attack is highest immediately following its onset with most deaths occurring within the first few hours.

Pain relief. This is generally with morphine-based drugs, e.g. diamorphine. These opiates have sedative as well as analgesic properties and may have direct beneficial effects on the circulation, e.g. by decreasing the heart's filling pressure. Opiates typically cause some nausea and even vomiting and an anti-emetic is usually given at the same time (e.g. prochlorperazine). Where pain is not an immediate problem simple sedation with diazepam may suffice to allay anxiety.

Complications. These are treated as they arise, e.g. arrhythmia, heart failure, and will be dealt with in other sections of this chapter.

Myocardial salvage. Intravenous beta-adrenergic blocking drugs limit infarct size. They should be used unless there is a clear contraindication such as heart failure or heart block.

Coronary artery patency. Clot lysing (thrombolytic) agents can restore patency to the vessels and may even prevent infarction if given early enough. They reduce myocardial damage and substantially lower death rates from MI. Aspirin is also effective in this context and, combined with thrombolytic agents, its effects are additive. Suspected infarct patients should be given aspirin as soon as possible.

Commonly used thrombolytic agents are streptokinase, anistreplase and tissue plasminogen activator (TPA). Streptokinase and anistreplase are much cheaper but because of antibody formation cannot be used again within 4 years. Under these circumstances TPA is then used.

Myocardial remodelling

Following an MI the heart may alter shape (remodelling). Angiotensin-converting enzyme (ACE) agents have been shown to modify this with long-term mortality and morbidity benefits, especially if there is cardiac impairment or failure.

Late care

Rehabilitation. Physical training and psychological help enable most MI patients to achieve a better quality, and possibly quantity, of life.

Secondary prevention. Risk factors such as hypertension, smoking and hypercholesterolaemia should be tackled to prevent recurrence.

Oral beta-blockers can also be used. There is good evidence that they are still effective at 1–3 years. All MI patients should be kept on lifelong aspirin treatment.

ARRHYTHMIAS

Rhythm disorders of the heart (arrhythmias) are extremely common.

1. Most arrhythmias are benign. Their importance lies in the symptoms they cause, e.g. palpitations.
2. Some arrhythmias are more serious and can even be life threatening.
3. Arrhythmias are often intermittent.
4. Some arrhythmias represent underlying heart disease, e.g. atrial flutter, whilst some are commonly associated with otherwise normal hearts, e.g. ventricular ectopic beats.

TACHYARRHYTHMIAS

With these arrhythmias the heart rate is fast. For convenience both ventricular and atrial ectopic beats are included in this group. The patients are usually aware of palpitations and may notice the arrhythmia switching on and off. They may notice sudden fatigue and dizziness and sometimes become breathless. They seldom lose consciousness although this often occurs with ventricular tachycardia and inevitably with ventricular fibrillation. They sometimes experience angina when the rate is very rapid and there is underlying IHD.

Often the cause of the arrhythmia is unknown but sometimes it can be brought on by excessive tea or coffee intake or by other cardiac stimulants such as cigarette smoking and alcohol.

Tachyarrhythmias are common with overactivity of the thyroid gland (thyrotoxicosis) or with valvular heart disease. They also occur with IHD and sometimes with high blood pressure. The tachyarrhythmias arising in the atria often occur for no known reason.

Sinus tachycardia

The rhythm is normal, the rate is in excess of 100 beats/min, and it is seen with exercise or excitement, when it is physiological.

Sinus arrhythmia

This is a variant of normal sinus rhythm where the heart rate increases with inspiration and decreases with expiration. The changes in rate can be particularly marked, especially in young people.

Supraventricular ectopic beats

Isolated beats arising from the atria are usually asymptomatic and generally benign. They need no treatment but can give rise to palpitations.

Paroxysmal supraventricular tachycardia (Fig. 1.8)

There are bursts of rapid regular atrial activity. The heart rate is up to 180 beats/min and it tends to occur in young people with basically healthy hearts.

Attacks may last from a few seconds to many days. When they occur

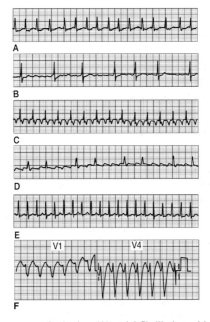

Fig. 1.8 Common arrhythmias: (A) atrial fibrillation with a rapid ventricular rate; (B) atrial fibrillation with a controlled ventricular response; (C) rapid atrial flutter with 2:1 ventricular response (block); (D) atrial flutter with variable block; (E) supraventricular tachycardia; (F) ventricular tachycardia.

frequently they can be a considerable nuisance and may require anti-arrhythmic treatment but more usually they are self-limiting and certain manoeuvres which the patients can carry out themselves may terminate an attack. These include Valsalva manoeuvre (forced expiration against a closed glottis), carotid sinus massage, rubbing an eyeball, taking a cold drink, and immersing the face in cold water. All of these cause activation of the vagus nerve but sometimes drug treatment and, very rarely, correction by means of an electric shock (cardioversion) are required. Few of these patients require long-term therapy. Arrythmias can sometimes be permanently abolished, e.g. by special cardiac catheter techniques (ablation).

Atrial fibrillation (AF) (Fig. 1.8)

AF is very common—approximately one person in ten over the age of 75 is permanently in this rhythm—and it increases in frequency with age.

The atria do not contract properly (fibrillate) and transmit impulses down to the ventricle in a totally irregular manner. Clinically, the major problem is with the rapid rate and treatment is aimed either at correcting the arrhythmia or controlling the heart rate, usually with digoxin. When AF arises in an apparently normal heart it should be converted back to normal sinus rhythm either by drugs or electrically (cardioversion).

AF resistant to drug treatment is often associated with thyrotoxicosis. Troublesome AF can be treated by ablation (destruction) of the atrio-ventricular node together with permanent pacemaker insertion. Over the age of 65, patients with AF should be anticoagulated to prevent embolic strokes.

Atrial flutter

This arrhythmia (Fig. 1.8) usually occurs in diseased hearts, e.g. in rheumatic heart disease. The atria are not contracting normally and again can transmit irregularly to the ventricles giving a clinical appearance similar to AF. However, the ECG shows much coarser waves in the atria called F waves.

Pre-excitation syndromes

Some people have abnormal tracts of tissue connecting the atria to the ventricles (bypass tracts). This allows the atrioventricular node and its heart rate modifying influence to be bypassed (pre-excitation). When these individuals develop atrial arrhythmias the resultant ventricular rate can be very fast and dangerous, e.g. 220–250 beats/min. Bypass tracts occur in the Wolff-Parkinson-White (Fig. 1.9) and Lown-Ganong-Levine syndromes.

Ventricular ectopic beats

Here abnormal (ectopic) beats arise from the ventricles. The pulse feels as though beats are being missed. In fact, the beats are premature (Fig. 1.9) and do not allow the heart enough time to fill; hence no pulse is transmitted peripherally. The heart usually makes up the lost ground with the following

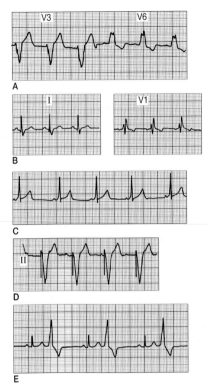

Fig. 1.9 Common ECG appearances: (A) left bundle branch block; (B) right bundle branch block; (C) Wolff-Parkinson-White syndrome, shows short PR interval and slurred upstroke to the QRS complex (delta wave); (D) pacing rhythm; (E) coupled ventricular ectopic beats.

beat so that the sensation to the patient can be one of pauses and thumps. In a small percentage these beats are caused by heart disease but generally they arise in an otherwise sound heart from one focus and, if of the benign variety, tend to go away with exercise. Those arising from diseased hearts tend to increase with the extra strain of exercise.

Benign ventricular ectopic beats seldom require treatment but they can occur up to 40 000 times per day in which case they can cause a lot of distress.

Ectopic beats arising near the T wave of the preceding QRS complex (R on T) or from several different foci can be associated with a risk of serious ventricular arrhythmias.

Ventricular tachycardia

Three or more ectopic beats occurring in rapid sequence is known as ventricular tachycardia (see Fig. 1.8). The rate is usually so rapid that cardiac output falls and ventricular tachycardia may deteriorate to ventricular fibrillation. All patients must be restored to normal rhythm by treatment and if the

Table 1.3. Classification of anti-arrhythmic drugs

Class I	Membrane-stabilising agents, e.g. lignocaine, mexiletene, disopyramide, flecainide, propafenone
Class II	Beta-adrenergic blocking agents
Class III	Prolong action potential duration, e.g. amiodarone, sotalol (also class II agent), bretylium
Class IV	Calcium channel blocking agents, e.g. verapamil, diltiazem

Knowledge of this classification allows a rational approach to drug therapy of arrhythmias, e.g. two agents in the same class would not be used together.

Note digoxin is not classified as an anti-arrhythmic agent in this classification.

episodes are short lived and self terminating, preventive therapy should be initiated either by drugs or an implantable defibrillator.

Ventricular fibrillation (VF)

This is one of the forms of cardiac arrest with the ventricles failing to contract. Cardiac output drops immediately. Within a few seconds the patient will be hypotensive and unconscious. Electrical cardioversion is required and preventive medical therapy (Table 1.3) instituted or an implantable defibrillator inserted where the arrhythmia has been survived and is likely to recur.

BRADYARRHYTHMIAS

These are rhythm disorders where the heart rate is excessively slow.

Sinus bradycardia

Usually defined as sinus rhythm slower than 50 beats/min, this can be quite normal in fit people, e.g. athletes. Drugs such as beta-blocking agents slow the heart rate but, in the elderly, sinus bradycardia often reflects underlying problems with the conduction tissue.

Heart block (Fig. 1.10)

First degree heart block occurs when the PR interval on the ECG is prolonged.

Second degree heart block occurs when there is some dissociation between atrial and ventricular activity, e.g. two atrial contractions for every ventricular one (Mobitz type II). One particular form of second degree heart block occurs when the PR interval progressively lengthens until eventually one P wave is not followed by a QRS complex (Wenckebach phenomenon or Mobitz type I).

Third degree heart block occurs when there is no association between atrial and ventricular activity.

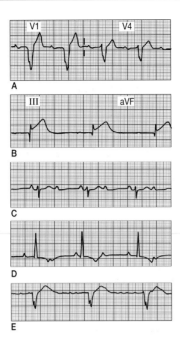

Fig. 1.10 Various types of conduction defect. (A) First degree heart block (long PR interval) with the QRS complexes showing left bundle branch block; (B) first degree heart block in acute inferior myocardial infarction; (C) second degree heart block (Mobitz type II); (D) third degree (complete) heart block; (E) complete heart block in AF. Note that here, despite the fibrillation, the QRS complexes occur at regular intervals.

All three types are usually associated with abnormalities of the conduction tissue with most occurring as part of a degenerative process. IHD is another common cause. Generally, first degree heart block and the Wenckebach phenomenon do not need treatment but second degree heart block otherwise and third degree heart block may need treatment with pacemaker implantation. There is a rare form of congenital complete heart block where the overall heart rate is usually a little faster and pacing may not be required.

Sick sinus syndrome

This syndrome is associated with periods of rapid heart rates and of slow heart rates. No intervention is required in asymptomatic patients but in some the rate is so slow that a pacemaker has to be inserted, or so rapid that drug treatment is needed. It is not uncommon for both forms of treatment to be required. Generally the prognosis in sick sinus syndrome is good.

Cardiac pacemakers

These may be temporary, where the electrodes are inserted into the right ventricle, or permanent, where the electrodes are inserted into the right atrium, the right ventricle or both.

Temporary pacemakers are used while awaiting permanent pacing, e.g. in hospitals with only temporary pacing facilities, or where the conduction defects may reverse, e.g. heart block following an acute inferior MI.

Permanent pacemakers are used in the treatment of irreversible conduction defects. Anti-tachycardia pacemakers can be used to control or terminate rapid arrythmias.

VALVULAR HEART DISEASE

Valvular heart disease (Table 1.4) occurs when the valves become stenosed or incompetent or both. Combinations of valve lesions can occur together but for learning purposes each lesion is best described separately.

Table 1.4. Aetiology of valvular heart disease

Mitral stenosis
  Rheumatic heart disease
  Congenital (very rare)
Mitral incompetence
  Rheumatic heart disease
  Ischaemic heart disease
    papillary muscle
    dysfunction/infarction
    ruptured chordae tendinae
  Prolapsing valve
  Myxomatous degeneration of the
    valve ring
  Secondary to left ventricular
    failure/dilatation
    (functional mitral incompetence)
  Rheumatic disease
    rheumatoid arthritis
    ankylosing spondylitis
  Rupture of the chordae tendinae
  Infective endocarditis
  Other rare causes
    ostium primum atrial septal
      defect
    hypertrophic cardiomyopathy
    Marfan's syndrome
Aortic stenosis
  Rheumatic heart disease
  Congenital (often bicuspid valves)
  Degenerative (usually biscuspid
    valves)

Aortic incompetence
  Rheumatic heart disease
  Congenital (often bicuspid valves)
  Hypertension
  Rheumatic diseases
    ankylosing spondylitis
    rheumatoid arthritis
  Infective endocarditis
  Marfan's syndrome
  Secondary to aortic dissection
  Syphilis and yaws
Tricuspid stenosis
  Rheumatic heart disease
Tricuspid incompetence
  Secondary to right heart failure
    (functional tricuspid
    incompetence)
  Rheumatic heart disease
  Infective endocarditis (notably
    drug addicts)
Pulmonary stenosis
  Congenital
Pulmonary incompetence
  Secondary to pulmonary
    hypertension
  Congenital

Table 1.5. Diagnosis of rheumatic fever. This is made if two major, or one major and two minor, criteria are present

Major criteria	Minor criteria
Chorea (Sydenham's—called St Vitus' dance) Carditis Migrating polyarthritis Subcutaneous nodules Erythema marginatum	Raised ASO titre Other evidence of recent streptococcal infection Fever Raised white cell count (leukocytosis) Arthralgia Elevated ESR or viscosity Increased C-reactive protein Prolonged PR interval on the ECG

MITRAL STENOSIS

Mitral stenosis usually develops many years after an attack of rheumatic fever (Table 1.5). It occurs more commonly in females but is now becoming rare as rheumatic fever dies out in developed countries. Rheumatic fever and subsequently rheumatic heart disease are still extremely common in under-developed countries.

Symptoms

1. Dyspnoea.
2. Palpitations, from atrial fibrillation which may be intermittent at first but usually becomes permanent.
3. Frequent winter chest infections.
4. Haemoptysis.
5. Effects of systemic emboli: clots form in the enlarged left atrium, especially if it is fibrillating, and may dislodge and result in strokes, ischaemic limbs, etc.

Signs

1. Malar flush (mitral facies), seen as a plethoric colour high on both cheeks.
2. The irregularly irregular pulse of atrial fibrillation.
3. Tapping apex beat. The stenosed mitral valve prevents blood from entering the left ventricle which is underfilled. As a result the apex beat feels like a tap on the chest wall.
4. A heave at the left sternal edge from right ventricular enlargement, found when pulmonary hypertension develops.
5. Loud first heart sound over the mitral area. It may even be palpable to the touch. There is also an opening snap audible in early diastole. Both are only heard if the valve is mobile and are lost when it becomes stiff and calcified.

6. Loud second heart sound in the pulmonary area when pulmonary hypertension develops.

7. Rumbling low pitched mid-diastolic murmur heard at the apex. It may be better heard after exercise or by turning the patient to the left. Later in diastole if the patient remains in sinus rhythm the murmur may be accentuated due to atrial contraction—so-called pre-systolic accentuation.

Investigations

ECG usually shows atrial fibrillation but there may be left atrial hypertrophy (P mitrale) if sinus rhythm persists. Sometimes right ventricular hypertrophy also occurs (R wave larger than S wave in V1 ± T wave inversion in leads V2 and V3).

Chest X-ray. There is usually cardiomegaly and left atrial enlargement, i.e. double shadow on the right heart border, enlargement of the left atrial appendage seen as a bulge below the left pulmonary artery (usually the border is concave here) and widening of the bifurcation of the trachea. The upper lobe blood vessels may become more prominent as pulmonary congestion develops.

Echocardiography, now the most useful investigation for confirming the diagnosis and assessing its severity (Fig. 1.11).

Cardiac catheterisation, now largely restricted to preoperative assessment.

Treatment

Complications are treated medically: digoxin for AF, diuretics for heart failure and anticoagulants to prevent clot formation and embolisation. The valve may be dilated surgically (mitral valvotomy) or replaced. It may also be stretched by a balloon–mitral valvuloplasty.

MITRAL INCOMPETENCE

Mitral incompetence has many causes (see Table 1.4) and is relatively common. It may develop rapidly, e.g. post-MI when a papillary muscle ruptures, or gradually, e.g. after rheumatic fever.

Symptoms

When acute dypsnoea and pulmonary congestion dominate. When chronic, the symptoms are similar to those of mitral stenosis (see p. 19), palpitations are less common and emboli occur but less often.

Signs

1. Collapsing pulse, less marked than with aortic incompetence and sometimes referred to as the 'mini collapsing' pulse.

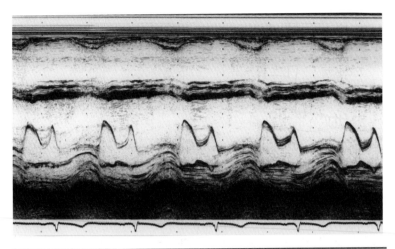

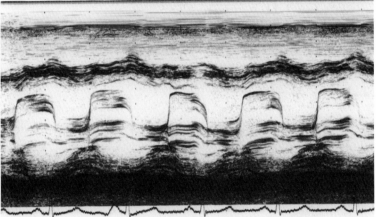

Fig. 1.11 Echocardiogram of normal mitral valve (top) showing the characteristic M shape. The lower trace is typical of mitral stenosis.

2. Sustained apex beat, often displaced towards the left.
3. Left parasternal heave of right ventricular hypertrophy develops with the onset of pulmonary hypertension.
4. Soft first heart sound at the apex as the cusps of the valve fail to come together properly.
5. Loud pulmonary second sound when pulmonary hypertension develops.
6. Pansystolic murmur heard at the apex and out towards the axilla and extending throughout the whole of systole.
7. As blood passes from the left atrium to the ventricle a further heart sound may be heard early in diastole over the apex (third heart sound).

Investigations

ECG usually shows sinus rhythm but can also show atrial fibrillation. Left atrial enlargement (P mitrale) occurs, as will left ventricular hypertrophy in more severe cases (S wave in V1 and R wave in V5 or V6 total > 35 mm).

Chest X-ray. Usually some degree of cardiomegaly is seen but signs of left atrial enlargement are less clearcut than they are with mitral stenosis. Upper lobe blood diversion may occur.

Echocardiography. Modern echocardiograms confirm the diagnosis and can give a good estimate of its severity.

Cardiac catheterisation. A left ventricular angiogram confirms the extent of the leak. It is largely restricted to preoperative assessment.

Treatment

Treatment may be medical, with digoxin for AF and diuretics for pulmonary congestion. Anticoagulants are used when there is evidence of left atrial enlargement and AF develops.

Surgery involves either replacing the valve (in most cases) or repairing it (in a few).

Functional mitral incompetence secondary to heart failure often improves as the heart failure is brought under control.

AORTIC STENOSIS

Aortic stenosis is usually degenerative, often occurring on previously bicuspid valves, and presentation is commonly in later life. Some are congenital and may present at any age. Those secondary to rheumatic fever often also have mitral valve involvement and present in middle age.

Symptoms

1. Angina. The left ventricle hypertrophies and outgrows its blood supply while the aortic pressure, and hence coronary artery pressure, gradually falls as the valve stenosis develops.
2. Syncope due to heart block which develops as the valve and surrounding tissue calcify. Syncope on exertion (effort syncope) also occurs.
3. Dyspnoea from pulmonary congestion.
4. Palpitations. Left atrial pressure may rise leading to atrial arrhythmias such as AF.
5. Occasionally sudden death occurs.

Patients with aortic stenosis are often asymptomatic because of the very considerable reserves of the left ventricle. The onset of symptoms is therefore very important and early investigation and treatment are indicated.

Signs

A slow rising pulse is present. The blood pressure is low for the age together with a low pulse pressure. A sustained powerful apex beat is not generally displaced until heart failure develops. A thrill can sometimes be felt over the aortic area, in the carotid arteries or in the suprasternal notch.

The second heart sound is soft over the aortic area, especially when the valve becomes calcified and immobile. In younger people there may be an early systolic sound—the so-called ejection click. The murmur is a harsh ejection systolic murmur best heard over the aortic area and lower left sternal edge. It radiates well to the carotid arteries.

Investigations

ECG usually shows left ventricular hypertrophy and may also show ischaemia (so-called left ventricular strain pattern).

Chest X-ray shows a bulky but not grossly enlarged heart (Fig. 1.12). There is dilatation of the early part of the ascending aorta (post-stenotic dilatation). The lateral chest X-ray may demonstrate calcification in the valve. When heart failure ensues the heart enlarges.

Echocardiography confirms the diagnosis and gives a reliable assessment of its severity.

Cardiac catheterisation is reserved for cases of doubt or for preoperative assessment.

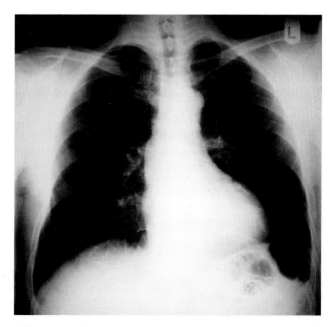

Fig. 1.12 Postero-anterior (PA) X-ray of the heart in aortic stenosis. The heart is not enlarged but looks bulky while the aorta is dilated just at its origin (post-stenotic dilatation).

Treatment

When the patient becomes symptomatic an aortic valve replacement is needed. In some younger patients the valve may be split (aortic valvotomy). In a few elderly patients, in the young, or in those too ill for surgery, balloon dilatation of the valve is occasionally performed (aortic valvuloplasty).

AORTIC INCOMPETENCE

Symptoms

The symptoms of aortic incompetence are similar to those of aortic stenosis except that syncope occurs much less often. The heart seems to be able to cope well with aortic incompetence and judging the timing of valve replacement can be very difficult. Aortic incompetence has many causes (see Table 1.4). Sometimes, there are also additional complicating features, such as aneurysms of the aorta in syphilis and in Marfan's syndrome.

Signs

1. Collapsing or 'waterhammer' pulse.
2. Prominent arterial pulsations, e.g. the carotid arteries (Corrigan's sign).
3. High systolic and low diastolic blood pressure, i.e. wide pulse pressure.
4. Often, it is not possible to determine Korotkoff's fifth sound.
5. Quincke's sign (nailbed capillary pulsation).
6. Dancing retinal arteries (pulsating retinal vessels) on fundoscopy.
7. Sustained apex beat which is displaced.
8. Soft aortic second sound.
9. High-pitched early diastolic murmur best heard at the lower left sternal edge and over the aortic area. It is classically described as blowing.
10. There may be an ejection systolic murmur over the same areas. This results from the large volume of blood having to be ejected at each systole and does not necessarily mean that the patient also has aortic stenosis.
11. Mid-diastolic murmur at the apex. The regurgitant jet of aortic blood may impinge upon the mitral valve resulting in a murmur there. This is the Austin-Flint murmur and, again, does not mean that the patient has mitral stenosis.

Investigations

ECG may show left ventricular hypertrophy and strain pattern.

Chest X-ray shows cardiomegaly together with dilatation of the whole of the ascending aorta. It is more extensive and prominent than the post-stenotic dilatation of aortic stenosis.

Echocardiography confirms the diagnosis and can assess the severity.

Cardiac catheterisation. An injection of contrast into the aorta (aortogram) at cardiac catheterisation can also quantify the leak in the valve.

Aortic incompetence is well tolerated but if symptoms develop an aortic valve replacement is required.

TRICUSPID STENOSIS

Tricuspid stenosis is almost invariably secondary to rheumatic fever and as such occurs with rheumatic mitral or aortic valve disease which tend to dominate the clinical picture. There may be disproportionate venous and hepatic congestion and the liver may pulsate. It is often discovered coincidentally at echocardiography or cardiac catheterisation when the other valves are being investigated. Right atrial hypertrophy may be seen on the ECG and enlargement on the chest X-ray. Treatment is by tricuspid valvotomy and insertion of a supporting ring (annuloplasty).

TRICUSPID INCOMPETENCE

Tricuspid incompetence is usually secondary to right heart failure; it occurs when the right ventricle enlarges sufficiently to stretch the valve ring. The clinical picture is of dilated neck veins with prominent 'V' waves, a pulsatile enlarged liver and peripheral and sacral oedema and, if severe, ascites may also develop. It can disappear dramatically with resolution of the heart failure but annuloplasty may be required. Occasionally valve replacement is needed.

PULMONARY STENOSIS

Pulmonary stenosis is usually congenital. It is often asymptomatic, detected at a medical examination. There may be a palpable thrill over the pulmonary area and a harsh ejection murmur radiating out into the lung fields. Even in mild cases the pulmonary arteries may be prominent on X-ray (from post-stenotic dilatation). In severe cases the ECG shows right atrial and right ventricular hypertrophy. Echocardiography and, if needed, cardiac catheterisation confirm the diagnosis and give a reliable measure of its severity. Balloon dilatation is the treatment of choice although surgery may be needed in some cases.

PULMONARY INCOMPETENCE

Pulmonary incompetence is caused by pulmonary hypertension. The latter and its cause dominate the clinical picture and the pulmonary incompetence is largely a coincidental finding. Loud second heart sounds and an early diastolic murmur are heard in the pulmonary area and high left sternal edge.

INFECTIVE ENDOCARDITIS

This term now includes subacute bacterial endocarditis (SBE) and acute bacterial endocarditis (ABE).

SUBACUTE BACTERIAL ENDOCARDITIS

Aetiology

Streptococcus viridans (the common dental organism). This now causes 30–50% of cases; in the past it was even more common. *Strep. epidermidis, Strep. faecalis, Staphylococcus aureus* and *Haemophilus influenzae* are other causative organisms.

In about 10% of cases the organism cannot be grown from the bloodstream and unusual infections, such as Q fever and those caused by chlamydia, anaerobes or fungi, should be sought. The latter are particularly important where prosthetic valves have been inserted.

Symptoms and signs

SBE usually presents very insidiously with weight loss, vague ill health, loss of appetite and energy and fever. Diagnosis is difficult but eventually some helpful physical signs may appear, such as finger clubbing, small linear haemorrhages in the nailbeds of the hands and toes (splinter haemorrhages), painful nodules on the fingers (Osler's nodes), splenomegaly, small haemorrhagic spots in the optic fundi and probably resulting from arteritis (Roth's spots) and subconjunctival haemorrhages.

Microscopic haematuria and proteinuria are present in about 60% of patients, usually reflecting immune-complex-mediated glomerulonephritis.

About 85% of the patients have a heart murmur, which may change in the course of the illness. Infective endocarditis typically develops on the valves of the heart but it may also occur on the heart wall, e.g. in the right ventricle opposite a ventricular septal defect (VSD).

Heart failure may result and can develop suddenly as valves perforate or are destroyed. SBE generally develops in relation to an underlying cardiac abnormality. It more usually occurs where there is high pressure turbulence, e.g. with a VSD or in aortic stenosis. It is, therefore, relatively rare in mitral stenosis and atrial septal defects. Patients with a patent ductus arteriosus are particularly at risk. There must be bacteraemia for endocarditis to occur and this is particularly liable to happen with dental work or gastrointestinal surgery.

Investigations

Blood cultures must be taken before antibiotic treatment is started. Usually six blood cultures are sufficient (i.e. two batches of three).

A full blood count viscosity and ESR. These patients usually have a normocytic normochromic anaemia and a raised ESR. There is often a raised white cell count.

Complement levels are low with increased complement degradation products, reflecting consumption.

Echocardiography detects vegetations on the valves. Absence of vegetations does not exclude infective endocarditis. Echocardiography can be extremely useful in monitoring progress of the condition and identifying the underlying cardiac abnormality.

Treatment

Antibiotics should be administered intravenously for up to 4 weeks. A switch to oral antibiotics can be made before this time if the organism is very sensitive. Often, both penicillin and an aminoglycoside are used to potentiate each other. The blood levels of the antibiotics should be checked and titrated against their cidal (i.e. effective killing) levels of the organism. With prosthetic valves up to 6 weeks of intravenous treatment is advocated. During treatment it may become apparent that the infection is progressing remorselessly or that the valves or renal function are deteriorating. All of these are indications for surgery.

ACUTE BACTERIAL ENDOCARDITIS (ABE)

This is a much rarer condition and tends to be seen in people who are either immunosuppressed or subjected to overwhelming infection, e.g. drug addicts. Infection often develops on normal valves and the tricuspid valve can be affected, which is unusual with SBE. *Staph. aureus* is a common organism; it is highly destructive and associated with a high overall mortality.

CARDIOMYOPATHY

These are conditions that primarily affect cardiac muscle itself.

DILATED CARDIOMYOPATHY

Some cases may follow a previous infection (myocarditis) of the heart muscle or may be due to end-stage hypertension. Other cases are alcohol induced or associated with thyrotoxicosis. In most people, congestive or dilated cardiomyopathy is of unknown aetiology; they usually present with severely dilated hearts and heart failure.

Treatment is that of heart failure and removal of the cause, if possible. The majority deteriorate steadily and die within a few years of diagnosis if transplantation is not possible.

HYPERTROPHIC CARDIOMYOPATHY

This used to be called hypertrophic obstructive cardiomyopathy (HOCM). The cardiac muscle hypertrophies in a disorganised way eventually obliterating the cardiac chamber. It may be due to autosomal dominant mutations in the beta myosin heavy chain gene, or sporadic. The patients present with rhythm disorders, breathlessness, heart failure, angina and syncope. The ECG is often grossly abnormal but the echocardiogram is characteristic showing asymmetrical hypertrophy, especially of the interventricular septum. This also results in a peculiar systolic anterior motion of the mitral valve. The aortic valve also closes early.

Treatment is with anti-arrhythmic agents, especially amiodarone. Beta-blockers and verapamil have also been used but when heart failure supervenes diuretics may be needed. In symptomatic patients, progress is often remorse-less and life expectancy poor unless heart transplantation is performed.

RESTRICTIVE CARDIOMYOPATHY

This rare form of cardiomyopathy is usually caused by amyloid infiltration of the heart. It restricts movement of the left ventricle, hence the name. Clinically, the differentiation from constrictive pericarditis is important as the latter can be treated surgically whereas restrictive cardiomyopathy cannot.

DISSECTION OF THE AORTA

In patients with high blood pressure or atheromatous plaques of the aorta, blood can track into the aortic wall, travelling for a variable distance and then re-entering the aorta itself. The outcome is decided by the distance, the re-entry point and the extent of the damage it causes en route. It may extend from just above the aortic valve all the way down beyond the renal arteries. Hypertension is the common predisposing factor but there are associations with Marfan's syndrome, coarctation of the aorta, bicuspid aortic valves and unfortunately with the third trimester of pregnancy. Three types have been described (Fig. 1.13):

1. Type 1 affects the ascending aorta and around the arch and is generally the most extensive.
2. Type 2 affects the ascending aorta.
3. Type 3 affects the descending aorta.

These are thoracic aneurysms but, of course, many aneurysms also occur in

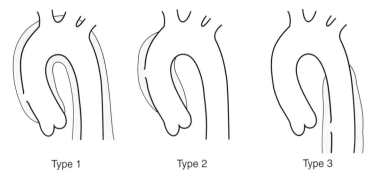

Type 1   Type 2   Type 3

Fig. 1.13 Types of aortic dissection.

the abdomen. The treatment of choice for descending thoracic dissections is medical but surgical repair is required for types 1 and 2 and intra-abdominal aneurysms.

On examination all the arteries coming off the arch should be checked, i.e. the radials and the carotids. Often the renal arteries are affected and the femoral arteries should also be checked. The dissection may cause the aortic valve to become incompetent and sometimes blood leaks into the pericardial sac or into the pleural space.

The chest X-ray shows a broad mediastinum and the various scanning techniques of the aorta such as ultrasound, computed tomography (CT) or magnetic resonance imaging (MRI) may delineate the exact extent of the problem. Aortograms can be dangerous in this situation but are occasionally needed.

In all cases treatment is initially medical with bedrest, pain relief and lowering of the blood pressure but surgery may be required urgently for dissections involving other major arteries or the ascending aorta.

CARDIAC TUMOURS

Cardiac tumours are very rare. Myxomas are the most common, usually occurring in the left atrium. Occasionally they occur elsewhere in the heart and sometimes recur after surgical removal. They are diagnosed by echocardiography. There is a high risk of embolisation and they should be removed by surgery as soon as possible.

MYOCARDITIS

Acute infection of the heart rarely leads to clinical problems. However, occasionally myocarditis mimics MI and it is thought that it can also progress to congestive or dilated cardiomyopathy in some patients.

In South America, Chagas' disease, caused by trypanosomiasis, is a common infection causing myocarditis and leading on to cardiomyopathy.

PERICARDITIS

Pericarditis may be acute or chronic. Acute pericarditis is usually the result of a viral infection and is self limiting. It can, however, be part of the clinical picture of MI and also occurs in uraemia.

Pericarditis causes a superficial scratching sound over the heart that occurs in time with the heartbeat. It may also vary with respiration.

The ECG may show ST segment elevation which is concave upwards and present in most, if not all, of the leads.

In benign pericarditis the condition tends to be self limiting although anti-inflammatory drugs may occasionally be needed to ease the pain.

CONSTRICTIVE PERICARDITIS

In this condition the pericardium is thick and stiff and impairs cardiac filling. It may even be calcified and it used to be largely secondary to tuberculous infection.

Impaired filling of the heart may give rise to physical signs such as ascites and hepatomegaly. The venous pressure is usually raised and increases with inspiration (Kussmaul's sign). The heart itself may be largely impalpable which is out of keeping with the other physical signs, and a loud third heart sound may be audible (the pericardial knock).

The ECG is usually of low voltage and the chest X-ray shows a round heart (Fig. 1.14) often with calcium in the pericardium, more easily seen on a lateral film.

Likewise, the echocardiogram may show dense echoes around the heart. Besides tuberculosis, other causes are trauma, rheumatoid arthritis, uraemia or secondary to neoplastic disease.

PERICARDIAL EFFUSION

Fluid may gather in the pericardial sac. This is most commonly seen in heart failure or secondary to neoplastic involvement. When fluid gathers, the

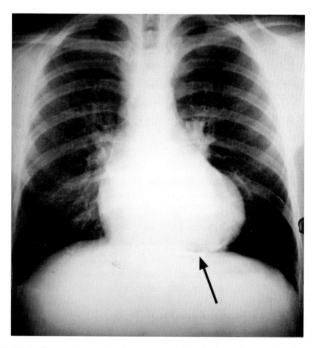

Fig. 1.14 Chest X-ray in constrictive pericarditis. The heart is large and very round in shape. Calcification (better seen on a lateral film) is noted on the diaphragmatic surface of the heart

heart becomes compressed, resulting in pericardial tamponade. The physical signs represent those of impaired cardiac filling with a raised jugular venous pressure (JVP), a large liver, ascites, peripheral oedema and 'pulsus paradoxus'—a fall in blood pressure during active inspiration of more than 10 mmHg (which is not in fact paradoxical, but an exaggeration of normal). The heart sounds are soft and distant.

The chest X-ray shows a round enlarged heart and there are low voltages on the ECG. Echocardiography is by far the best way of detecting and quantifying pericardial effusions. An echo-free space is seen behind the heart and also anteriorly if the effusion is large. Because of the risk of infection, effusions should not be drained unless they are causing acute hypotension ('cardiac tamponade'). If the effusion is caused by neoplastic disease, tapping the effusion may be required to help with the diagnosis.

HEART FAILURE

Heart failure occurs when the output of the heart is incapable of meeting the demands of the tissues. There may, therefore, be high output failure when the demands are excessive, e.g. in thyrotoxicosis and anaemia, or low output failure where the heart itself is defective, e.g. following an MI. Many other terms have been used to describe heart failure, e.g. left heart failure, right heart failure, congestive cardiac failure, backward failure, forward failure, etc. In practice when either ventricle is failing, the other is seldom left unaffected. Failure of the left ventricle causes pressure increases upstream, i.e. in the lungs, which ultimately affect the right ventricle and may cause it to fail. When the heart fails, several endocrine and renal compensatory mechanisms are set in force.

Salt and water retention. Patients with heart failure retain fluid, which gives rise to many of the physical signs, e.g. peripheral oedema or pulmonary crepitations and pulmonary oedema. The renin–angiotensin system is activated and aldosterone and vasopressin levels increase.

Vasoconstriction. In order to preserve the blood supply to the vital organs, the blood supply to the less important areas, i.e. the skin and muscles, may be reduced. Therefore the patient often looks very pale or even cyanosed. This is due to activation of the sympathetic nervous system. Knowledge of these various compensatory mechanisms, many of which in the long term can be disadvantageous, has allowed a rational approach to therapy.

Aetiology (Table 1.6)

Certain drugs depress myocardial contractility; for example beta-blockers can cause an impaired heart to fail. Others can cause fluid retention (e.g. corticosteroids) or even damage the heart (e.g. some anti-cancer drugs).

Heart failure may also be secondary to other conditions such as hypothyroidism, hyperthyroidism, anaemia, diabetes, hypertension and obesity.

Table 1.6. Aetiology of heart failure (low output)

Heart muscle disease	Arrhythmias*
Myocardial infarction/ischaemia	Atrial fibrillation
Cardiomyopathy	Atrial flutter
Myocarditis	Complete heart block
Pressure overload	Other causes
Hypertension	Constrictive pericarditis
Aortic stenosis	Pericardial tamponade
Volume overload	
Mitral incompetence	
Aortic incompetence	

*If they persist, even benign arrhythmias such as supraventricular tachycardia (SVT) can lead to heart failure.

However, ischaemic and valvular heart disease are by far the most common causes.

Symptoms and signs

The symptoms and signs depend very much on whether failure predominantly affects the left or right side of the heart.

Left-sided heart failure is associated with dyspnoea, tachycardia, low blood pressure and thready low volume pulse. The patient is often pale, clammy and sweaty but in compensated or treated heart failure most of these physical signs are absent.

There may be crepitations in the lung fields and examination of the heart may reveal a cause for the failure, e.g. aortic stenosis. In other cases the heart may be enlarged, the quality of the heart sounds is generally poor, and there may be additional heart sounds, e.g. a third or fourth heart sound.

If failure is predominantly right sided, or if right-sided failure is present in addition to left-sided failure, venous pressure is usually elevated and can be seen as a raised JVP in the neck.

The liver may be enlarged and may be pulsatile. There is usually peripheral oedema in the lower limbs if the patient is upright and over the lower end of the back if the patient is confined to bed (sacral oedema).

Ultimately fluid may gather in the abdomen (ascites); this is a sign of very severe heart failure. Enlargement and congestion of the liver may cause nausea, tenderness over the liver, and jaundice.

Investigations

These patients are often unwell and investigation commonly follows treatment.

ECG. This is helpful in determining whether the patient may have had an

MI and also for showing any abnormal rhythm patterns. It may also demonstrate hypertrophy as occurs in hypertension or aortic stenosis. The ECG is seldom normal in heart failure.

Chest X-ray (Fig. 1.15) is occasionally helpful in determining the cause of heart failure but more usually simply confirms an enlarged heart with the appearance of fluid in the lung fields. Pleural effusions may be present.

Echocardiography is particularly useful in the assessment of left ventricular function and may also identify any valvular abnormality.

Cardiac catheterisation is needed in some cases, e.g. to exclude a left ventricular aneurysm.

Treatment

Treatment depends upon whether the onset of the heart failure is acute or chronic. In all forms of heart failure, symptomatic treatment is initiated to be followed by treatment of the underlying cause.

ACUTE LEFT VENTRICULAR FAILURE (LVF)

The onset of LVF is often extremely sudden. It may first occur in the middle of the night when redistribution of blood from the lower limbs to the chest is the final straw for the failing heart. Likewise, an acute onset of a rhythm disorder or undue physical exertion may be the precipitating

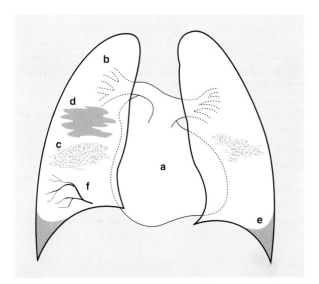

Fig. 1.15 The postero-anterior (PA) chest X-ray findings in heart failure. (**a**) An enlarged heart; (**b**) upper lobe blood diversion, i.e. prominent upper lobe pulmonary vessels; (**c**) fluid in the lung fields; (**d**) fluid in the lung fissures; (**e**) pleural effusions; (**f**) prominent lung lymphatics—Kerley B lines.

factor. The patient is usually acutely breathless, very distressed and unable to communicate.

Treatment

1. The patient should be sat upright and 100% oxygen administered. The upright position reduces venous return to the heart and also takes pressure off the diaphragm.
2. A loop diuretic, e.g. frusemide, is given intravenously.
3. Intravenous opiates, e.g. morphine; in addition to the psychological relief they bring, these drugs also benefit left ventricular function.
4. Digoxin. The use of digoxin in acute heart failure is controversial. It has a slow onset of action and can cause arrhythmias.
5. Some patients do not respond to the above measures and vasodilators can then be used. Glyceryl trinitrate (GTN) reduces both preload and afterload and can be used both sublingually or intravenously. Other drugs used occasionally in this context are sodium nitroprusside, hydralazine and prazosin.
6. Aminophylline has been used to dilate the airways. It also increases both heart rate and myocardial contractility but it may induce arrhythmias and has to be used carefully, if at all.

CHRONIC LEFT VENTRICULAR FAILURE

Chronic LVF can range from mild to very severe. The former is often simply managed by diuretics, but recently the ACE inhibitors have been used at this stage as are oral nitrates. The arterial vasodilators hydralazine and prazosin can be substituted where ACE inhibitors are contraindicated.

Bedrest is very important. All patients are well advised to have a siesta and in more severe cases a few days in bed often reduces the work of the heart enough for it to at least partially recover. Reduction of sodium and water intake may be necessary.

The treatment of the causes of LVF is described under the various headings, i.e. arrhythmia, MI, valvular heart disease, etc.

RIGHT VENTRICULAR FAILURE

Right ventricular failure (RVF) is almost always secondary to LVF although it can occur in its own right with pulmonary hypertension or pulmonary valve disease. Treatment is essentially similar to that of LVF.

HYPERTENSION

In Western societies blood pressure increases with age. In young women it is generally a little lower than in young men but crossover occurs in middle age so that elderly females have higher blood pressures than elderly men.

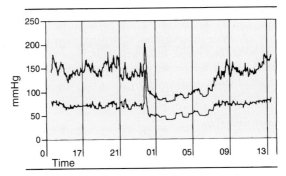

Fig. 1.16 Ambulatory intra-arterial blood pressure recording showing systolic and diastolic pressures over a 24-hour period. Note the wide variations in pressure that occur over this period with the characteristic fall during sleep.

Except for extremely low blood pressures, there is a linear relationship between the level of blood pressure and cardiovascular risk.

Blood pressure is very labile (Fig. 1.16). Anxiety (the alerting response) can artificially elevate the blood pressure and it is well known that doctors can induce this response—white coat hypertension.

Many blood pressure measurements have to be taken before classifying a patient as hypertensive. As treatment for high blood pressure is generally life-long, the diagnosis has to be secure before starting treatment.

Except for the malignant phase, hypertension is an asymptomatic disorder so when treatment is instituted it is important that it causes no symptoms. Lack of compliance is one of the great difficulties in managing hypertension. It is thought that about 10% of the population have significantly elevated blood pressures; many of these are undetected and many are detected but not managed properly. The quality of care in hypertension is all important to the outcome.

IDIOPATHIC HIGH BLOOD PRESSURE

In most people, no cause can be found for the high blood pressure. This is called primary or essential hypertension and there is often a family history.

Obesity. Obese people have higher blood pressures in the main than slim people and worthwhile reductions in blood pressure can be obtained by weight loss.

Alcohol. There is a roughly linear relationship between alcohol intake in units and blood pressure.

Salt intake. People with high blood pressure should be discouraged from adding salt to their food.

Exercise. Exercise is anti-hypertensive and a combination of increased exercise and weight loss can be very effective in reducing blood pressure.

A cause can be found for hypertension in 2–3% of middle-aged people. Even then, the treatment is very much as for essential hypertension with the result that extensive investigation of hypertension in middle and later life has largely been abandoned. In 20-year-olds, however, there is a 50% chance of detecting one of the causes of secondary hypertension and they should be investigated more exhaustively.

Symptoms and signs

History taking and physical examination are very important. Certain drugs can cause hypertension and enquiries should be made about them, e.g. the oral contraceptive pill. Absence of a family history of hypertension, a rapid increase in blood pressure over 1–2 years, and abnormal urinalysis all suggest secondary hypertension.

The influence of high blood pressure on the target organs, e.g. the heart, blood vessels, kidneys and brain, should be sought. The risk to the cardio-vascular system of any given level of blood pressure is increased 4- or 5-fold in the presence of target organ damage.

Hypertension is usually asymptomatic, except in malignant hypertension (rare) where fibrinoid necrosis of small blood vessels occurs. This gives rise to a systemic illness with weight loss, loss of appetite and general malaise. These patients have protein and blood in the urine with changes in the optic fundi and, untreated, their outlook is poor.

In the remainder of hypertensives, the physical signs are more subtle.

1. The heart may be enlarged clinically but generally in pressure overload the heart hypertrophies concentrically inwards so that the apex is left ventricular in type but not displaced.
2. The optic fundi should always be examined as this is the only place in the body where arteries can be viewed directly. The classification of Keith and Wagener is used to describe them (Table 1.7).
3. The abdomen should be examined for masses (phaeochromocytoma), the kidneys palpated, and the urine tested for protein and blood.
4. Renal artery bruits may be heard on either side of the umbilicus or just below the ribs at the back in renal artery stenosis.
5. Femoral arteries should be palpated and in coarctation of the aorta the femoral arteries are diminished and the pulse delayed. Abnormal blood vessels in coarctation may be detected over the back near the scapulae where they may be both felt and pulsations heard. In coarctation the blood pressure should be checked in both upper and lower limbs.

Investigations

Investigation of a middle-aged patient with hypertension is limited to chest X-ray, ECG, electrolytes, creatinine, urinalysis, full blood count and lipid profile. Much of this will show any target organ damage, e.g. left ventricular hypertrophy on the ECG. Where a secondary cause for hypertension is suspected, there are specific tests as discussed below.

Table 1.7. Retinal changes in hypertension (Keith–Wagener classification)

Grade 1	Arteries become straighter and reflect light due to thickening of their walls (silver wiring). They may also show some variation in calibre
Grade 2	In addition, the arteries (because they are thickened) compress the veins at points where they cross each other (arteriovenous (AV) nipping)
Grade 3	In addition, flame-shaped haemorrhages are seen as are soft (cotton wool) white exudates
Grade 4	In addition, swelling (papilloedema) of the optic disc occurs

Points to note

Grades 1 and 2 may appear with advancing years. It is their premature appearance that is important

Grades 3 and 4 represent severe hypertensive change and often occur with malignant hypertension

Even in grade 4 hypertension there may be minimal or no upset in vision

Grades 3 and 4 changes usually resolve within a few weeks of successful anti-hypertensive treatment

In a younger patient, routine investigation would also include assessment of urinary catecholamines and renal imaging, looking for reflux nephropathy or evidence of renal artery stenosis.

SECONDARY CAUSES OF HYPERTENSION

Coarctation of aorta

In any young person presenting with high blood pressure, coarctation of the aorta should be suspected (see under Congenital heart disease, p. 47).

Endocrine causes

Cushing's syndrome
These patients usually present with the clinical picture of Cushing's syndrome and the hypertension is simply part of that picture (see p. 179).

Primary hyperaldosteronism (Conn's syndrome)
Excessive production of aldosterone may be due to an adrenal adenoma or to increased activity of both glands and causes sodium retention and potassium loss. It causes hypertension which may be refractory to treatment with conventional antihypertensive treatment, but responds well to the aldosterone antagonist spironolactone. Hypokalaemia may occur, but may also be caused by thiazide diuretics and is not universal. The diagnosis is made by finding a raised plasma aldosterone : renin ratio and confirmed by CT scanning and selective venous sampling.

Phaeochromocytoma

This tumour usually arises in the adrenal glands but in 10% is found in sympathetic nervous tissue elsewhere. Approximately 10% are malignant. Phaeochromocytomas may occur in association with other endocrine tumours or with neurofibromatosis. They should be suspected in patients with severe or rapid-onset hypertension, particularly with episodic symptoms suggestive of sympathetic overactivity (e.g. tremor, pallor, sweating, panic), and the diagnosis should be excluded in all hypertensive patients under the age of 40. Hypertension may be episodic or, more commonly, sustained.

Urinary excretion of catecholamines or metanephrines should be measured in an acidified 24-hour sample. Measurement of plasma catecholamines is seldom useful. Occasionally the tumour can be palpated (though repeated palpation should be avoided as it can cause massive catecholamine release). The tumour is located using CT and, occasionally, MIBG isotope scanning, and removed surgically following alpha- and beta-blockade.

Renal causes

Most renal diseases can cause high blood pressure. Chronic pyelonephritis or glomerulonephritis and polycystic kidney disease are common causes.

Renal artery stenosis

Renal artery stenosis should be suspected with relatively recent onset of hypertension. A bruit may be heard in the abdomen but often there are no physical signs. In the younger patient fibromuscular dysplasia is the cause while in the older patient atheroma narrows the renal artery. In these older patients there may be evidence of atheroma elsewhere. Renal ultrasound will show a smaller kidney on the affected side. An intravenous pyelogram (IVP) may show a delay in contrast medium appearance and clearance on the affected side. A renal arteriogram is performed to assess the anatomy, and renal vein renin levels may be elevated on the affected side.

In older patients the only reason for operating on renal artery stenosis is to preserve renal function but in younger patients either surgical correction of the stenosis is performed or dilatation by means of balloon angioplasty may be attempted. About 50% of such people will have their hypertension cured by the procedure and another 35% will be easier to control medically.

Pregnancy

Pre-eclampsia is a disease usually of first pregnancies in which hypertension, proteinuria and oedema occur in the third trimester, with thrombocytopenia and hyperuricaemia. It is thought to be due to placental hypoperfusion, causing activation of the clotting system and endothelial dysfunction. It may progress to eclampsia (convulsions) unless the fetus is delivered, even if antihypertensive treatment is given.

Treatment of hypertension during pregnancy is controversial, as many antihypertensive drugs may affect fetal blood supply and some interfere with embyrogenesis. If treatment is thought warranted, methyldopa and labetalol are the drugs of first choice.

Drugs

The contraceptive pill
This is the most common drug causing high blood pressure. Usually this is only a matter of a few mmHg but in some patients it can be greater.

Corticosteroids
Usually steroids have to be given for important reasons, e.g. asthma, arthritis, etc., and cannot be stopped. The dose should certainly be titrated down to the lowest level possible and then the blood pressure treated if need be.

Liquorice derivatives
Carbenoxolone, which was used to treat peptic ulcers, can increase blood pressure.

Other drugs, e.g. the non-steroidal anti-inflammatory agents, can interfere with the action of some anti-hypertensive agents.

PATHOLOGICAL CONSEQUENCES OF HIGH BLOOD PRESSURE

High blood pressure predisposes to damage in the target organs. Before effective treatment, heart failure was the most common end point; now, it is MI and IHD. Good blood pressure management has only reduced modestly the high incidence of IHD. The pathological sequelae of hypertension are myocardial ischaemia/infarction, cerebrovascular accident, renal failure, heart failure, and aneurysm formation with subsequent dissection or rupture.

Treatment

Treating people with severe hypertension is very effective in preventing subsequent morbid events. In the mild to moderate range of blood pressures, there is greater debate and the benefits are less clear cut.

Irrespective of the cause of high blood pressure, all hypertensive patients (except for those with very severe or malignant hypertension) should be encouraged to take more exercise, lose weight if obese, and minimise their alcohol and salt intake.

With drug therapy, if one agent does not work, another should be substituted rather than added. The commonly used first-choice drugs are thiazide diuretics, beta-adrenergic blocking agents, calcium channel blocking agents and ACE inhibitors. To these may be added in due course alpha-adrenergic blocking agents and angiotensin II blocking drugs.

Thiazide diuretics (e.g. bendrofluazide, cyclopenthiazide, hydrochlorothiazide). These drugs are all effective anti-hypertensive agents. Hypokalaemia is the major side-effect but they also have adverse effects on blood lipids, blood glucose and uric acid levels. They may also cause excessive loss of sodium particularly in the elderly. Despite this they have been shown in general to be safe and effective in hypertension.

Beta-adrenergic blocking agents. Wherever possible, cardioselective (i.e. largely working on the heart) agents should be used, e.g. atenolol, metoprolol. Beta-blocking agents can provoke bronchospasm and are contraindicated in asthma. They may also worsen heart failure and because of the drop in cardiac output can cause fatigue. Cold hands and feet and impotence occur as may bad dreams. Again, in most patients they cause no problems and are good and effective anti-hypertensive agents.

Calcium channel blocking drugs. These constitute several different chemical types but basically all act as vasodilators. Some, e.g. verapamil, have a negative effect on heart rate while nifedipine may even increase the rate. The side-effects include fluid retention, constipation, headaches and flushing.

ACE inhibitors are well tolerated and seem to be safe. In people with high renin levels they can cause a precipitous fall in blood pressure. This is more likely to occur in people already on diuretics. They also inhibit kinin breakdown, causing dry cough (common, but harmless) and angioneurotic oedema (rare, but life-threatening).

Alpha-adrenergic blocking agents are effective and may improve dyslipidaemia. Long-acting agents (e.g. doxazosin, terazosin) seldom cause postural hypotension; they also relax the bladder sphincter, which can be beneficial in men with bladder outflow obstruction.

Other anti-hypertensive agents. After these first-choice drugs, which can be used in practically any combination, additional drugs available include systemic arterial vasodilators, e.g. hydralazine, and centrally acting drugs such as methyldopa, clonidine and reserpine. All centrally acting drugs tend to have central side-effects such as sedation but clonidine can cause marked rebound hypertension after it is withdrawn while reserpine is said to cause depression. Impotence may also occur with these drugs. Angiotensin II antagonists have recently been introduced and seem to be relatively free of side-effects.

Minoxidil is a potent vasodilator which is generally best reserved for hospital use. Its principal side-effect is unsightly hirsutism.

Labetalol is a combined alpha- and beta-blocking drug which is predominantly alpha when used intravenously and beta when used orally. It is used in pregnancy and in the management of malignant hypertension.

MALIGNANT HYPERTENSION

In about 1% of patients with hypertension the blood pressure follows an accelerated and worsening course. When necrosis of the small blood vessels (fibrinoid necrosis) occurs, severe changes are found in the optic fundi and proteinuria and haematuria result. This is malignant hypertension and if untreated will lead to death, usually within 1 year.

Malignant hypertension may also present with hypertensive encephalopathy, in which there is raised intracranial pressure and the patient is confused and disorientated. LVF and dissection of the aorta can also result from malignant hypertension.

In all forms of malignant hypertension the first essential is to reduce the blood pressure but not to normal levels. Any reduction in blood pressure is a move in the right direction and initially a systolic pressure of around 200 mmHg and a diastolic pressure of around 110 mmHg is an acceptable target. In the ensuing days and weeks the blood pressure can be titrated further downwards. With dissection of the aorta, more vigorous treatment is required, possibly using intravenous drugs and monitoring in an intensive care unit. All patients with malignant hypertension should be admitted to hospital for treatment.

PERIPHERAL VASCULAR DISEASE

Aetiology

Smoking, hyperlipidaemia, hypertension and diabetes are the major causes.

Symptoms and signs

Cramp-like discomfort, usually in the calves or buttocks, on exertion. If disease is severe, the pain can occur at rest. If ulcers are present they can be very painful. There is coldness in the legs distally. The major signs are cold limbs (often a difference between the two sides), hair loss, shiny pale skin, absent or poor pulses and possible ulcers or gangrene.

Management

The risk factors must be reduced, and the patient started on regular aspirin. Good skin and foot care, e.g. by a chiropodist, are essential. Regular exercise to encourage development of collateral (new) vessels should be encouraged. Treatment may be by balloon dilatation or surgical.

RAYNAUD'S DISEASE AND RAYNAUD'S PHENOMENON

Spasm occurs in the digital arteries, and the fingers become white and bloodless. It is much worse in colder weather and occurs in up to 5% of the population. It is more common in females and occasionally secondary to other diseases (Raynaud's phenomenon) but is usually of unknown aetiology (Raynaud's disease).

TEMPORAL ARTERITIS

Inflammation of the temporal arteries presents as headache with tenderness over the vessels. It may lead to sudden blindness and needs immediate treatment with large doses of corticosteroids, e.g. 60–80 mg prednisolone daily.

The blood viscosity and ESR are raised when the disease process is active.

TAKAYASU'S ARTERITIS

Arteritis of the vessels arising from and including the aortic arch eventually leads to loss of pulses (pulseless disease) and hypertension.

SYPHILIS

Syphilis causes aortitis which, in turn, may lead to aortic aneurysms, aortic valve incompetence and narrowing of the ostia of the coronary arteries.

VARICOSE VEINS

Seen in the lower limbs, varicose veins are usually of cosmetic importance only. Occasionally they cause pain and discomfort and may lead to ulcer formation. Treatment is by sclerosing injection or surgical removal.

SUPERFICIAL THROMBOPHLEBITIS

This usually occurs in the legs but may also involve the veins of the arms. The vein is inflamed and thrombosed and can be very painful and tender. It feels like a hard cord and is frequently seen at sites of intravenous infusions. Thrombophlebitis responds to simple symptomatic therapy, e.g. pain relief or anti-inflammatory drugs.

DEEP VENOUS THROMBOSIS (DVT)

There are several predisposing factors to DVT, including immobility (especially in hospital), increasing age, obesity, surgery, varicose veins, pregnancy, family history, contraceptive pill use and thrombophilia (p. 350). Malignancy also predisposes to DVT and should be suspected if the DVT is recurrent.

The patient may be asymptomatic but will often have calf pain, swelling of the leg with prominence of superficial veins and discoloration (cyanosis). The affected limb is usually warm and there is a risk of pulmonary embolism. DVT can be detected by ultrasound but more usually a venogram is performed. Anticoagulation is required for 3 months although if recurrent it may be for life. Support stockings and occasionally, if the thrombosis is massive, thrombolysis may be used (streptokinase).

CONGENITAL HEART DISEASE

Congenital heart disease is found in 8 out of every 1000 children born. Many aborted fetuses are also found to have malformed hearts. If a couple already has one child with congenital heart disease then the chances of the next or subsequent children being affected is increased to 25 per 1000 live births.

The aetiology of congenital heart disease is largely unknown but there are some associations:

1. chromosome abnormalities such as occur with Turner or Down syndromes
2. exposure to rubella virus in early pregnancy
3. drug exposure in the first trimester of pregnancy
4. ionising radiation.

NEONATAL CONGENITAL HEART DISEASE

The incidence and type of congenital heart disorders are quite different in this age group from those in the older child. These young patients present either with signs of heart failure or with cyanosis. They should all be referred for specialist investigation and treatment as soon as anything is suspected.

CONGENITAL HEART DISEASE IN OLDER CHILDREN

This is usually classified as cyanotic or acyanotic. The acyanotic forms greatly exceed cyanotic forms.

ACYANOTIC CONGENITAL HEART DISEASE

Ventricular septal defect (VSD) (Fig. 1.17)

This is a defect (sometimes multiple defects) in the interventricular septum. Overall, VSDs constitute 25% of all cases of congenital heart disease and

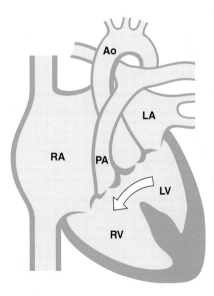

Fig. 1.17 Ventricular septal defect.

are the most common malformation. Because the left side of the heart has higher pressures than the right, the flow through the defect is in a left-to-right direction. The high-pressure left ventricle can pump large quantities of blood through a VSD and it is the quantity of such flow (or shunt) that determines the outcome; 30–40% of VSDs will close spontaneously, usually in the first year of life, but possibly up to the fourth decade.

Symptoms and signs

At any age, large VSDs can cause heart failure with dyspnoea, fatigue, failure to gain weight or to thrive.

Most children are asymptomatic but are closely followed up in case they develop heart failure or the pressure in their lungs starts to rise (pulmonary hypertension).

Unless heart failure has resulted, these patients appear normal but the heart may be enlarged clinically. The heart sounds are usually normal but if pulmonary hypertension is developing, the pulmonary second sound (P2) is loud. There is a pansystolic murmur, best heard at the left sternal edge in the third and fourth intercostal spaces. A systolic thrill can often be felt in the same area.

Investigations

Chest X-ray shows an enlarged heart with increased lung markings due to the increased pulmonary blood flow, i.e. plethoric lung fields.

ECG is usually normal but T wave changes in lead V1 in particular may indicate the onset of pulmonary hypertension in young children, i.e. the T waves become flat or upright being normally inverted.

Echocardiography often demonstrates the defect in the interventricular septum and quantifies the size of the shunt.

Cardiac catheterisation can quantify the shunt and injection of contrast medium can identify its site.

Treatment. This should be medical if at all possible because of the possibility that the VSD may close spontaneously but some do need to be closed surgically.

Atrial septal defect (ASD) (Fig. 1.18)

There are two major types: ostium secundum defect, which is usually an isolated defect, and ostium primum defect, which forms part of the spectrum of abnormalities occurring when there is defective development of the endocardial cushions in the heart and as well as the atrial septum, the ventricular septum and both mitral and tricuspid valves may be defective.

Symptoms and signs

These patients are usually asymptomatic and the ASD is found coincidentally when a murmur is noticed. The second heart sound remains split either

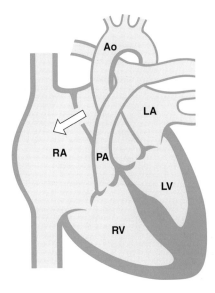

Fig. 1.18 Atrial septal defect.

widely with some respiratory variation or more classically fixed splitting occurs.

Increased blood flow over the normal pulmonary valve results in an ejection systolic murmur. With ostium primum defects, there may be pansystolic murmurs of mitral reflux or of a VSD or both. If pulmonary hypertension develops the P2 may be loud.

Investigations

Chest X-ray shows a characteristic peardrop appearance. This arises because the aorta is small and the pulmonary artery is large. The lung fields look plethoric and the heart is slightly enlarged (Fig. 1.19).

ECG usually shows a partial right bundle branch block (RBBB) pattern. There is a shift of the heart's electrical axis to the left in ostium primum defects (left axis deviation) and to the right in ostium secundum defects (right axis deviation). The PR interval may be prolonged in primum but not secundum defects.

Echocardiography identifies and quantifies the defect and is able to differentiate the two types.

Cardiac catheterisation can confirm the defect and quantify the degree of shunting.

Treatment

Large ASDs need to be closed if the pulmonary to systemic blood flow ratio is 2 : 1 or greater. Spontaneous closure does not occur. Small ASDs are best

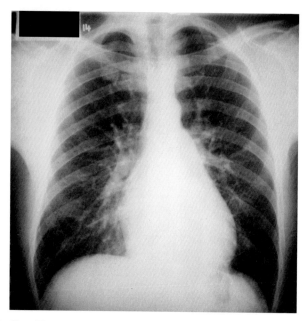

Fig. 1.19 Chest X-ray in ASD showing the typical appearance of small aorta, enlarged pulmonary artery, increased heart size and lung vascularity (plethoric lung fields).

left alone. All patients with ASDs, whether open or operated upon, are liable to develop atrial arrhythmias, e.g. atrial fibrillation, in later life.

Patent ductus arteriosus (PDA) (Fig. 1.20)

In utero the ductus arteriosus carries oxygenated blood from the placenta through into the aorta, bypassing the lungs. It normally closes at birth. When it remains open, it allows blood from the high-pressure aorta to flow through into the pulmonary artery. The duct can vary in size from trivial to very large in which case it can cause heart failure early in life. It sometimes closes in response to indomethacin but surgical closure is simple and safe and this is often needed. In very young children the physical signs are limited to an ejection systolic murmur over the upper left sternal edge and there are usually prominent bounding pulses.

Older children are usually symptom-free and the ductus is found on routine examination. Physical findings include large volume pulses and the characteristic 'machinery' murmur which has systolic and diastolic compoents because of the continuous pressure gradient between the aorta and pulmonary artery.

The ECG and chest X-ray are often normal although the lung fields may be plethoric and the heart enlarged when the patent ductus is itself large. In this latter case the ECG may show right ventricular hypertrophy. Echo-cardiography can demonstrate the ductus and quantify the shunt. Cardiac

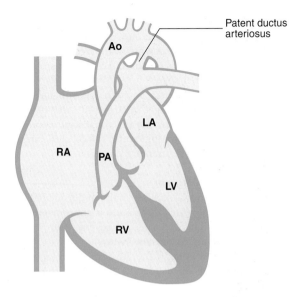

Fig. 1.20 Patent ductus arteriosus.

catheterisation is seldom necessary. This lesion carries a high risk of infection (infective endocarditis) and is usually closed unless very small.

Aortic stenosis

These patients may present with heart failure in the neonatal period but aortic stenosis is detected much more commonly later in life when a murmur is heard. These abnormal valves often have only two cusps.

Symptoms and signs
1. Usually asymptomatic and normal.
2. Unlike adult cases, angina and heart failure are uncommon.
3. Occasionally effort syncope occurs.
4. Low volume pulse.
5. Coarse ejection systolic murmur over the aortic area radiating to the neck. There may be a systolic thrill.
6. The chest X-ray is often normal, as is the ECG.
7. The diagnosis is confirmed at echocardiography.

Treatment is surgical in severe cases, by either splitting the valve (valvotomy) or replacing it. Balloon dilatation may be possible.

Rare forms of aortic stenosis occur where the narrowing is either above the valve (supravalvular) or below it (subvalvular).

Coarctation of the aorta

This may present early in life with heart failure or be picked up later in well children. The aorta is narrowed just below the left subclavian artery. The pulses in the arms and legs are of different quality and the femoral pulses may be delayed and weak when compared with the radial pulses. Blood pressure in the upper limbs is elevated. An ejection systolic murmur is heard over the upper left sternal edge.

Collateral blood vessels may be both felt and heard over the scapula. These are blood vessels that have enlarged to carry blood by an alternative route to the lower limbs, bypassing the constricted aorta.

Sometimes, associated bicuspid aortic valves, aortic stenosis or aneurysms of the circle of Willis in the brain are present.

Investigations and treatment

The chest X-ray may show notching on the underside of the ribs from erosion by intercostal collateral vessels. The aorta is abnormal in shape, showing two bulges—the '3' sign. The opposite, the reverse 3 or 'E' sign, is seen in the oesophagus using a barium swallow X-ray.

Echocardiography may show the site of the coarctation. Cardiac catheterisation is often still needed to identify the site of the collateral vessels and establish whether significant aortic stenosis is present and to demonstrate the site of the coarctation itself. Treatment is surgical but up to 50% of patients will still need anti-hypertensive therapy. If significant hypertension does not develop in the upper limbs then the coarctation is best left alone.

Pulmonary stenosis

This lesion is relatively common and may affect the pulmonary valve, or the stenosis may be just below the valve in the right ventricle. There is an ejection systolic murmur over the pulmonary area that radiates out clearly to the lung fields over the back. There is often a thrill at the second left intercostal space and with valvular stenosis a systolic sound (ejection click) may be heard. The pulmonary second sound is widely split. If severe enough, balloon dilatation is the treatment of choice although surgery may sometimes be necessary.

Ebstein's anomaly

The tricuspid valve is seated low in the right ventricle so that part of the ventricle is atrialised (i.e. incorporated into the right atrium). The degree of this determines the functional end result, i.e. mild with no disability to severe with intractable heart failure from the inadequate right-sided structures.

CYANOTIC CONGENITAL HEART DISEASE

Tetralogy of Fallot

The tetralogy comprises pulmonary stenosis, VSD, right ventricular hypertrophy and overriding of the aorta. It is the most common form of cyanotic congenital heart disease after the first year of life. Much more rarely, there

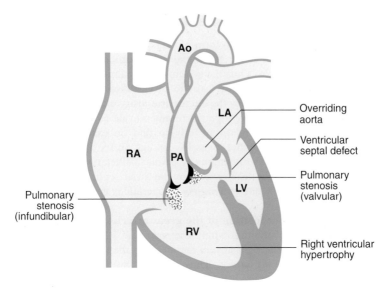

Fig. 1.21 Tetralogy of Fallot.

is an associated ASD—Fallot's pentalogy. As with pure pulmonary stenosis, the pulmonary narrowing may either affect the valve, be just below the valve in the right ventricle or both (Fig. 1.21).

Symptoms and signs
Cyanosis, the degree of which may come and go, is present. Severe cyanotic episodes are known as 'spells' and are probably caused by spasm occurring in the narrow part of the right ventricle. Cyanotic spells may be precipitated by exertion or crying.

These children may frequently squat, especially after exercise. Cerebral thrombosis or abscesses may occur. The heart is not usually greatly enlarged and a pulmonary stenotic murmur is heard. A systolic thrill may be present in the pulmonary area.

Investigations
The chest X-ray shows a boot-shaped heart. There is a relative absence of the pulmonary arteries, and the lungs show diminished vascular markings (i.e. oligaemic lung fields). The ECG shows right ventricular hypertrophy. Echocardiography is diagnostic, showing the features of the tetralogy and especially the overriding by the aorta of the interventricular septum. Cardiac catheterisation may be needed to confirm the anatomy.

Treatment
Cyanotic spells are a medical emergency. These respond to morphine and also to beta-adrenergic blocking drugs. Digoxin should be avoided as it increases myocardial contractility and excitability. Surgery is eventually indicated in most patients.

Transposition of the great arteries

This is the most common form of cyanotic congenital heart disease in neonates. The aorta is connected to the right ventricle and the pulmonary artery to the left ventricle. Thus the systemic and pulmonary circulations are completely separate and for the baby to survive there must be some connection between the two. Usually the ductus arteriosus remains patent although these children also often have a patent foramen ovale or associated VSD.

There is usually relatively little to find on examination but the chest X-ray shows a heart that looks like an egg on its side and the diagnosis is confirmed by echocardiography or cardiac catheterisation.

The cardiologist tears a hole in the atrial septum to allow the child to survive and, later, one of a variety of operations is carried out.

Corrected transposition of the great arteries

This is a rare condition where the right and left ventricles have switched over such that the right atrium empties into the left ventricle which empties into the pulmonary artery. Thus the transposition has become corrected. Not surprisingly, there is a high incidence of associated defects, e.g. VSD.

PULMONARY HYPERTENSION

Elevation of the pulmonary artery pressure (pulmonary hypertension) occurs where there is increased pulmonary blood flow, caused by an ASD, VSD or PDA (i.e. left-to-right intracardiac shunting of blood), increased pulmonary capillary pressure caused by increased back pressure from left heart disease, e.g. LVF, mitral valve disease, or increased pulmonary vascular resistance from chronic lung disease (e.g. chronic bronchitis, emphysema), recurrent pulmonary thromboembolism or primary pulmonary hypertension (see below).

The physical signs reflect the increased pulmonary and right heart pressures: loud pulmonary second sound, right ventricular enlargement, right heart failure, and a pulmonary valve incompetence (early diastolic) murmur may be audible.

The chest X-ray may reveal the cause, e.g. mitral stenosis, emphysema. In addition, the proximal pulmonary arteries are enlarged and the peripheral pulmonary arteries small and depleted in number. The ECG may show right atrial and right ventricular hypertrophy. Treatment is that of the underlying cause.

PRIMARY PULMONARY HYPERTENSION

This is a rare condition of unknown aetiology but it may lead to recurrent thrombosis of the pulmonary arteries. It predominantly affects young adult females and is remorselessly progressive leading to death within a few years. There is no effective treatment but anticoagulants are usually started and vasodilators have had limited success.

PULMONARY EMBOLISM

Pulmonary embolism ranges from small, with no clinical effect, to massive with sudden death (10%). The emboli usually arise from the leg or pelvic veins in people who have been immobile or had recent surgery/childbirth. There may be clinically apparent deep vein thrombosis.

Symptoms and signs

Clinical features include chest pain or choking sensation, dyspnoea, syncope or collapse, haemoptysis and tachycardia and other signs of circulatory compromise, e.g. low blood pressure.

Investigations

The chest X-ray and ECG are often normal initially. Ventilation/perfusion (V/Q) scans are helpful (the lung is ventilated but not perfused). Venograms are sometimes performed to establish the source of the emboli; rarely, pulmonary angiography is required but this itself can be dangerous.

Treatment

1. Anticoagulation for 6 months in mild to moderate cases.
2. Clot lysis (thrombolysis) with streptokinase in moderate lesions causing some circulatory deficit.
3. Surgical removal of the embolus in severe cases with circulatory compromise or collapse.

If pulmonary emboli are recurrent then lifelong anticoagulation is required with or without surgical plication of the inferior vena cava or the insertion of a filter.

COR PULMONALE

Cor pulmonale is defined as right heart failure resulting from chronic lung disease or chest deformity, e.g. chronic bronchitis and emphysema, pulmonary fibrosis (fibrosing alveolitis), recurrent pulmonary thromboembolism, severe kyphoscoliosis, and rarely neuromuscular disease such as myasthenia gravis.

Treatment is that of the cause and of heart failure.

2

RESPIRATORY MEDICINE

Gabriel Laszlo, James R. Catterall

Diseases of the upper respiratory tract affect the nose, nasal sinuses, pharynx, larynx, and lymph nodes draining these. Infections of the upper respiratory tract are generally minor but are common and inconvenient. Bronchial and pulmonary disease is second only to heart disease as a cause of death in industrialised countries and is a major cause of morbidity and loss of earnings. Cigarette smoking causes carcinoma of the bronchus and contributes significantly to chronic obstructive airways disease (COAD). Both tuberculosis and asthma are increasing in prevalence worldwide.

ACUTE INFECTIONS OF THE AIR PASSAGES

MINOR RESPIRATORY INFECTIONS

Virus infections of the upper respiratory tract
Viruses cause the common cold, pharyngitis and tonsillitis (sore throat, fever and neck stiffness from enlarged cervical glands), laryngo-tracheitis (hoarseness, painful cough, laryngeal obstruction in children ('croup')) and conjunctivitis (sore eyes).

Spread is by droplet infection, the incubation period is short, infectivity high in the early stages and serious complications may occur in susceptible individuals. The virus may be isolated for up to 96 hours.

Complications include middle ear pain from eustachian tube obstruction with the retention of serous fluid, while *Streptococcus pneumoniae*, *Haemophilus influenzae* and *Strep. pyogenes* may cause secondary bacterial otitis media. Osteomyelitis of the mastoid bones (mastoiditis) is now rare. Recurrent otitis media can result in minor deafness with learning difficulties.

Tonsillitis
Streptococcal tonsillitis causes an intense sore throat with pain, fever and malaise. It must be distinguished from infectious mononucleosis (p. 418). Post-streptococcal complications, including glomerulonephritis, rheumatic fever, chorea, scarlet fever and peritonsillar abscess, are now rare.

Oropharyngeal thrush

Candida albicans causes white plaques of fungus on the pharynx and palate which peel easily (thrush). Rare in healthy individuals, thrush complicates treatment with broad-spectrum antibiotics and oral and inhaled corticosteroid drugs, and is also found when immunity is defective. The infection may spread to the oesophagus or lungs. Eradication from the mouth and gastrointestinal (GI) tract is by oral non-absorbed antifungal antibiotics.

POTENTIALLY SERIOUS UPPER RESPIRATORY INFECTIONS

Diphtheria (see page 415)

Epiglottitis

Epiglottitis is a rare epidemic infection of children and adults with capsulated type B *H. influenzae* which invades and causes swelling of the epiglottis and epiglottic folds. There are microabscesses in the epiglottis. After minor respiratory symptoms, the patient rapidly develops a sore throat, dribbling, dysphagia for saliva, muffling of the voice, restlessness and prostration. Depression of the tongue for examination is dangerous in children as it may cause complete airway obstruction. Parenteral antibiotics are needed, with intravenous hydration in severe cases. The significant mortality rate is reduced by early treatment. Preventive vaccination is now available.

Bronchiolitis

This occurs mainly in children and is an acute infection of the respiratory tract with obstructive inflammation of the bronchioles. Most cases are caused by the respiratory syncytial virus. Presentation is with coughing, signs of airways obstruction, hyperinflation of the chest and limpness. Treatment consists of hydration and oxygenation with ventitatory support if the PCO_2 rises.

Whooping cough (pertussis) (see page 416)

Influenza

This is an endemic, epidemic and occasionally pandemic illness causing fever, rigors and muscle pains with upper and lower respiratory symptoms of varying severity. The incubation period is 24–48 hours and the virus is excreted for up to 7 days. Complications include pneumonia, myocarditis, polyneuritis, myelopathy and encephalitis. There are three major strains (A, B, C) with epidemics of A and B occurring every 2–3 years. There is little crossimmunity between strains; vaccination is only partially effective.

PNEUMONIA

Pneumonia is inflammation of the lung parenchyma resulting from infection. The term pneumonitis is reserved for lung inflammation caused by physical or chemical injury, e.g. irradiation.

Pneumonia remains an important cause of morbidity and mortality. In the UK, it causes ten times as many deaths as all other infectious diseases together, and in developing countries it is the most common cause of hospital admission in both adults and children.

The alveoli are normally kept sterile by local and humoral defences. Pneumonia occurs when these defences are overwhelmed by a sufficient number of virulent organisms or when the defences are impaired.

Community-acquired pneumonia usually occurs in previously healthy people or in patients with only slight impairment of lung defences. It is almost always caused by one of a small range of virulent organisms of which *Strep. pneumoniae* is the most common (Table 2.1). Pneumonias caused by *Mycoplasma pneumoniae, Legionella pneumophilia* and influenza virus often occur in epidemics.

Hospital-acquired pneumonia complicates many medical conditions and surgical operations and is usually from aspiration of gram-negative oropharyngeal organisms, especially in patients undergoing intensive care. Predisposing factors are intubation and the use of H_2-receptor antagonists.

Aspiration pneumonia occurs when large numbers of oropharyngeal flora reach the lower respiratory tract in patients with impaired upper airway defences. It is usually polymicrobial with gram-negative bacteria, gram-positive cocci and anaerobes all contributing.

Table 2.1. Community-acquired pneumonia. Clinical, radiological and haematological features associated with the most common causative organisms

Streptococcus pneumoniae	By far the most common cause at any age
	Rigors, herpes labialis; lobar consolidation
Staphylococcus aureus	Influenza epidemics, drug addicts
	Bilateral cavitating pneumonia
Klebsiella pneumoniae	Alcoholics, elderly
	May have more gradual onset than pneumococcal pneumonia in some patients
	Upper lobes, 'bulging' out on X-ray
Mycoplasma pneumoniae	Epidemic, especially in closed communities
	Cold agglutinins positive in 50%
Chlamydia spp	Contact with sick birds not always elicited
Legionella spp	Outbreaks in hotels and hospitals (water-cooled air conditioning); also spontaneous
Influenza virus	In epidemics
	Diffuse bilateral shadowing on chest X-ray
	May be complicated by superinfection with *Staph. aureus*

N.B. Although these features are typical, no clinical or radiological abnormality is specific for a particular organism.

Table 2.2. Pneumonia in the immunocompromised host. Common causative organisms associated with different defects in host defences

Neutropenia (e.g. cytotoxic chemotherapy, aplastic anaemia)	Bacteria Fungi
Defect in antibody production (e.g. splenectomy, myeloma, chronic lymphatic leukaemia)	Encapsulated bacteria, especially *Streptococcus pneumoniae*
Defect in cell-mediated immunity (e.g. Hodgkin's disease, AIDS, immunosuppressive therapy)	Viruses (CMV, HS, VZ) *Pneumocystis carinii* Fungi *Mycobacterium tuberculosis*, *M. avium-intracellulare* (in AIDS)

CMV = cytomegalovirus; HS = herpes simplex; VZ = varicella zoster

Pneumonia in the immunocompromised patient. Patients with AIDS or haematological malignancies and patients receiving cytotoxic/immunosuppressive therapy are at greatly increased risk. Different forms of immunodeficiency predispose to different organisms. The range of pathogens is wide and includes fungi (Table 2.2).

Pathology

The organisms are usually inhaled. They excite an inflammatory response in the bronchioles and alveoli, which become filled with organisms, fluid and inflammatory cells, the bronchi remaining patent (consolidation). A whole lobe or segment may be densely consolidated (lobar/segmental pneumonia) or the inflammation may be patchy, affecting mainly the lower lobes (broncho-pneumonia).

Symptoms

Systemic symptoms include fever, rigors, sweating, malaise, myalgia and headaches. Respiratory symptoms are cough, sputum (purulent when a pyogenic organism is present; absent, mucoid or watery in other patients), haemoptysis (often absent, and rarely marked; classically rusty in pyogenic infections), dyspnoea at rest, confusion (most common in the elderly, usually associated with hypoxaemia) and pleuritic pain (common in bacterial cases). Diaphragmatic pleurisy may mimic acute surgical conditions of the abdomen and may also be referred to the shoulder (C4 dermatome).

Signs

The patient is usually ill, pyrexial and tachypnoeic, and sometimes cyanosed. There may be pleuritic pain. Blisters of labial herpes simplex may be present (reactivation of latent infection by fever).

Localising chest signs are not always present, especially in non-bacterial pneumonia and in early bacterial pneumonia, but in established pneumonia they result from bronchiolo-alveolar inflammation (fine/medium inspiratory crackles), consolidation (diminished chest movement on affected side, dullness to percussion, bronchial breathing, increased vocal resonance, whispering pectoriloquy) and pleural inflammation (pleural rub or effusion).

Investigations

Chest X-ray

The chest X-ray shows opacification without loss of volume. Any loss of volume of a lobe or lung affected by pneumonia should arouse suspicion of proximal bronchial obstruction (Fig. 2.1).

The pattern of opacification on chest X-ray indicates the extent of lung involvement and may give clues to the likely causal organism.

Lobar or segmental pneumonia. Dense opacification of a whole lobe or segment, sometimes more than one, may indicate *Strep. pneumoniae* or *Klebsiella pneumoniae.*

Bronchopneumonia. Bilateral patchy opacification, mainly in the lower zones, often indicates a mixed infection with *Strep. pneumoniae* and *H. influenzae* although bronchopneumonia can also occur with other organisms.

Diffuse bilateral shadowing is typical of viral and other non-pyogenic pneumonias, e.g. *M. pneumoniae, Pneumocystis carinii.*

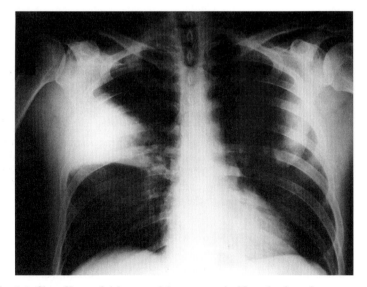

Fig. 2.1 Chest X-ray of right upper lobe pneumonia. Note the dense homogeneous opacification limited at its lower border by the horizontal fissure.

Cavities are typically seen in pneumonia due to *Staph. aureus* or *Klebsiella pneumoniae* and also in tuberculosis.

Other investigations

Arterial blood gas tensions are measured to determine the severity of hypoxaemia; $PaCO_2$ is usually low.

Differential blood count. Neutrophil leucocytosis often occurs in bacterial infections but the white cell count may be normal or low in the severely ill. A low white cell count is typical of non-bacterial infections and in immuno-compromised patients.

Identification of the causative organism. Blood culture is positive in 50% of fulminating bacterial pneumonias. Sputum culture is more sensitive than blood culture but less specific. Acute and convalescent serum for anti-bodies to viruses, *Legionella*, *Mycoplasma* and *Chlamydia* can be used to make a retrospective diagnosis. Bronchoalveolar lavage, with microscopy and cul-ture of the fluid, is used in seriously ill patients who have not responded to standard treatment and in immunosuppressed patients, in whom the range of possible organisms is wide.

Differential diagnosis

Other causes of consolidation are pulmonary infarct, pulmonary eosinophilia, pulmonary tuberculosis and malignancy. Non-infective causes of pneumonia are listed in Table 2.3. Bronchopneumonia can be confused with acute pul-monary oedema due to heart failure or adult respiratory distress syndrome.

Table 2.3. Non-infective causes of pneumonia

	Cause	Course
Eosinophilic pneumonia (synonym: pulmonary eosinophilia)	Aspergillosis, hypersensitivity to drugs or cryptogenic	Recurrent, responds to oral corticosteroids
Cryptogenic organising pneumonia	Variant of cryptogenic fibrosing alveolitis	Recurrent, responds to oral corticosteroids
Acute chemical burns	Inhalation injury by toxic chemical fumes	Bronchial hyperreactivity May heal with bronchiolar fibrosis, chronic airflow obstruction
Radiation	Radiotherapy	Subacute 1–20 weeks after treatment Lasts several weeks Good resolution, functional impairment
Exogenous lipid pneumonia	Inhalation of oily droplets	Chronic

In immunocompromised patients, the usual clues to infection (e.g. pyrexia, leucocytosis) may be absent. Non-infectious causes of pulmonary infiltrates in these patients include extension of the primary disease (e.g. in haematological malignancies), intrapulmonary bleeding in thrombocytopenia and lung damage caused by cytotoxic drugs/irradiation.

Complications

Pleurisy and serous pleural effusion are much more common after bacterial than viral pneumonia. Empyema (pus in the pleural cavity) should be evacuated, if necessary surgically. Resolution of pneumonia may be poor, leading to abscess formation or fibrosis.

Treatment

Antibiotics
Treatment should be started without delay, i.e. before the results of cultures are known. In severe pneumonia, antibiotics should be given parenterally. The choice of antibiotic will depend on the likely organism, taking into account the clinical, radiological and haematological findings.

In community-acquired pneumonia, macrolides (erythromycin, clarithromycin) cover most of the causative organisms, though ampicillin or a cephalosporin is usually added if the infection is severe. If staphylococcal pneumonia is suspected (especially common during epidemics of influenza), flucloxacillin is added.

Aspiration pneumonia usually responds to a combination of ampicillin (or a cephalosporin) and metronidazole.

Hospital-acquired pneumonia is usually treated with an antipseudomonal β-lactam, e.g. azlocillin or ceftazidime, often combined with an aminoglycoside.

In the immunocompromised patient, the choice of antibiotic depends on the nature of the immune defect (e.g. azlocillin and gentamicin in neutropenia; high-dose co-trimoxazole for suspected *P. carinii* in AIDS).

Supportive treatment
Oxygen (to keep the PaO_2 > 60 mmHg; 8 kPa), fluids (parenteral if necessary, to maintain adequate hydration) and analgesia for pleuritic pain are important.

Prognosis

Prognosis depends on the underlying health and age of the patient, the causative organism and whether bacteraemia or complications such as hypotension, leucopenia and renal failure occur. The overall mortality for pneumococcal pneumonia is 5–13%. In most patients who survive, resolution is remarkably complete.

Prevention

Vaccines against influenza viruses and *Strep. pneumoniae* are recommended for patients at increased risk, including chronic respiratory disease, chronic heart failure, chronic renal failure, diabetes mellitus and defective immunity, e.g. asplenia.

LUNG ABSCESS

A necrotic area of lung, secondary to aspiration of anaerobic and aerobic bacteria often from the mouth. Differential diagnosis: tuberculosis, carcinoma.

TUBERCULOSIS

This is caused by an infection of the tubercle bacillus (*Mycobacterium tuberculosis*) in the lungs and elsewhere. Tuberculosis is characterised by granulomatous lesions which tend to become necrotic and heal by fibrosis.

New cases are now notified in England and Wales at a rate of 10–20/ 100 000 per year with a low mortality, deaths occurring mainly in the elderly and in occasional undiagnosed cases.

Patients with HIV infection (p. 419) are particularly susceptible to a wide variety of mycobacterial strains. Where overcrowding and poor nutrition and alcoholism persist, the incidence and mortality remain high and tuberculosis is a significant cause of mortality in the young worldwide (India, South East Asia, Africa, the Pacific Islands). Resistance to infection and to reactivation is lowered by malnutrition, alcoholism, diabetes mellitus, smoking, corticosteroids given in high doses long term, immuno-suppression, silicosis, pregnancy, old age and diseases associated with reduced immunity.

Microbiology

The organism, an acid–alcohol-fast bacillus, may be stained in smears of sputum or bronchial lavage fluid, concentrated urine and CSF and may be cultured on special media in 6 weeks. Rapid identification by DNA amplification can be used to detect person-to-person spread of organisms.

PRIMARY TUBERCULOUS INFECTION

This usually occurs in childhood in places where the disease is common. There is a minor inflammatory reaction at the site of entry (lungs, tonsils, small intestine) with rapid spread to regional lymph nodes. Most commonly there is a small area of consolidation (Ghon focus) in the periphery of the middle and lower lobes of the lungs with hilar adenopathy. Cervical and mesenteric node tuberculosis are less common than formerly. Clinical manifestations may be absent or include mild malaise, weight loss or failure to grow, a brief febrile illness, cough, erythema nodosum or phlyctenular conjunctivitis. In the great majority of cases uncomplicated healing and calcification occur.

Complications of primary tuberculous infection
Complications include: obstruction of lobar bronchi by enlarged nodes, bronchial seeding with confluent pneumonia, pleural effusion (a common cause of unexplained pleural effusion in patients under 30 years old), pericardial effusion and blood-borne spread to the kidneys, bone, meninges and adrenals. Widespread macroscopic lesions throughout the body are called **miliary tuberculosis**. These phenomena occur within 12 weeks to 1 year of primary infection (or when immunity is impaired).

Post-primary tuberculosis

Post-primary tuberculosis arises by direct progression of a primary lesion (rarely before puberty in Europeans), reactivation of a dormant lesion, haematogenous spread to the lungs or reinfection. The illness has a slowly progressive course.

Pathology
Usually the upper lobes are affected. The organisms are contained within caseating granulomata surrounded by areas of inflammation. Healing is by fibrosis. Disease may spread to the pleura, the larynx, the tongue and the intestines, or cause miliary tuberculosis.

Symptoms and signs
These may be inconspicuous initially. There is lassitude, loss of weight, pyrexia 37–39°C, anorexia, cough (dry or with purulent sputum), haemoptysis and amenorrhoea.

The patient may look wasted but with high colour. In advanced cases there are signs of cavitation with amphoric breathing, consolidation, collapse and fibrosis with post-tussive inspiratory crackles.

Investigations
1. Chest X-ray appearances depend on severity and include patchy irregular opacities centred on one or both upper lobes, cavities within such lesions, streaks of fibrosis radiating from the hilum, calcification and solitary round shadows (Fig. 2.2).
2. Search for *M. tuberculosis* in sputum, or in bronchoscopic aspirate if sputum is not available or not informative.
3. Tuberculin test (e.g. *Mantoux* or *Heaf* test) detects previous BCG (Bacille Calmette–Guerin) vaccination or previous or present tuberculosis infection. Tests are very occasionally negative with active disease.
4. Advanced cases show anaemia, raised plasma viscosity, raised erythrocyte sedimentation rate (ESR) and acute phase proteins. Leucocytosis is unusual.

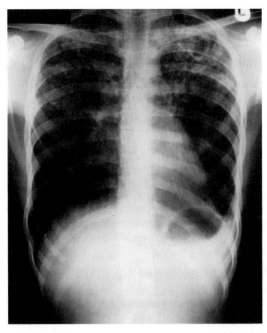

Fig. 2.2 Chest X-ray of pulmonary tuberculosis, showing bilateral nodular upper zone opacification. There is a cavity on the left.

Complications
These include hyponatraemia, tuberculous empyema or pericarditis, tuberculous pneumonia, miliary tuberculosis, massive haemoptysis and amyloidosis.

Differential diagnosis
Bronchial asthma, pyogenic lung abscess, pneumonia, drug-induced lung infiltrates, Wegener's granuloma, resolving pulmonary oedema.

Treatment of infection with M. tuberculosis
Combinations of antimycobacterial chemotherapeutic agents are given to prevent the emergence of resistant strains. A regimen consisting of rifampicin, isoniazid and pyrazinamide for 2 months, followed by rifampicin and isoniazid for 4 months has been shown to sterilise most infections. Other drugs are available. The best regimens result in a relapse rate of less than 1%; results are worse if compliance is poor.

Miliary tuberculosis

This usually presents with pyrexia and weight loss. Miliary shadowing on chest radiology and tubercles on the choroid, visible on ophthalmoscopy, are classic hallmarks. Usually there are no localising features, so diagnosis is difficult. Liver biopsy may show granulomata, and mycobacteria may be isolated from bronchial secretions, urine or bone marrow culture. A therapeutic trial of anti-tuberculous therapy may be necessary.

Prevention of tuberculosis

1. Screening. Infective cases are identified by screening individuals from high risk areas and contacts of cases using chest X-rays and tuberculin tests.

2. BCG vaccination. BCG is an attenuated tubercle bacillus used as a vaccine against tuberculosis. It was highly effective in England and Wales from 1965 to 1970 in reducing the incidence from 5% to 0.5% in the under 20s age group, with the virtual abolition of life-threatening miliary or meningeal tuberculosis. High-risk individuals, including healthcare and social workers and travellers, are vaccinated. BCG vaccination is ineffective in many parts of the world, including India and the USA; the reasons are unknown but probably related to genetic and nutritional differences. BCG vaccination produces a moderately positive tuberculin test (e.g. Heaf test grade 1 or 2). A strongly positive tuberculin test (e.g. Heaf test grade 3 or 4) indicates current or previous infection: chemotherapy may be advisable.

OTHER CHRONIC BACTERIAL INFECTIONS

Non-tuberculous mycobacteria

Some non-tuberculous myocobacteria (e.g. *M. kansasii, M. xenopi, M. avium-intracellulare*) cause chronic pulmonary infection, leading to fibrosis and cavitation. These infections often occur in pre-existing chronic lung disease. Weight loss, cough, sputum, dyspnoea and sometimes haemoptysis may occur, but the clinical findings are sometimes dominated by underlying disease. Progression of disease is generally more indolent than in tuberculosis, but the organisms are more resistant to treatment. The patients are not infectious.

Actinomycosis and nocardiosis

Originally classified as fungi, *Actinomyces* and *Nocardia* are now known to be bacteria. They are uncommon causes of chronic pneumonia, which may mimic tuberculosis, bronchogenic carcinoma or lung abscess. In actinomy-cosis, sinuses may develop and discharge through the chest wall. They are often diagnosed at thoracotomy. Prolonged treatment of at least 6 months is necessary. *Actinomyces* respond to penicillin, *Nocardia* to sulphonamides.

SOME PULMONARY MYCOSES

Aspergillosis

Aspergillus, mostly *A. fumigatus*, is by far the most common fungal cause of respiratory disease in the UK. In some patients, disease is due to an immune hypersensitivity to the spores. In others, the organism grows and forms hyphae in the respiratory tract, often with co-existence of immune hypersensitivity. Culture of *Aspergillus* from sputum does not necessarily indicate disease, as it may be caused by inhalation of spores or by contamination of culture plates. However, a heavy growth should be considered suspicious of disease. The presence of actual fungal hyphae in smears of sputum or bronchial washings is always significant. The syndromes caused by *Aspergillus* are as follows.

1. Asthma. Some patients with asthma have evidence of type 1 hypersensitivity (e.g. positive immediate skin prick tests or specific IgE) to *A. fumigatus*. Serum precipitins to *A. fumigatus* may also be present. Treatment of the asthma is not affected by these findings.

2. Allergic bronchopulmonary aspergillosis. This usually occurs in patients with asthma. It may present as:

(a) fleeting lung shadows with eosinophilia
(b) recurrent lobar collapse with *Aspergillus* growing in bronchi or mucus plugs
(c) bronchiectasis, usually in the proximal airways and usually in the upper lobes.

A positive skin prick test to *A. fumigatus* is found in all cases, and serum precipitins to *A. fumigatus* in most. Treatment is with oral corticosteroids. Physiotherapy may also help when lobar collapse or bronchiectasis is found.

3. Mycetoma. This is a ball of fungal hyphae growing in an existing lung cavity. Serum precipitins to the causative fungus are positive in nearly all cases. Skin prick tests and IgE to *A. fumigatus* are usually negative. Most aspergillomata are asymptomatic and most require no treatment. The most common symptom is haemoptysis, which is occasionally massive and fatal. Resection is sometimes practicable. Corticosteroids in low doses can be used to suppress systemic symptoms.

4. Invasive aspergillosis. Invasion of *Aspergillus* into normal lung occurs almost exclusively in immunocompromised patients. The condition is fatal unless treated, and may involve spread to the blood and other organs. Treatment is with intravenous amphotericin B.

Histoplasmosis

Endemic in central and northern USA, *Histoplasma capsulatum* is a dimorphic fungus causing acute and chronic granulomatous disease, similar to primary tuberculosis and chronic sarcoidosis. The condition responds to intravenous amphotericin B given for 14 days. Adrenal failure is common in the disseminated form of the disease. Serological tests are available.

Cryptococcosis

Cryptococcus neoformans, a ubiquitous yeast, causes chronic pulmonary disease and infects skin and bones. Acute or subacute meningitis is the most common syndrome, often presenting as obscure pyrexia. Amphotericin B is given for several weeks.

CHRONIC AIRFLOW OBSTRUCTION

Chronic diffuse airflow obstruction occurs in chronic bronchitis and emphysema, chronic bronchial asthma, obliterative bronchiolitis and bronchiectasis (including cystic fibrosis).

These conditions are characterised by chronic inflammation and damage to the bronchi and lungs, with reduction of expiratory flow rate and breathlessness. In some, usually older, patients, these conditions coexist or become indistinguishable from each other, and the general terms chronic obstructive lung disease (COLD), chronic obstructive pulmonary disease (COPD) and chronic obstructive airways disease (COAD) are used.

CHRONIC BRONCHITIS AND EMPHYSEMA

Chronic bronchitis consists of chronic mucus hypersecretion, causing regular expectoration of sputum, especially in the winter months, and narrowing and obliteration of small airways. Emphysema is a pathological term meaning dilatation of the air spaces distal to the terminal bronchioles with destruction of their walls.

These conditions usually coexist and are almost always caused by smoking. Chronic bronchitis alone is occasionally caused by occupational dusts and by the use of irritant fuels indoors. Emphysema with or without chronic bronchitis is occasionally caused by alpha-1-antitrypsin deficiency.

Pathology

Bronchial mucous glands are hypertrophied and goblet cell numbers increased. There is no excessive secretion of mucus. Squamous metaplasia, with desquamation and loss of the ciliated columnar epithelium, results in pooling of sputum and retention of inhaled organisms. Damage to the intact airways results in first colonisation and then invasion of the lower respiratory tract by upper respiratory organisms, notably *H. influenzae* and *Strep. pneumoniae*. Inflammatory cells accumulate within respiratory bronchioles and cause breakdown of adjacent alveolar walls by the liberation of proteases.

Pathophysiology

Physiological consequences of bronchiolar and alveolar damage consist of reduction in airflow during forced expiration, gas trapping and hyperinflation. This causes:

1. increased work of breathing
2. impaired gas exchange with alveolar hypoxia

3. secondary changes in pulmonary arteries leading to pulmonary hypertension
4. right ventricular hypertrophy—'cor pulmonale'—in which fluid retention further damages the lungs with worsening of pulmonary gas exchange
5. secondary polycythaemia, with predisposition to pulmonary artery and vascular thrombosis.

Epidemiology

Epidemiological studies have shown:

1. a major effect of cigarette smoking, related to dose
2. a marked interaction between smoking and living in towns
3. a rise in mortality associated with severe air pollution
4. decreased mortality in privileged sections of the community
5. predisposition caused by neonatal and childhood respiratory infection, prematurity, asthma and certain occupations.

Fifty per cent of smokers admit to morning cough and sputum; 25% of these develop progressive dyspnoea caused by chronic airflow obstruction. For a lifelong smoker, symptoms become important at the age of 50, and mortality is advanced to a median of 65 years.

Symptoms and signs

In patients with predominantly chronic bronchitis the main symptoms are cough and sputum which precede dyspnoea. When emphysema is dominant, patients present with dyspnoea on effort, inexorably progressive over several years. Very breathless patients often lose weight.

The main signs are a large chest with horizontal ribs, low diaphragm, reduced cricosternal distance and symmetrical reduction of chest expansion, absent cardiac and hepatic dullness, increased use of accessory muscles of respiration, expiration through pursed lips, quiet breath sounds, and rhonchi.

Some patients with severe chronic airflow limitation are able to maintain relatively normal oxygenation by hyperventilating. These patients are constantly very breathless and tend to lose weight but they are not cyanosed and do not develop cor pulmonale or secondary polycythaemia. In contrast, other patients develop central cyanosis, hypoxaemia, CO_2 retention, secondary polycythaemia and cor pulmonale with elevation of the jugular venous pressure and peripheral oedema. The reasons for these different clinical patterns are poorly understood and most patients lie within these two extremes, which are sometimes referred to as 'pink puffers' and 'blue bloaters'.

Investigations

1. Respiratory function tests. PEF, FEV1 and FEV1/VC are low. Residual volume is increased, and total lung capacity is normal or high (Fig. 2.3). In emphysema, gas transfer (measured as carbon monoxide transfer factor) is reduced. FEV1 response after bronchodilator therapy is < 20%. VC, blood gases and exercise tolerance vary with the clinical state.
2. Chest X-ray to exclude other diseases.

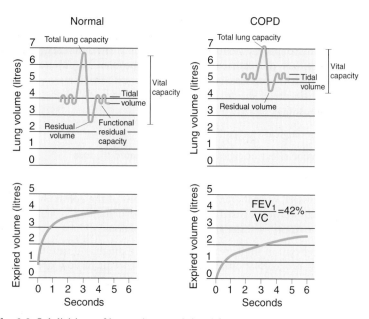

Fig. 2.3 Subdivisions of lung volume and timed forced expiratory volume in a patient with COPD, compared with the average normal values for a subject of the same sex, age and height. The lung volume traces (upper panels) illustrate the movement of the spirometer as the subject breathes first tidally, then to full inspiration (total lung capacity, TLC) and then to full expiration (residual volume, RV). Normal breathing is then resumed, at the resting lung volume (functional residual capacity, FRC). Residual air is measured indirectly, usually by the dilution of an insoluble gas such as helium, which is introduced in tracer quantities into the spirometer. The forced expiration curves (lower panels) are obtained by exhaling a full breath as fast as possible into the spirometer. When air flow is normal, the volume of air forcibly expired in the first second (FEV1) is greater than 75% of the total volume exhaled (FVC, forced vital capacity). In this example of COPD, the lung volumes are increased because of (1) reduced elasticity of the alveoli (due to pulmonary emphysema) and (2) trapping of air (because, although *normal* airways are patent at the resting lung volume, narrowed airways are closed and they only open as the lung expands). Residual volume is increased because closure of narrowed airways prevents further expiration. It follows that vital capacity is usually reduced. Total lung capacity may be normal, or may be increased when the loss of elasticity is severe. The forced expiratory trace shows that air flow is diminished.

3. CT scan demonstrates thick-walled bronchi and the macroscopic lesions of emphysema.
4. Right ventricular hypertrophy may be detected on ECG or echo-cardiography.
5. Alpha-1-antitrypsin estimation to detect hereditary deficiency.

CHRONIC BRONCHIAL ASTHMA (see p. 69)

Patients with asthma, especially those who smoke, are prone to develop irreversible progressive bronchiolar obliteration. The prognosis is said to be better if these patients take prophylactic medication and do not smoke. They may be identified by a diagnosis of asthma prior to the development of chronic changes, by a history of variability of symptoms unrelated to infective episodes, the presence of other atopic disorders, by physiological tests and by the lack of characteristic emphysematous changes on CT scan.

The degree of shortness of breath is related to airflow obstruction. Hypoxaemia and secondary pulmonary hypertension occur late in the disease. Wheezing is common, especially after exertion, and partially relieved by the inhalation of bronchodilator drugs.

OBLITERATIVE BRONCHIOLITIS

This is a rare cause of irreversible airflow obstruction characterised by fibrosis and obliteration of bronchioles without asthma or emphysema. It sometimes complicates rheumatoid arthritis, severe viral bronchiolitis or inhalation of chemicals and is a manifestation of rejection after lung transplantation.

Some patients with fibrosing lung diseases, notably sarcoidosis and extrinsic allergic alveolitis, develop bronchial inflammation and narrowing. The course and progress is similar to that of chronic bronchitis, except that associated lung fibrosis results in reduced lung volumes for the same degree of airflow limitation. Characteristic radiographic changes are generally present, and thick-walled, distorted bronchi are particularly well seen on CT scans.

TREATMENT OF CHRONIC AIRFLOW OBSTRUCTION

1. *Assessment of reversibility*. Irreversible chronic bronchitis is difficult to distinguish from untreated or partially treated asthma. Response to a 3-week trial of oral prednisolone, with serial tests of ventilatory function, identifies these patients.
2. Symptomatic improvement in respiratory discomfort and walking distance may follow the use of bronchodilators, even when simple ventilatory tests are not improved.
3. Peripheral oedema indicates generalised fluid retention, and diuretics may relieve dyspnoea as well as oedema.
4. In patients with chronic airflow obstruction, with FEV1 < 1.0 litre and $PaO_2 < 55$ mmHg (7.5 kPa), long-term oxygen therapy at home (2.0 l/min via a nasal cannula for at least 15 hours daily) may improve quality of life and reduce hospital admissions.
5. Benefits may be obtained from supervised exercise re-training and endurance may be increased by portable oxygen therapy.
6. In cases of severe dyspnoea at rest, the use of respiratory depressants and continuous oxygen may provide relief in the terminal phase of the illness.
7. Some patients benefit symptomatically from antimicrobial treatment of lower respiratory infection identified by culture of purulent sputum.

EXACERBATIONS OF CHRONIC AIRFLOW OBSTRUCTION

Minor respiratory infections may result in worsening of lung function, respiratory distress, increased wheezing and shortness of breath, worsening pulmonary gas exchange and the development of respiratory muscle fatigue. In patients with fluid retention, exacerbations may be precipitated by an increase in lung water. In either case, proliferation of lower respiratory organisms follows with the development of purulent sputum.

Treatment is with antibiotics active against *H. influenzae* and *Strep. pneumoniae*, the usual respiratory pathogens. Regular bronchodilators relieve dyspnoea. Systemic corticosteroids may have an anti-inflammatory effect during acute exacerbations but must be withdrawn if not shown to have long-term benefit. Oxygen therapy and the treatment of respiratory failure are discussed on page 101.

BRONCHIECTASIS

This is a localised or generalised dilatation of the bronchi with susceptibility to increased sputum production and recurrent bronchopulmonary infection.

Most cases result from chest infections in childhood (notably measles, whooping cough or adenovirus infections), allergic asthma, allergic broncho-pulmonary aspergillosis, cystic fibrosis, defective cilia (rare), obstruction to a bronchus, extrinsically (e.g. tuberculous lymphadenopathy) or intrinsically (e.g. inhaled foreign body), or as a complication of congenital or acquired IgG_2 deficiency.

Pathology

Lung fibrosis causes traction on adjacent bronchial walls. The dilated bronchi lack cilia, leading to pooling of secretions and chronic bronchial infection. *H. influenzae*, *Staph. aureus* and *Pseudomonas aeuruginosa* are common pathogens. Bronchopulmonary vascular anastomoses may rupture causing haemorrhage.

Symptoms and signs

Severe. Sputum greater than 30 ml per 24 hours, purulent and offensive; cough on lying down or exercise; haemoptysis of fresh blood; dyspnoea with restrictive or obstructive ventilatory disturbance; episodes of pneumonia with fever, pleuritic pain and sometimes vomiting during expectoration; clubbing of fingers and toes; coarse expiratory crackles over the affected lobes heard throughout inspiration; cyanosis and respiratory failure when ventilatory function is reduced.

Mild. The patient may have no signs between chest colds or have a tendency to expectorate sputum in small volumes daily. There may be a few persistent crackles but no clubbing or gross pulmonary dysfunction.

Investigations

1. Sputum culture for antimicrobial sensitivity.

2. In severe cases, bronchiectasis can be seen on the plain chest X-ray as cystic changes and/or 'tramline shadows' of thickened bronchial walls. In most patients, however, CT scanning is required.
3. Vital capacity and FEV1, with PaO_2 and $PaCO_2$ in severe exacerbations, are guides to the effectiveness of treatment.
4. Immunoglobulin levels.

Complications

Major haemoptysis, cerebral abscess, secondary (AA) amyloidosis.

Differential diagnosis

Congenital abnormalities of the respiratory tract.

Treatment

Exercise and postural drainage help to reduce the volume of retained sputum and resident organisms. Antibiotics, if necessary in high doses, are given until lung function is optimised. Relapsing infections sometimes respond to regular maintenance chemotherapy if they relapse immediately. Inhaled steroids may be helpful when there is associated asthma. Localised disease may be resectable surgically. Life-threatening haemoptysis may require bronchial artery embolisation.

Prognosis

Severe cases progress to respiratory failure and chronic obstruction in the fifth or sixth decade, regardless of any remission as a result of surgical treatment. Mild or moderate cases have a normal lifespan.

ASTHMA

Bronchial asthma is defined as widespread narrowing of the airways which changes in severity over short periods of time either spontaneously or with treatment. It is common and increasingly reported, affecting 5–10% of children and 2–5% of adults.

Asthmatic airways differ fundamentally from non-asthmatic airways in showing bronchial hyperreactivity, i.e. airway narrowing in response to a variety of stimuli (trigger factors) which cause little or no narrowing in normal subjects.

The pathological basis of bronchial hyperreactivity is infiltration of the airways with inflammatory cells, mainly neutrophils and eosinophils. These appearances improve in parallel with symptoms when asthmatics are treated with inhaled corticosteroids.

Many asthmatics, especially those with juvenile-onset asthma, are atopic or have a family history of atopy. However, the relationship between asthma and atopy is complex, because:

1. not all atopic individuals develop asthma
2. not all asthmatics are atopic
3. the pathological appearances of atopic and non-atopic asthma are very similar.

Non-atopic ('intrinsic') asthmatics sometimes suffer from vasomotor rhinitis and nasal polyps.

Rarely, asthma is a manifestation of autoimmune disease, e.g. the Churg–Strauss syndrome (p. 93).

Trigger factors

Although many trigger factors can be shown to provoke asthma, most patients are affected by only a few, and usually no definite trigger can be identified. The trigger factors affecting an individual may also change over time. In two-thirds of patients, asthma worsens in the early hours of the morning (Fig. 2.4). The reasons are not fully understood but include overnight falls in circulating adrenaline and cortisol levels, and increases in airway vagal tone.

In clinical practice, attacks of varying duration are most commonly precipitated by:

1. airborne allergens, which may be seasonal (e.g. grass pollen), non-seasonal (e.g. house dust mite) or occupational (e.g. urinary proteins from laboratory animals)
2. viral infections of the upper or lower respiratory tract
3. exercise (worse in cold air) (Fig. 2.5)
4. cold air (worse with exercise) and changes in humidity
5. cigarette smoke, inert dusts, aerosols and other irritants.

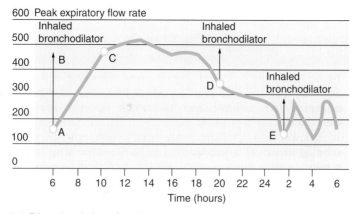

Fig. 2.4 Diurnal variation of peak expiratory flow (PEF) in an asthmatic. Exercise-induced asthma may be superimposed upon this variability which occurs spontaneously. (**A**) Morning dips; (**B**) relief by bronchodilator; (**C**) near normality during the day; (**D**) fall during the evening; (**E**) nocturnal awakening.

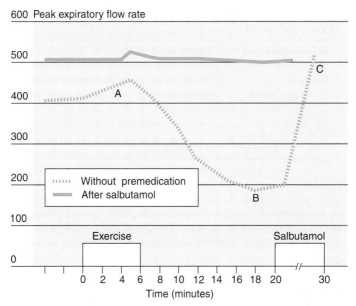

Fig. 2.5 Measurement of PEF before, during and after exercise-induced asthma. (**A**) Transient rise of PEF at start of exercise; (**B**) fall after exercise. This fall takes place more rapidly in children than in adults and is shown here beginning to resolve spontaneously after 20 minutes; (**C**) the attack is terminated rapidly by the administration of a bronchodilator aerosol.

Rarer triggers include:

1. salicylates and non-steroidal anti-inflammatory drugs
2. tartrazine food colourings
3. ingested allergens
4. psychological stress and emotional shocks
5. occupational factors (see below).

Occupational asthma

Exposure to allergens or chemicals at work can cause asthma. It can occur in atopic or non-atopic individuals, and it is not clear why some individuals develop asthma while others involved in the same work do not. The term occupational asthma is used when the allergen or chemical at work is believed to be the underlying cause of the bronchial hyperreactivity. It does not apply to patients with pre-existing asthma who have exacerbations at work due to non-specific irritants. The number of recognised causes of occupational asthma is increasing (Table 2.4).

Pathology

Airway narrowing is caused by constriction of airway smooth muscle, oedema

Table 2.4. Some causes of occupational asthma

Sensitising agent	Found in:
Isocyanates	Spray paints, varnishes, plastics, packing, printing
Epoxy resins	Hardeners in plastic adhesives
Colophony fumes (pine resin)	Soldering
Animal urine and insect droppings	Research laboratories
Flour and grain	Milling, baking

of the bronchial wall, and tenacious sputum (mucus plugs) in the airway lumen. Inflammatory cells are present, especially eosinophils and T lymphocytes, and the ciliated airway epithelium is disrupted.

Symptoms

Symptoms consist of episodic wheeze and/or dyspnoea and/or cough. In many patients symptoms resolve between asthma attacks but in chronic asthma it is common for symptoms to persist in a less severe form between exacerbations. Points to note in the history include the following:

1. Symptoms are usually worse at night or in the early morning. This is often the first evidence of an impending severe attack.
2. Cough is common and may be the only symptom.
3. Trigger factors cannot always be identified.
4. Intolerance of cigarette smoke is common. However, some asthmatics smoke.
5. Sputum is typically thick and jelly-like, sometimes with thick plugs or small spirals.
6. A family history of atopy (i.e. asthma, hay fever and/or eczema) is common.
7. Occupational asthma should be suspected when symptoms improve at weekends and/or on holiday.

Signs

Between attacks there may be no abnormal findings, although some patients may have coexistent nasal obstruction or eczema.

During periods of bronchoconstriction, wheeze (usually multiple, sometimes audible without a stethoscope, sometimes only heard on forced expiration), prolongation of expiration, hyperinflation of the lungs and tachycardia may be present.

In severe attacks, increasing tachycardia, often > 120/min, pulsus paradoxus from large swings of intrathoracic pressure, increasing distress, often with marked agitation, use of accessory muscles, and eventually exhaustion are seen. The latter is an ominous sign, leading to diminished breath sounds (as less air is moved with each breath), confusion and coma caused by hypoxaemia and CO_2 retention.

Investigations

Demonstration of reversible airflow obstruction is critical to the diagnosis of asthma. Airflow obstruction shows reversibility to bronchodilators and spontaneous variability. Reversibility to bronchodilators shows as a 15% rise in peak flow, FEVI or VC 10–20 minutes after inhaling a beta-adrenergic agent (Fig. 2.6). Spontaneous variability is best demonstrated by peak flow measurements at home 2–3 times daily, including a measurement on waking. Most patients with asthma show a 'morning dip' in peak flow (Fig. 2.7). In suspected occupational asthma, measurements may need to be made more frequently.

Skin prick tests to common allergens help to identify atopic individuals and occasionally point to specific allergens. Nasal, bronchial and food challenge may help the expert in difficult cases.

Chest X-ray, performed mainly to exclude other disease, is often normal, although it may show hyperinflation. A chest X-ray is crucial in acute severe asthma to exclude pneumothorax.

Arterial blood gas tensions are usually normal and measured only in severe asthma. $PaCO_2$ should be low during acute attacks. A 'high normal' $PaCO_2$ is a very serious sign, suggesting the onset of ventilatory failure.

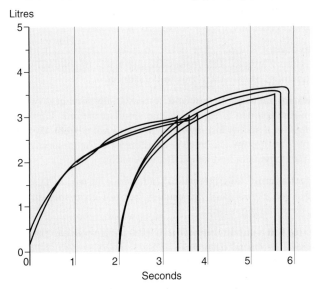

Fig. 2.6 Timed forced expiratory traces in an asthmatic subject before and after administration of a bronchodilator. In this subject both the FEV1 and vital capacity rise after use of the bronchodilator.

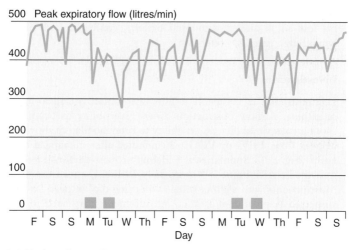

Fig. 2.7 Peak expiratory flow measurements in an asthmatic subject. Note the spontaneous variability in peak flow, with 'morning dips'. In this example the asthma was aggravated by the use of isocyanate paint sprays.

A blood count may show eosinophilia which is suppressed by systemic steroids.

Differential diagnosis

Chronic bronchitis and emphysema. Most patients with chronic bronchitis and emphysema have irreversible airflow obstruction. Those who do show reversibility should be treated in the same way as asthmatics.

Infection. Wheeze may occur in chest infections, and purulent sputum in asthma attacks. The main difficulty arises in children in whom 'recurrent bronchitis' usually turns out to be asthma.

Central airway obstruction. Occasionally laryngeal or tracheal tumours, or aspiration of a foreign body, can simulate asthma. However, the main sign is stridor, a mainly inspiratory sound, and not wheeze which is mainly expiratory. The spirometric trace is characteristic. Acute laryngeal oedema occurs as part of generalised anaphylactic reactions.

Psychogenic 'laryngospasm' (adduction of true or false cords) may cause difficulty. Blood gases are usually, but not invariably, normal. Diagnosis is by direct laryngoscopy.

Acute left ventricular failure. This can mimic (or exacerbate) asthma by causing nocturnal dyspnoea.

Complications

These include ventilatory failure, pneumothorax, pneumomediastinum, and allergic bronchopulmonary aspergillosis.

Treatment

Routine treatment

Avoidance. Beta-blockers should be avoided by all patients, as should occupational chemicals known to cause asthma. Allergens, foodstuffs and drugs to which there is an idiosyncratic reaction (e.g. aspirin) need be avoided only if they cause symptoms. Patients with occupational asthma may be entitled to compensation.

Medication. This involves:

1. Suppression of inflammation by the regular inhalation of corticosteroids, using the minimum dose to optimise lung function. This dose may vary. Inhaled corticosteroids (or, in some children, disodium cromoglycate) is required in all patients except those whose attacks are infrequent and who respond rapidly to inhaled beta-agonists. A variety of inhaler devices are available (Fig. 2.8).
2. Relief of bronchoconstriction by inhaled beta-agonists.
3. Treatment of exacerbations with high-dose inhaled steroids, or oral steroids, according to severity (see below).
4. Some patients who are receiving the above treatment obtain additional relief from long-acting inhaled beta-agonists, inhaled anticholinergic bronchodilators, or long-acting oral aminophylline.

Education

This takes time and should include simple explanation of asthma, correct use of inhaler device and peak flow meter, principles of drug therapy, especially prophylactic versus symptomatic treatment, and recognition of worsening asthma and specific instructions on appropriate action

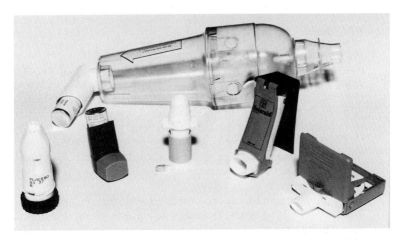

Fig. 2.8 A selection of devices for the administration of inhaled bronchodilators.

Recognition and management of worsening asthma

Recognition. Patients should be aware that the following are warning signs of an impending attack:

1. increase in nocturnal waking due to asthma
2. failure of symptoms to resolve by midmorning
3. progressive deterioration day by day
4. a cold which 'goes down to the chest'.

Treatment. Prompt action can often abort an asthma attack. Mild exacerbations (morning PEF > 70% predicted) can usually be managed by doubling the dose of inhaled steroid, but more severe attacks (morning PEF 50–70% predicted) should be treated with oral prednisolone.

Recognition and management of acute severe asthma

Recognition. In a distressed or exhausted asthmatic patient, indications for emergency hospital treatment are inability to speak in full sentences, pulse rate >120/min (140/min in a child), central cyanosis, PEF well below the patient's usual value, and no relief from the patient's usual or beta-agonist therapy. Exhaustion, diminished breath sounds, mental confusion and a low PaO_2 with a high or high–normal $PaCO_2$ are signs of life-threatening asthma.

Treatment. As soon as possible (in the house or ambulance) the patient should receive oxygen, a beta-agonist, ideally via a nebuliser or large-volume spacer device, and hydrocortisone 200 mg i.v. or prednisolone 40 mg p.o. Lung function is monitored, and treatment reduced according to response. Some patients require additional bronchodilators, e.g. inhaled anticholinergic agents or i.v. aminophylline. Exhaustion, failure to respond promptly to emergency treatments and inability to maintain adequate oxygenation are the main indications for transfer to the ITU, where assisted ventilation may be needed.

Prognosis

Most patients have a normal lifespan and controllable symptoms with exacerbations of asthma occurring at unpredictable intervals. Some adults with chronic asthma develop irreversible or partially irreversible airflow obstruction, with symptoms even between exacerbations. Decline of lung function over time is greater in adult-onset asthma. A few patients need maintenance oral prednisolone with consequent side-effects.

Children with asthma often become symptom-free at puberty but at least 50% have asthma in adult life. Children at greatest risk of having adult asthma are those with severe disease, those whose asthma started at an early age and those with severe infantile eczema.

Death from asthma is uncommon considering the prevalence of the disease. Some 1500 deaths from asthma occur in England and Wales each year. Most deaths occur outside hospital, half resulting from underestimation of the severity of attacks by patients and doctors.

CYSTIC FIBROSIS

Cystic fibrosis (CF) is an autosomal recessive condition caused by one of a number of mutations on chromosome 7. One individual in 25 is a carrier. A defective membrane transfer protein affects chloride ion transport in mucosa. Many of the symptoms are explicable by obstruction of tubules by mucus. Pancreas, lung, sinuses, bile ducts and seminiferous tubules are affected. Presentation is with intestinal obstruction in infancy, failure to thrive, steatorrhoea and associated vitamin deficiency, or with recurrent respiratory infection leading to bronchiectasis and progressive respiratory impairment. Hepatic cirrhosis, sinusitis and pneumothorax are frequent problems. Diabetes mellitus occurs. Most males have azoospermia but girls are fertile (Fig. 2.9).

It is now the most common serious Mendelian genetic disorder in

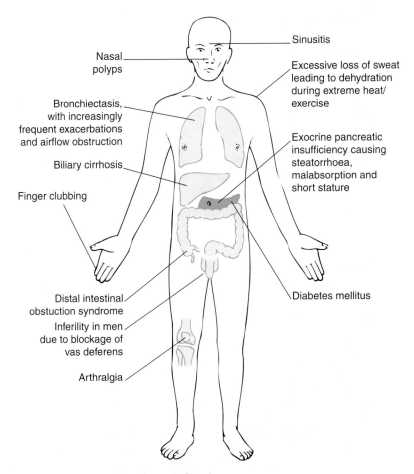

Fig. 2.9 Clinical problems in cystic fibrosis.

Caucasians, although it is rare in Asians and Africans. To date, some 80 mutations have been identified in different individuals. The most common is ΔF508, which occurs in 70% of CF genes. Approximately 50% (70% × 70%) are homozygous for this mutation, the remaining 50% having ΔF508 and another, less common, mutation, or two of the less common mutations. Discovery of these mutations has enabled more accurate identification of carriers, with implications for genetic counselling and, potentially, for population screening. This raises many ethical issues.

Symptoms and signs

Failure to thrive, steatorrhoea, recurrent or chronic bronchial infection with purulent sputum, progressive shortness of breath, and haemoptysis, often severe.

Clubbing of fingers and toes is nearly always present. Chest deformity, usually hyperinflation, sometimes restrictive, respiratory crackles over the upper lobes, and respiratory failure are seen.

Investigations

Sweat [Na^+]. In children, > 59 mmol/l is diagnostic. In adults, 70–90 mmol/l is borderline, > 90 mmol/l is diagnostic.

Chest X-ray. Bronchiectasis, cysts and nodular changes in upper and middle zones, fibrosis and recurrent consolidation, and abscess formation are present.

Sputum. *H. influenzae, Staph. aureus* and *Ps. aeruginosa* are the common pathogens occurring in that order during the lifetime of the patient, unless eradicated by antibiotic treatment.

Pancreatic function is impaired (p. 270). Adequacy of pancreatic replacement is monitored in children by stool fats and by height and weight, and in adults by serum levels of fat-soluble vitamins (A, E and D) and calcium.

Lung function. Airflow obstruction is progressive, with falling FEV1 and usually hyperinflation. PaO_2 is reduced during exacerbations. Elevation of $PaCO_2$ occurs late. Infective pulmonary exacerbations cause transient falls of VC.

Complications

These include heat exhaustion (loss of sodium in sweat), pneumothorax, haemoptysis, abdominal pain, constipation and intestinal obstruction (meconium ileus equivalent, also known as distal intestinal obstruction syndrome).

Treatment

Adequate calorie intake must be ensured. Oral pancreatic supplements are given before meals and snacks in doses sufficient to control steatorrhoea.

H_2 antagonists reduce gastric breakdown of pancreatic enzymes. Vitamins A, D and E supplements are needed.

Exercise is beneficial, postural drainage and forced expiratory physiotherapy aid expectoration. Long-term flucloxacillin, up to 4 g per 24 hours, prevents staphylococcal lung infection. Vaccination against influenza and pneumococcal infection is recommended. In some patients, lung function and symptoms can be improved with daily nebulised DNase, which reduces sputum viscosity by lysing the DNA released by dead inflammatory cells in the airways.

Acute exacerbations are treated for as long as necessary with appropriate antibiotics. Frequent recurrences are treated with nebulised antibiotics. Indwelling intravenous lines may be needed. Antibiotics are given for fever, acute pneumonic illness, increasing sputum or progressively falling VC. Consistent carefully explained management by a skilful team and easy access to expert care are essential.

Bilateral lung or heart/lung transplantation is available for patients with severe disease (FEV1 < 30% predicted) and is increasingly successful. It has offered hope to many patients who previously had none. However, because of the limited availability of donor organs, only one in four patients accepted for transplantation survive to receive a transplant.

Prognosis

Life expectancy is improving. It is dependent on the severity of the respiratory disease. The median duration of survival is currently around 30 years. By the year 2000 it is estimated that there will be more adults with CF than children.

SARCOIDOSIS

Sarcoidosis is a systemic disease of unknown cause with non-caseating granulomata in lymph nodes and other sites, usually having a benign course. Its prevalence varies according to population, ranging from 27 to 200 per 100 000. Clinically indistinguishable disorders may be caused by chronic exposure to industrial beryllium (berylliosis) and by tattooing. The characteristic pathological lesion is the granuloma, a reaction to an insoluble antigen, which may heal with no residue or with fibrosis. CD4 (helper) T lymphocytes are concentrated in active sites such as the lung, which results in reduced immunoreactivity elsewhere (delayed hypersensitivity tests may become negative). T cell function is normal, as is resistance to infection.

Symptoms and signs

Acute sarcoidosis presents with a febrile illness, erythema nodosum and bilateral enlargement of the hilar lymph nodes in the chest. Prognosis is good with more than 80% recovering spontaneously. A few patients develop pulmonary infiltrations and may become breathless. The lung changes may

Table 2.5. Systemic manifestations of chronic sarcoidosis

Eye	Anterior uveitis, glaucoma
	Posterior uveitis
	Kerato-conjunctivitis (occasionally dryness)
	Lachrymal gland enlargement
Salivary exocrine glands	Parotid and other salivary glandular enlargement, dry mouth
Skin	Recurrent erythema nodosum (rare)
	Papules and nodules: 'lupus pernio'
	Hypertrophic scars are common
Joints	Polyarthralgia, polyarthritis
	Bone cysts (accompanied by skin changes)
Central nervous system	Neuropathy, especially cranial
	Meningomyelitis
	Posterior pituitary lesions, diabetes insipidus
Gastrointestinal tract	Hepatomegaly, splenomegaly with portal hypertension
Ear, nose and throat	Nasal, laryngeal granuloma
Lung	Bronchial inflammation, stenosis
	Lung granuloma and fibrosis, rarely pleural
	Hilar adenopathy
Heart	Cardiomyopathy
	Heart block
	Sudden death
Kidney	Granulomatous interstitial nephritis
General	Hypercalcaemia and renal complications
	Enlarged lymph nodes
	Fever (rare)

progress to a chronic destructive fibrotic disease which may occasionally be fatal. Afro-Caribbeans are more commonly prone to severe forms.

Chronic sarcoidosis may present in a variety of ways (Table 2.5). Pulmonary sarcoidosis presents with rapid or slow progression of cough, dyspnoea or chest pain, and may be detected at a routine chest X-ray. Cardiac sarcoidosis (rare) causes arrhythmias, sudden death and congestive cardiomyopathy.

Examination reveals some of the manifestations listed. Inspiratory crackles are usually scanty or absent. Cor pulmonale may result from progression to severe pulmonary fibrosis.

Investigations

1. Characteristic histology of affected node or site—liver, bronchus, lung, labial gland—is diagnostic.
2. Kveim test. Installation of 0.1 ml of antigen from sarcoid spleen intra-dermally will result in a granuloma in 6 weeks (confirmed by biopsy).
3. Chest X-ray may show bilateral hilar lymphadenopathy and diffuse lung shadows, especially in upper and middle zones. Later, upper zone or

generalised pulmonary fibrosis will be seen with generalised cyst formation (honeycomb lung) and 'eggshell' calcification of hilar nodes. CT and magnetic resonance scans will show the extent of adenopathy and pulmonary involvement.

4. Blood. Raised ESR and plasma viscosity occur in most patients with erythema nodosum. Serum calcium levels are elevated in 10%. Abnormal liver function and elevated angiotensin-converting enzyme level may be detected. Most patients with lone pulmonary sarcoid have no blood abnormality.

5. Lung function tests do not mirror exactly the severity of radiological granulomatosis but show good correlation with the degree of dyspnoea. Reductions of VC and gas transfer (measured as carbon monoxide transfer factor) occur with alveolar wall fibrosis. Fibrotic disease or bronchial stenosis causes chronic airways obstruction. Hypoxaemia and respiratory failure occur late.

6. Bronchoscopy may show granulomata, bronchial stenosis and characteristic histology.

7. Hand X-rays show cysts in bone.

Differential diagnosis

Tuberculosis may also cause bilateral hilar lymphadenopathy and erythema nodosum. All organs may be involved in sarcoidosis.

Prognosis

Prognosis is variable: 50% remit, 50% become chronic with a marginally reduced life expectancy, and a few progress rapidly. The disease is more aggressive in patients of African descent.

Treatment

Active pulmonary sarcoidosis responds to corticosteroids which, given early, suppress granuloma formation and prevent progression to fibrosis but do not alter the prognosis for eventual remission or relapse. Control is sustained if necessary with moderate doses of prednisolone (5–17.5 mg daily for 4 weeks). There is no known radical cure.

Absolute indications for corticosteroid therapy include anterior uveitis (drops are effective), posterior uveitis, hypercalcaemia, dyspnoea, and cardiac and CNS involvement (efficacy variable).

Corticosteroids should be considered where skin lesions are disfiguring, for nasal disease and symptomatic lymphatic or glandular swellings or for drying of salivary secretions.

TUMOURS OF THE LUNG

Almost all tumours of the lung are malignant or potentially malignant. By far the most common is bronchial carcinoma.

BRONCHIAL CARCINOMA

Bronchial carcinoma is responsible for more male deaths in the developed world than any other cancer, with more than 30 000 deaths/year in the UK. The principal cause is cigarette smoking. The death rate in the UK seems to have reached a plateau in men. It is less common but rising in women and now rivals breast carcinoma as the most common malignant disease, reflecting a 4-fold rise in cigarette consumption by women between 1940 and 1975. The excess risk approximately halves every 5 years after smoking is stopped. Pipe and cigar smokers have a smaller increased risk. Passive smoking may carry a significant risk. Patients with asbestosis also have an increased risk of bronchial carcinoma.

Pathology

Most tumours originate in the larger bronchi where they may cause partial or total obstruction. They spread to the mediastinum, pleura and chest wall by direct invasion, and to the hilar, mediastinal and supraclavicular lymph nodes via the lymphatics. The most common sites for blood-borne metastases are the brain, liver and bones. The histological subtypes (Table 2.6) vary in prognosis.

Symptoms and signs

Local effects of tumour in a bronchus
1. Cough (frequently ignored because most smokers regard a morning cough as normal), sometimes changing in character.
2. Haemoptysis, which should always be investigated.
3. Bronchial narrowing—dyspnoea, stridor (if the narrowing affects the trachea or main bronchi), fixed rhonchus, distal infection with peripheral obstruction.
4. Distal collapse—dyspnoea, mediastinal shift to the affected side, diminished expansion, dullness to percussion, diminished breath sounds and diminished vocal resonance all on the affected side.
5. Weight loss, usually with anorexia.

Table 2.6. Characteristics of different cell types in primary bronchial carcinoma

Cell type	Frequency	Growth	Metastases
Squamous	40%	Slow	Early
Small cell	25%	Rapid	Early
Large cell undifferentiated	20%	Intermediate	Intermediate
Adenocarcinoma	15%	Intermediate	Intermediate
Alveolar cell carcinoma	<1%	Rapid	Late

6. Finger clubbing is seen in 30% of patients. Note that chronic bronchitis and emphysema do not cause finger clubbing.

Spread to mediastinum (Fig. 2.10)

1. Left recurrent laryngeal nerve paralysis leads to hoarse voice, bovine cough.
2. Superior vena caval obstruction causes headache, sometimes aggravated by bending forward, plethora and peripheral cyanosis of the face and conjunctivae, engorged non-pulsatile neck veins, and distended collateral veins on the chest wall.
3. Dysphagia from compression of the oesophagus by either the tumour or lymph nodes.
4. Phrenic nerve paralysis results in elevation and paradoxical movement of the diaphragm; this causes dullness and diminished breath sounds but is usually easier to detect radiologically than clinically.
5. Pericardial invasion causes a blood-stained pericardial effusion and arrhythmias.

Spread to pleura and chest wall

1. Malignant pleural effusions are usually blood-stained. Pleural effusion in bronchogenic carcinoma is not always the result of local invasion but may be secondary to infection.
2. Chest wall pain—constant and often severe.
3. Apical (superior sulcus, Pancoast) tumours often erode the first rib and involve the brachial plexus and cervical sympathetic nerves. They may

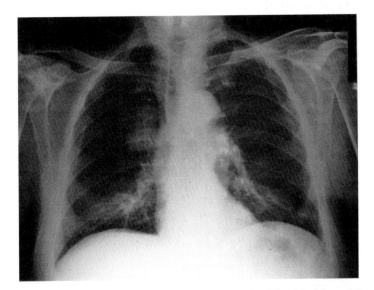

Fig. 2.10 Chest X-ray showing tumour at the upper pole of the right hilum. (There is also a cavitating opacity in the right lower zone, which may have been due to infection or neoplasia but was not investigated because of the patient's general condition.)

cause pain in the inner aspect of the arm (T1 dermatome), wasting of the small muscles of the hand and Horner's syndrome.

Spread to lymph nodes

1. Hilar lymphadenopathy can cause bronchial narrowing by extrinsic compression. Enlarged hilar lymph nodes can also cause retrograde obstruction of pulmonary lymphatics—lymphangitis carcinomatosis—which presents with cough and dyspnoea.
2. Mediastinal lymphadenopathy can compress and invade other mediastinal structures.
3. Supraclavicular lymphadenopathy is detectable clinically and should always be sought on examination.

Distant blood-borne metastases

1. Bone—pain, pathological fractures, including vertebral collapse, and hypercalcaemia. Hypercalcaemia can also result from squamous growths. Symptoms include malaise, nausea, confusion, thirst, polyuria and constipation.
2. Liver—hard, irregular hepatomegaly, sometimes tender.
3. Brain—epilepsy, localising neurological defects, headache, papilloedema.
4. Adrenal glands—usually asymptomatic but can rarely cause Addison's disease.
5. Skin—painless nodules.

Non-metastatic (paraneoplastic) complications

1. Pulmonary hypertrophic osteoarthropathy—painful wrists or ankles.
2. Endocrine syndromes caused by products of tumour cells which mimic hormones—Cushing's syndrome (ACTH), dilutional hyponatraemia (ADH), hypercalcaemia (parathyroid hormone-related peptide), gynaecomastia (oestrogens).
3. Neuromuscular syndromes—peripheral neuropathy, cerebellar dysfunction, dermatomyositis and a form of myasthenia (Eaton-Lambert syndrome).

Investigations

Chest X-ray is the most common clue to diagnosis. Sometimes the tumour is detected on routine X-ray. Radiological appearances include slight enlargement or distortion of a hilar shadow or an obvious hilar mass, an area of pulmonary collapse with or without a hilar shadow, unresolved pneumonia, pleural effusion, lung abscess, a peripheral mass and occasionally lymphangitis carcinomatosa.

The sputum can be examined cytologically but a negative result does not exclude the diagnosis.

Bronchoscopy with biopsy establishes the diagnosis and the position of the tumour in the bronchial tree in over 70%.

Screening for liver and bone metastases is by determining alkaline phosphatase, aspartate aminotransferase and serum calcium levels. Liver scan (ultrasound or CT) and radiological investigation for bone metastases (plain

X-rays with or without an isotope bone scan) or brain metastases (CT scan) are indicated only if there is a clinical or biochemical suspicion of metastases.

CT or MRI of the thorax determines the extent of a bronchial carcinoma, demonstrating invasion of the mediastinum and chest wall, enlargement of hilar and mediastinal lymph nodes, and other pulmonary lesions.

Mediastinoscopy is required to biopsy enlarged mediastinal lymph nodes, and pleural biopsy and cytology of the pleural fluid to diagnose most malignant effusions.

FEV1, VC and effort tolerance need to be determined. Respiratory failure will probably ensue if, after resection of the tumour, FEV1 is less than 1.0 litre.

Surgical excision may be necessary for diagnosis of resectable peripheral masses of uncertain cause.

Differential diagnosis

The differential diagnosis is wide and depends on the mode of presentation. The respiratory diseases that resemble bronchogenic carcinoma radiographically are pneumonia, lung abscess, tuberculosis, pulmonary infarction and pulmonary metastases. For lymphatic carcinomatosis and alveolar cell carcinoma, the differential diagnosis also includes cryptogenic fibrosing alveolitis and other causes of diffuse pulmonary fibrosis.

Treatment

Surgery. Removal of the affected lobe or lung is the treatment of choice, as it provides the best chance of cure in all cell types. However, most patients are unsuitable for surgery at the time of presentation, either because the tumour has spread to the pleura, mediastinum or beyond, or because the patient is generally unfit for major thoracic surgery owing to cardiorespiratory disease or advanced age. Approximately 20% of patients are considered suitable for surgery, and of these 25–50% survive 5 years, the best results being obtained with squamous carcinoma. Resection of an apparently localised small cell tumour is usually followed by chemotherapy because of the likelihood of undetected metastases being present at diagnosis.

Radiotherapy. Occasionally localised lung cancer can be cured by high-dose radiotherapy. Palliative low-dose radiotherapy can greatly improve the quality of life, whatever the cell type. It is particularly useful for localised bone pain caused by either local spread or metastases, superior vena caval obstruction, stridor and impending bronchial obstruction, dysphagia from oesophageal compression, severe haemoptysis or cough and cerebral metastases.

Chemotherapy. In small cell lung cancer, combination chemotherapy can prolong life (currently by 6–12 months in the 70% of patients who respond) and relieve symptoms. Large clinical trials are essential to document the effectiveness of different regimens. In non-small cell lung cancer, chemotherapy is much less effective, and its place is not yet established.

Palliation. Palliation is sometimes achieved by radiotherapy or chemotherapy (see above). For pain, regular analgesia is an alternative, with non-steroidal anti-inflammatory drugs and opiates. Occlusion of major airways by the tumour can be relieved by laser therapy and/or the insertion of a stent. Malignant pleural effusions causing breathlessness may be aspirated, followed by chemical pleurodesis. Hypercalcaemia is treated with fluids ± diphosphonates.

Counselling and continuing care by doctors and nurses is essential.

OTHER PRIMARY LUNG TUMOURS

Bronchial adenomas

These uncommon tumours usually present with haemoptysis, recurrent infection or lobar/segmental collapse. The majority can be seen at broncho-scopy; 90% are **carcinoid tumours**, the remainder being **cylindromata**. Malignant change and local invasion are uncommon, metastases and the carcinoid syndrome rare. The treatment of choice is surgical excision unless there is evidence of metastasis. The outlook is excellent unless there is malignant change in the excised tumour.

Hamartomas

These rare benign tumours are fetal rests which grow in middle life. They may calcify. They resemble peripheral carcinomas and are usually removed by segmental resection.

Lymphomas

Occasionally, a lymphoma arises in the lung in the absence of disease elsewhere. More often, however, pulmonary involvement occurs when there is generalised disease with involvement of other organs.

SECONDARY TUMOURS OF THE LUNG

Blood-borne pulmonary metastases are common and can arise from malignant tumours anywhere in the body. The most common primary sites are breast, kidney, ovary, testes and GI tract. They are usually multiple and sometimes appear as well defined round opacities, so-called cannonball secondaries. They usually cause few respiratory symptoms unless lung tissue is extensively replaced by tumour or pleural effusion develops. Lymphangitis carcinomatosis (see p. 84) can also occur as a result of metastases, often from breast carcinoma.

DIFFUSE PULMONARY INFILTRATION AND FIBROSIS

Several conditions cause diffuse infiltration of the alveolar walls with inflammatory cells, with or without alveolar exudate and fibrosis. The bronchioles

Table 2.7. Disorders leading to diffuse pulmonary fibrosis

Cryptogenic fibrosing alveolitis and fibrosing alveolitis associated with connective tissue disorders, e.g. scleroderma

Sarcoidosis

Extrinsic allergic alveolitis

Pneumoconioses
   Asbestosis
   Silicosis
   Coal workers' pneumoconiosis

Radiation fibrosis

Drugs, e.g. amiodarone, cytotoxic drugs, nitrofurantoin, sulphasalazine

Paraquat poisoning

Recurrent pulmonary oedema, e.g. secondary to mitral valve disease

may be involved. These present either as acute illnesses or insidiously, with breathlessness. Fine basal crackles are often present and some patients have finger clubbing. VC and lung volumes and/or gas transfer are reduced and there is variable hypoxaemia with hyperventilation. They progress to 'honeycomb lung' in which areas of the lung are replaced by cysts formed from dilated bronchioles surrounded by fibrosed and obliterated alveoli. Radiological change may be obvious but is not necessarily proportional to the functional abnormality.

Some causes are listed in Table 2.7. Most of these conditions are uncommon.

CRYPTOGENIC FIBROSING ALVEOLITIS (SYNONYM: INTERSTITIAL PNEUMONIA)

This is a progressive condition of unknown cause characterised by acute or insidious inflammation of the alveolar wall leading to fibrosis.

Pathology

In acute cases, there is desquamation of type II alveolar cells with macrophages into the alveolar spaces and lymphocytic infiltration of alveolar walls. There may be obliteration of bronchioles and patchy consolidation. In chronic cases, fibrosis within alveolar walls may obliterate whole lobules.

There is overlap with the systemic autoimmune diseases and conditions resembling cryptogenic fibrosing alveolitis occur in rheumatoid arthritis, systemic sclerosis, chronic active hepatitis, Sjögren's syndrome and renal tubular acidosis.

Symptoms and signs

Most patients present between the ages of 40 and 70. The acute form presents with rapid onset of dyspnoea at rest or on slight exertion with a non-productive cough. Fine inspiratory crackles are heard at the bases. Cyanosis or clubbing is present in the minority. Over half remit or respond to corticosteroids.

The more common chronic form presents with an insidious onset of exertional dyspnoea and variable, and usually, non-productive cough. Examination reveals fine inspiratory crackles, sometimes localised, heard at the end of inspiration. Clubbing occurs in over 50%. Only 10% respond to corticosteroids; more than half will die within 5 years of diagnosis.

Complications

These include bronchial infection, respiratory failure, pulmonary hypertension and pulmonary thromboembolic disease.

Investigations

Chest X-ray and high-resolution CT scans show progressively, fine nodulation, basal fibrosis and generalised 'honeycombing' (Fig. 2.11).

VC and residual lung volumes are low, expiratory flow rates normal (Fig. 2.12), and CO transfer factor reduced (the earliest abnormality in insidious cases). PaO_2 varies with clinical state but may be only slightly reduced in early cases. $PaCO_2$ is low except terminally.

Bronchoalveolar lavage and transbronchial biopsy show all types of inflammatory cells, including lymphocytes, neutrophils and eosinophils,

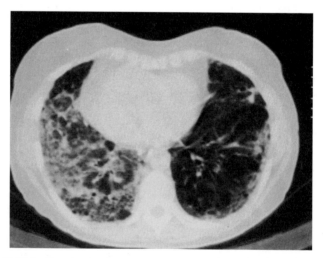

Fig. 2.11 Thin slice computed tomographic scan of cryptogenic fibrosing alveolitis (supine). The right side illustrates early abnormalities with fibrosis and cystic changes in a characteristic subpleural distribution. On the left the abnormalities are more advanced, showing complete disruption of the lung architecture by fibrosis, with secondary cystic changes.

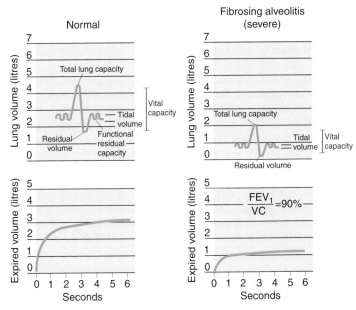

Fig. 2.12 Subdivisions of lung volume (upper panels) and timed forced expiratory volumes (lower panels) in a patient with severe fibrosing alveolitis, compared with average normal values for a subject of the same sex, age and height. (For definitions, see Fig. 2.3.) In this example of fibrosing alveolitis, all the subdivisions of lung volume are reduced, because the excess fibrous tissue limits expansion, increases the elasticity of the lung thus reducing the resting lung volume, and reduces the number of patent alveoli, thus reducing residual volume. The spirometer trace obtained by forced expiration shows that more than 75% of the total volume exhaled is exhaled within 1 second, indicating that air flow is not affected.

to be present in excess. (Lymphocytosis is said to be associated with steroid responsiveness; neutrophilia and eosinophilia with a poor prognosis.) Histology of small samples is unreliable because of the patchy nature of the disease but characteristic changes may be detected.

Thoracotomy and lung biopsy are employed when the diagnosis remains uncertain.

Differential diagnosis (see Table 2.7)

Acute cryptogenic fibrosing alveolitis has to be distinguished from viral pneumonia.

Treatment

Treatment is currently unsatisfactory. Corticosteroids in high doses generally improve function in acute cases and are reduced to maintenance doses as clinical improvement occurs. Relapse is common. In a few cases, steroid doses may be reduced by the concomitant use of immunosuppressant agents such as cyclophosphamide. Most patients respond only transiently.

EXTRINSIC ALLERGIC ALVEOLITIS

Numerous organic agents may cause acute or chronic bronchial and pulmonary lymphocytic infiltration, granulomas and fibrosis in susceptible subjects (Table 2.8).

Acute exposure leads to fever, malaise, cough and dyspnoea within 48 hours. The symptoms of chronic exposure are similar to those of chronic airflow obstruction, often without a history of preceding acute episodes. Lung function tests show a predominantly restrictive pattern with hypoxaemia. Stippling, diffuse lung fibrosis, often apical, will be seen on chest X-ray.

DISEASES CAUSED BY MINERAL DUSTS (PNEUMOCONIOSES)

Minerals inhaled at work or as a result of environmental pollution may cause clinical disease and/or radiographic change. Inhaled dust is transported out of the lungs by the mucociliary escalator and the alveolar macrophage system which transports the dust to the bronchi or to the lymph nodes. Toxic dusts damage macrophages with the liberation of cytokines resulting in an inflammatory response reflected in radiographic and functional changes. Molecular weight determines radiodensity (iron oxide, barium sulphate, tin oxide are opaque but inert). With heavy exposure, the lymphatics become blocked so that highly fibrogenic dusts are more toxic when mixed with inert particles.

Pneumoconioses result from a fibrous reaction to dusts retained in the lung, the severity of the condition depending on the inhaled dose, the size of the particles and their toxicity to macrophages.

Chronic bronchitis and emphysema are additional hazards, although their industrial incidence has been difficult to evaluate because of the small numbers of non-smoking men working in the industries concerned.

Table 2.8. Examples of extrinsic allergic alveolitis

Disease	Cause	Serum precipitin test
Farmer's lung ⎫ Mushroom worker's lung ⎭	Spores of thermophilic actinomycetes	Usually positive but 10% false negative, 20% false positive among farmers
Pigeon fancier's lung	Pigeon serum in excreta	20% false positive among breeders
Budgerigar fancier's lung	Budgerigar droppings	Usually positive
Malt worker's lung	*Aspergillus clavatus* spores	Usually positive
Grain handler's lung	Grain weevil	Numerous antigens, no test available
Pituitary snuff taker's lung	Animal antigens	No test available
Humidifier fever	Thermophilic actinomycetes ⎫ Saprophytic amoebae ⎭	Poor correlation between presence of antibodies and disease

Coalworkers' pneumoconiosis

Simple pneumoconiosis refers to the nodular lesions affecting the lungs of coalminers caused by carbon deposition and associated with focal emphysema. The lesions are situated near the respiratory bronchioles and have a minor effect on lung function. *Complicated pneumoconiosis*: In this condition sheets of fibrous tissue, known as progressive massive fibrosis, are deposited in the lungs. These can resemble lung tumours on X-ray and cause dyspnoea. Miners with rheumatoid arthritis are especially prone to rheumatoid nodules within the lung (Caplan's syndrome).

The prevalence of the disease among coalminers led to an extensive system for identification and compensation of these cases. Improved mining methods have drastically reduced the incidence of this disorder.

Silicosis

This pneumoconiosis, caused by the inhalation of finely particulate silica, complicates mining of precious metals, tin, copper, graphite, mica and anthracite, quarrying and dressing of slate, granite and sandstone, road drilling and sandblasting, pottery and ceramics manufacture, boiler scraping, and grinding (new techniques avoid silica). Silica is more fibrogenic than coal. Progressive fibrosis may occur.

Silicosis causes dyspnoea with recurrent respiratory infections. Characteristic chest X-ray changes include multiple fine nodules in the upper and middle zones, with peripheral 'eggshell' calcification of mediastinal lymph nodes. Massive fibrosis within the lungs may cavitate and the right ventricle may enlarge.

Functional changes include reduction of the VC and preservation of the FEV1/VC ratio. The differential diagnosis includes sarcoidosis, miliary tuberculosis and other causes of diffuse pulmonary mottling.

Diseases related to asbestos exposure

Asbestos (*Gr.* 'indestructible') is a natural fibre consisting of aluminium, calcium, iron, nickel and magnesium silicates. It resists high temperatures. Several forms exist, mainly chrysolite (white asbestos) and the amphiboles particularly crocidolite and tremolite (blue asbestos).

Asbestos fibres measure 20×3 μm. They are distributed axially in the airstream to the lower lobes and deposited subpleurally, being transported through lymphatic channels to the parietal pleura.

Conditions caused by asbestos are:

1. **Asbestosis** is a form of diffuse mainly basal pulmonary fibrosis clinically and radiologically similar to fibrosing alveolitis but with pleural involvement. It usually occurs 10–30 years or more after first exposure, the risk being related to the amount and duration of exposure.
2. **Pleural plaques,** which may calcify. Usually painless, they do not affect lung function.
3. **Non-malignant recurrent pleural effusion** with dense pleural thickening.

4. **Mesothelioma of pleura.** This is a malignant pleural tumour presenting with chest wall pain or pleural effusion. Local spread is more common than metastasis. It is usually fatal within 2 years; 90% of cases have been exposed to asbestos but in some cases the exposure has been low. Crocidolite is particularly implicated. The *peritoneum* may be involved.
5. **Carcinoma of the bronchus.** There is a marked interaction between cigarette smoking and asbestos in causing bronchial carcinoma.

Compensation

In many countries, compensation is available and litigation is commonplace. Until 1975 there was widespread ignorance among employers as to the necessary precautions; this is surprising because legal measures to control exposure were first introduced around 1930.

PULMONARY OEDEMA

The presence of oedema fluid in the pulmonary alveoli is caused by either transudation (cardiogenic, related to altered vascular pressure) or exudation (non-cardiogenic, related to vascular permeability).

Pulmonary transudation is usually caused by left ventricular failure or mitral stenosis. High altitude travel and raised intracranial pressure (ICP), which are rarer causes of pulmonary oedema, operate by altering vascular pressures in the presence of normal cardiac function.

Acute non-cardiogenic pulmonary oedema occurs in intensive care units (adult respiratory distress syndrome, ARDS). This complicates hypotension, oxygen toxicity, trauma and blood loss, fat embolism, lung contusion and haemorrhage, viral pneumonias and inhalation or injection of certain toxic or therapeutic agents.

Management involves oxygenation and artificial ventilation (p. 107) as well as treatment of the underlying condition with circulatory support when necessary.

PULMONARY INVOLVEMENT IN SYSTEMIC DISEASES

Rheumatoid arthritis (see p. 360)

Lung involvement includes fibrosing alveolitis (characterised by inspiratory crackles, gas transfer defect and respiratory symptoms in a proportion of such patients), 'necrobiotic' nodules which can cavitate and may be single or multiple, pleural effusion or painful pleural inflammation, recurrent broncho-pulmonary infection, acute pleuropericarditis, pulmonary hypertension and obliterative bronchiolitis.

Systemic lupus erythematosus (SLE) (see p. 375)

Acute manifestations which respond to steroids are recurrent pleural effusions, a syndrome like acute pulmonary oedema, small volume lungs, dyspnoea with reduced VC and CO transfer (possibly related to pulmonary vasculitis), diffuse pulmonary fibrosis (rarely typical fibrosing alveolitis), and respiratory muscle weakness, including impairment of diaphragm function in chronic SLE. Several of these conditions may coexist. There is generally a good symptomatic response to treatment with steroids and other agents, but some residual damage is usually detected by lung function tests.

Scleroderma (systemic sclerosis) (see p. 378)

Advanced cases show progressive basal alveolar and pulmonary vascular fibrosis, sometimes progressing to pulmonary hypertension. Dyspnoea and defects of pulmonary gas transfer precede X-ray changes. Respiratory muscles may be involved. Chest expansion may be affected by thickening of the skin.

Systemic vasculitis (see p. 379)

Each specific variant of this group of disorders shows several pulmonary manifestations. Wegener's granuloma is an acute multisystem disease, classically causing malaise with a destructive vasculitis and granulomatosis of the nose, sinuses and lungs, associated with glomerulonephritis. Pulmonary changes may mimic pneumonia or pulmonary tuberculosis, or may consist of widespread infiltrates or solitary nodules resembling tumours. Secondary infection occurs with *Staph. aureus*. Diagnosis is by histology and the presence of anti-neutrophil cytoplasmic antibody in serum. Treatment is with corticosteroids and immunosuppressants and has reduced the mortality from 100% to a small fraction.

Churg–Strauss syndrome consists of tumours within the lung, head and neck showing a characteristic granulomatous histology, associated with sinusitis, allergic rhinitis and bronchial asthma. The kidneys are not involved. The condition responds to corticosteroids. Asthma, eosinophilic pneumonia, pleurisy and pericarditis may form part of polyarteritis nodosa. Bronchial asthma and chronic airways obstruction occur in association with cranial arteritis.

All these disorders may affect blood vessels in the skin, peripheral nerves, heart, skeletal muscle and elsewhere.

Thyroid disease

Breathlessness in thyrotoxicosis may be caused by severe respiratory muscle weakness or by impaired cardiac function. Pleural effusions occur in severe hypothyroidism.

DRUG-INDUCED LUNG DISEASE

Various syndromes are produced by drugs (Table 2.9).

Table 2.9. Drug-induced lung disease. Various syndromes are produced by drugs. This list is incomplete. Some regimens are obsolete and are indicated with★

Bronchoconstriction	Beta-blockers
Asthma–anaphylaxis	Aspirin and non-steroidal anti-inflammatory agents
	Penicillin
	Sera (e.g. antitetanus)★, desensitising courses of pollen and other extracts (rarely)
Pulmonary eosinophilia	Nitrofurantoin (with small pleural effusions)
	Sulphonamides (usually without pleural effusions)
	Minocycline
Drug-induced systemic lupus erythematosus (SLE)	Hydralazine in high doses★
	Phenytoin
	Procainamide
Diffuse pulmonary fibrosis, acute and chronic	Amiodarone
	Nitrofurantoin
	Azapropazone, other non-steroidal anti-inflammatory drugs
	Gold
	Busulphan, bleomycin, other cytotoxic agents especially with radiotherapy
Pleuro-pulmonary fibrosis	Long-term practolol★
	Methysergide

Paraquat poisoning

Ingestion of paraquat leads to painful oropharyngeal and oesophageal ulceration, renal failure and progressive bronchopulmonary fibrosis.

THORACIC CAGE DISEASE

Kyphoscoliosis

Impaired expansion of the thoracic cage causes increased work of breathing and maldistribution of pulmonary ventilation and perfusion. Scoliosis causes greater impairment than kyphosis. Ventilatory failure, with cor pulmonale and congestive heart failure, may occur between the ages of 30 and 50 but most patients survive into old age. The prognosis correlates with VC and depends not only on the degree of kyphoscoliosis but also on the condition of the underlying lung and whether there is associated neurological disease.

Ankylosing spondylitis

Fusion of costovertebral joints yields a fixed chest with diaphragmatic ventilation. Inspiratory capacity is reduced by up to 30% but this does not cause blood gas disturbance or dyspnoea. Bilateral upper zone fibrosis complicates this condition (cause unknown). Patients may develop respiratory failure when diaphragm function is impaired, e.g. after abdominal surgery or if they smoke or develop other lung diseases.

Paresis of respiratory muscles

Causes include acute polyneuritis, poliomyelitis, spinal cord injury and many chronic neuromuscular disorders.

Patients present with recurrent chest infections, orthopnoea and nocturnal dyspnoea. Paralysis of the diaphragm with intact intercostal muscles causes a 50% reduction of VC, worse on lying down. Loss of respiratory innervation below C2, with preservation of sternomastoids, yields a VC of under 1 litre with a loss of automatic breathing during sleep. In general, reduction of VC below 2 litres results in dyspnoea and below 1 litre is associated with a risk of ventilatory failure, especially if PaO_2 is reduced by lung damage, e.g. repeated aspiration. Muscular weakness causes impairment of coughing.

In patients who develop chronic ventilatory failure, from kyphoscoliosis or respiratory muscle weakness, the outlook has been improved by assisted nocturnal ventilation via a nasal mask.

PLEURAL DISEASE

Spontaneous pneumothorax

This is the entry of air into a pleural cavity through a spontaneous rupture of the pleural surface of a lung. Partial or complete retraction of the lung, hyperinflation of the hemithorax and movement of the mediastinum towards the normal side follows entry of air into the pleural cavity. If the defect on the surface of the lung is small, it seals with spontaneous resolution. If the tear acts as a check valve allowing more air to enter the pleural space during inspiration, positive pressure builds up thus causing 'tension pneumothorax'.

Most cases occur in healthy young men who are often tall and thin. Most older patients have emphysema or have previously had tuberculosis. Rare predisposing causes include Marfan's syndrome, cystic fibrosis, 'honeycomb lung', lung abscesses, infarcts and ectopic endometriosis.

Symptoms and signs

Sudden chest pain, usually on the side of the pneumothorax but occasionally central, with shortness of breath in some instances, is the main symptom.

Signs may include diminished breath sounds on the affected side, increased respiratory rate, diminished movement on the affected side which may be larger than the other, increased resonance to percussion on the affected side, and a precordial sound in time with the heart beat.

Tension pneumothorax causes very severe breathlessness, distended neck veins and hypotension, secondary to the obstruction to the venous circulation.

Investigations

Chest X-ray shows the pneumothorax. The pleural edge is separated from the rib cage and lung markings are absent peripherally.

Complications

These include tension pneumothorax, bilateral pneumothorax, haemothorax, mediastinal air in pneumothorax (pneumomediastinum), persistent broncho-pleural fistula and chronic pneumothorax.

Treatment

Small pneumothoraces may be left to resolve spontaneously; this process is speeded by breathing 28% oxygen for 2–3 days.

Large pneumothoraces or those causing dyspnoea are aspirated. One attempt may be made with an intravenous cannula and a 3-way tap. Other-wise an intercostal catheter (16 French gauge or larger) is connected to an underwater seal. Excessively rapid expansion causes transient pulmonary oedema. This procedure is carried out in the ward or in the accident department as an emergency, but premedication with atropine and an opiate is advisable and good pleural analgesia is essential.

Intercostal catheters are usually inserted in the axilla, but the second anterior space may be convenient. Haemothoraces should be drained and anti-staphylococcal chemotherapy given.

After resolution, the intercostal tube is clamped and removed if there is no recurrence. Large bronchopleural fistulae may benefit from suction with a special pump that, for safety, cannot generate more than 30–40 cm of negative pressure above the water-seal and thus within the pleural cavity. Occasionally, pleurodesis or pleurectomy is necessary for persistent or recurrent pneumothorax.

Tension pneumothorax is a medical emergency requiring the insertion of a wide-bore needle into the pleural space to relieve compression of the great veins, followed by intercostal drainage.

Traumatic pneumothorax follows penetrating stab wounds, fracture of the ribs with penetration of the lung, chest operations and artificial ventilation with high pressures. Haemothorax is common and may rarely complicate spontaneous pneumothorax. Up to 3 litres of blood may be lost into a haemothorax.

Pleural effusion and pleurisy

'Pleurisy' is the term used when any condition involves the pleura resulting in pleuritic pain or a pleural friction rub. 'Pleural effusion' refers to the presence of fluid in the pleural space. The fluid usually consists of serum, but blood, pus and occasionally lymph may be found. Pleural effusions complicate several conditions, of which they may be the principal manifestation.

Serous effusions may be transudates caused by alterations in the balance of colloid osmotic pressure and lymphatic and vascular pressures. These pressures favour resorption under normal conditions. The protein content of these effusions is low (typically < 20 g/l). Transudates are caused by congestive cardiac failure or left ventricular failure of any cause and hypoproteinaemia, especially the nephrotic syndrome. Rare causes include myxoedema and ovarian fibroma (Meigs syndrome).

Inflammation or neoplasia of the pleural lining may result in pleural exudates in which capillary permeability is high and protein content approaches that of serum (typically > 35 g/l). Inflamed pleural surfaces not separated by effusion result in the typical pain of pleurisy.

Exudates may be caused by acute infection, e.g. bacterial pneumonia which may be serous or purulent (empyema), chronic infection (e.g. tuberculosis), subphrenic infection, pulmonary infarction, malignant disease (bronchial carcinoma, metastatic pleural carcinoma or pleural mesothelioma) and autoimmune disease (rheumatoid arthritis, SLE, systemic vasculitis).

Chylous effusions contain fat and lymphocytes. They are rare and caused by lymphatic obstruction or trauma to the thoracic duct.

Symptoms and signs

Symptoms are pleural pain and dyspnoea, the former usually being relieved by separation of the pleural surfaces when the effusion enlarges.

Signs are increased respiratory rate, shift of mediastinum towards the unaffected side, stony dullness on percussion, diminished breath sounds and signs of consolidation adjacent to the effusion.

Investigations

Chest X-ray will be required. Needle aspiration shows the presence and nature of fluid (Fig. 2.13). Blood-stained effusions are usually malignant or thromboembolic. Cytology and culture may reveal the cause. Malignant cells or pus cells may be diagnostic and specific organisms may be isolated. Lymphocytes and mesothelial cells are non-specific.

Pleural biopsy is best performed using a special needle at the time of the first chest aspiration. It is valuable in cases of suspected malignancy and tuberculosis.

Treatment

The underlying cause is treated. Large effusions may be drained through an intercostal tube if they cause breathlessness or discomfort. Large infected effusions should be drained promptly and treated surgically if they loculate.

Malignant effusions may be arrested by instilling sclerosant or cytotoxic agents (e.g. tetracycline, bleomycin) into the drained pleural cavity.

LUNG COLLAPSE

Pulmonary collapse usually occurs because of the obstruction of a lobar bronchus. Air or fluid in the pleura causes a reduction of lung volume. Absorption collapse then occurs as alveolar oxygen is absorbed. Nitrogen follows more slowly. Shrinkage of the lung volume leads to a rise in the diaphragm on the affected side, overdistension of the rest of the lung, mediastinal shift towards the affected side and flattening and diminished

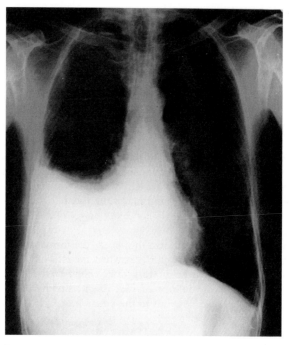

Fig. 2.13 Chest X-ray showing right pleural effusion. Note the characteristic appearance of a meniscus. In this example, the heart is central, indicating that there is underlying collapse of part of the right lung. The diagnosis was bronchogenic carcinoma.

movement of the affected side. The main causes are bronchial carcinoma, inhaled foreign body, compression of a bronchus by enlarged lymph nodes (e.g. lymphoma, primary tuberculosis), aspergillosis and viscid inspissated mucus which is not expectorated. The latter occurs postoperatively and in bronchial asthma.

Air or fluid in the pleural cavity also causes a reduction of volume of the lungs which resolves when they are drained (p. 96).

Symptoms and signs

Symptoms include breathlessness and sometimes pleural pain. Signs are increased respiratory rate, diminished chest wall movement, partial loss of resonance to percussion, diminished breath sounds on the affected side and diminished voice sounds.

Investigations

Some collapsed lobes are difficult to detect on chest X-ray. Bronchoscopy will reveal the nature of the bronchial obstruction.

Complications

These are bronchiectasis and lung abscess.

Differential diagnosis
Pneumonia, pulmonary infarction and pleural effusion.

Treatment
Obstruction to the bronchus needs to be relieved if possible. Foreign bodies are removed at bronchoscopy. Physiotherapy may aid expectoration of mucus plugs. Corticosteroids are given in asthma and allergic aspergillosis.

OBSTRUCTIVE SLEEP APNOEA SYNDROME

Obstructive sleep apnoea is upper airway obstruction during sleep. Sleep hypopnoea is upper airway narrowing during sleep without frank obstruction. When apnoea and/or hypopnoea occur repeatedly during sleep (usually > 10 times/hour) they may disrupt sleep and cause poor sleep quality, leading to daytime somnolence. The syndrome of daytime somnolence caused by repeated apnoea/hypopnoea during sleep is the sleep apnoea/hypopnoea syndrome. The daytime somnolence interferes with work, school performance and driving. Severe sleep apnoea syndrome carries a 3–4 times increased risk of road traffic accidents. It is a relatively common condition. In men aged 35–65 years, the group most affected, the prevalence of severe sleep apnoea is 3 per 1000. Mild and moderate forms occur more frequently.

Pathophysiology
The pharyngeal and laryngeal muscles normally maintain the patency of the upper airway during inspiration. However, during sleep these muscles are less active, and there is an increased tendency for the upper airway to be sucked in. Apnoea and hypopnoea occur when the pharyngeal muscles fail to maintain full patency of the airway. This most commonly occurs in middle-aged men with thick necks. Retrognathia, enlargement of the tongue (e.g. in acromegaly, hypothyroidism or trisomy 21) and enlargement of the tonsils and adenoids (mainly in children) also predispose to the condition. However, a substantial minority of affected individuals have no obvious anatomical predisposition.

Sleep disruption, which can be detected by electroencephalography, is thought to be caused by swings in intrathoracic pressure resulting from the changes in upper airway resistance. The transient hypoxaemia that often accompanies the apnoea and hypopnoea aids diagnosis but does not contribute to the sleep disturbance. The loud snoring that invariably accompanies the condition is due to increased vibration of the uvula and other loose tissue in the airway, resulting from the turbulent airflow.

Symptoms and signs
The major symptom is daytime somnolence. Partners report loud snoring and, sometimes, apnoea, though only 10% of patients wake with nocturnal choking. Nocturia occurs in one-third of patients.

There are no specific signs. Most patients have a large collar size and a minority have obvious anatomical crowding of the oropharynx. The blood pressure should be checked, as there is an association with systemic hypertension.

Investigation
Sleep apnoea syndrome is confirmed by demonstration of transient hypoxaemia (using transcutaneous oximetry) and of transient cessation of oronasal airflow or respiratory movement during sleep.

Differential diagnosis
Other causes of daytime sleepiness include narcolepsy, depression, and sleep disturbance from restless legs syndrome.

Treatment
Weight reduction may help, as may avoidance of alcohol and of hypnotics. Most patients will respond to the application of positive pressure to the upper airway via a nasal mask at night, though this has to be continued long term. Drivers with severe somnolence should inform the licensing authority, and avoid driving until the symptoms are controlled.

ACUTE UPPER AIRWAY OBSTRUCTION

Acute obstruction of the larynx or trachea leads to progressive hypoxaemia and CO_2 retention, resulting in bradycardia and cardiac arrest within 4–8 minutes. Whatever the cause, treatment involves clearing the airway and administering artificial ventilation with the highest possible concentration of oxygen by the most efficient route available (endotracheal intubation, mask ventilation, and airway or mouth-to-mouth respiration). False teeth should be removed and obstructing material such as regurgitated food hooked out from the back of the tongue before positive pressure ventilation begins. Cardiopulmonary resuscitation is given if the carotid pulse is absent.

Sudden death in restaurants is usually caused by the inhalation of large pieces of food, usually meat. Talking while eating, coupled with impaired coordination of swallowing, are responsible. Supraglottic obstruction may be relieved manually. Food in the trachea cannot be coughed up; emergency treatment consists of a vigorous upward push on the upper abdomen in the hope of displacing the diaphragm upwards and dislodging the wedged material (Heimlich manoeuvre).

Causes of laryngeal obstruction include angio-oedema, epiglottitis, diphtheria (rare), inhaled foreign body (e.g. child's dummy), and also croup or pertussis (p. 416). Laryngoscopy and intubation are performed when available. Needle tracheostomy or, in adults, cricothyroid puncture may be life-saving.

RESPIRATORY FAILURE

Respiratory failure is the inability of the respiratory system to oxygenate the blood to a normal level. It is arbitrarily said to be present when the arterial oxygen tension is less than 60 mmHg (8 kPa), when breathing air at sea level. It can occur with or without carbon dioxide retention ($PaCO_2$ > 50 mmHg; 6.7 kPa).

Central cyanosis is the only reliable clinical sign of hypoxaemia. However, it is often not detected until the SaO_2 falls well below 90%. The detection of hypoxaemia has been greatly improved by the routine use of pulse oximetry.

Carbon dioxide retention is also difficult to detect clinically, and any suspicion should lead to measurement of arterial blood gas tensions. Physical signs include mood disturbance, confusion or aggression, coma, flapping tremor of the hands, warm hands with dilated veins, papilloedema and raised intracranial pressure mimicking cerebral tumour.

TYPE I RESPIRATORY FAILURE

Hypoxaemia with a normal or low $PaCO_2$ is the most common form of respiratory failure. It is caused by ventilation/perfusion imbalance and occurs in a wide range of pulmonary disorders. Treatment is with oxygen, which should be given in high concentrations if necessary, since there is no risk of CO_2 retention.

TYPE II RESPIRATORY FAILURE (VENTILATORY FAILURE)

Hypoxaemia with an elevated $PaCO_2$ is caused by inadequate ventilation. It occurs in:

1. Blockage of the main airways. Acute ventilatory failure can result from acute obstruction of the larynx or trachea, drowning, and occasionally in acute severe asthma or acute bronchiolitis.

2. Disorders of the respiratory muscle and thoracic cage. Acute paralytic disorders such as myasthenia, polyneuritis and poliomyelitis may cause respiratory insufficiency. In the early stages, breathlessness results in a low PCO_2, but when the VC falls below 1 litre there is a risk of hypoventilation. Assisted ventilation is used.

Chronic neuromuscular weakness (e.g. muscular dystrophies, post-poliomyelitis syndrome) and thoracic cage disorders (e.g. kyphoscoliosis) can also lead to ventilatory failure. It is now possible to treat these patients long-term with positive pressure ventilation at night using a nasal mask. These patients are susceptible to acute on chronic ventilatory failure during respiratory tract infections or in the presence of heart failure.

3. Pulmonary insufficiency: chronic and acute on chronic respiratory failure. Severe lung diseases are accompanied by an increased work of breathing and disturbance of the pulmonary gas exchange mechanism. These result in hypoxaemia, with or without CO_2 retention, and patients may acclimatise to quite severe abnormalities of blood gases. When such patients develop acute bronchial infections or fluid retention, they suffer severe rises of PCO_2 and deterioration of arterial PO_2 and pH. Relief of hypoxaemia and sedation further reduce respiratory drive without improving the underlying condition and cause progressive underventilation and acute respiratory acidosis.

All patients with such exacerbations of pre-existing respiratory disease need arterial blood gas analysis. Artificial ventilation is indicated for worsening blood gases and respiratory muscle fatigue. The following measures may postpone the need for this:

1. controlled oxygen therapy (not more than 24–28%)
2. regular arousal
3. assisted coughing
4. measures to improve lung function, e.g. bronchodilators, diuretics and corticosteroids
5. infusion of respiratory stimulants may help if respiratory depression is reversible, e.g. after injudicious administration of oxygen or sedation.

Assisted ventilation is used if the patient becomes unconscious, uncooperative, unable to cough or exhausted. Inability to maintain the PO_2 greater than 55 mmHg (7.2 kPa) and a pH greater than 7.25 is a guide to the need for ventilation.

Oxygen therapy

Previously healthy patients, not acclimatised to hypoxaemia, urgently require restoration of PO_2 to normal levels to maintain cerebral and renal function. This can generally be achieved by means of a suitable mask, except in the presence of very severe diffuse lung or pulmonary vascular impairment, hypotension or an anatomical shunt.

High concentrations of oxygen, approaching 100%, can be administered only by systems that involve a valve and reservoir. Generous oxygen therapy is used for acute severe dyspnoea with hyperventilation (type I respiratory failure), e.g. left ventricular failure, bronchial asthma, pulmonary embolism, pneumonia. A firm plastic mask with holes capable of taking 12 litres per minute of oxygen flow is used. Oxygen concentration delivered to the patient depends on flow rate and the rate of depth of breathing, though flow rates of 6–8 litres per minute will usually deliver 40–60%.

Controlled oxygen therapy aims to increase PO_2 to around 60 mmHg (8 kPa), using masks employing the Venturi principle. The inflowing oxygen entrains large volumes of air, delivering a draught of fixed oxygen concentration.

Nasal cannulae are used when continuous oxygen therapy is required but exact concentration is not critical. The patient can eat and talk. This is well tolerated by convalescent subjects and those with chronic lung disease.

Home oxygen. Chronic respiratory insufficiency may be improved in selected patients by prolonged inhalation (15 hours or more daily) of oxygen at 2–4 litres per minute via a nasal cannula to achieve 95% saturation in the arterial blood: longevity is increased, polycythaemia is reduced and there are fewer episodes of oedema, fluid retention and infective exacerbations requiring admission to hospital. Long-term oxygen therapy is known to benefit patients with chronic airflow obstruction (FEV1 below 1 litre) who have a resting arterial PO_2 below 55 mmHg (7.2 kPa), and documented episodes of heart failure. Patients must give up smoking, and must be assessed to verify improvement, but can avoid a progressive rise in PCO_2 with this form of treatment.

Home oxygen can be delivered by means of a concentrator, which extracts nitrogen from room air.

Some patients who develop arterial desaturation during exercise benefit from portable oxygen therapy which prolongs effort tolerance.

Palliative oxygen therapy relieves hypoxaemia in end-stage fibrotic obstruction and malignant lung disorders and may relieve Cheyne–Stokes respiration in heart failure. Life expectancy is not improved.

3

INTENSIVE CARE
John Vann Jones, David P. Coates

Most hospitals have a high dependency unit (HDU) or an intensive therapy unit (ITU) for the management of particularly ill patients. Although some units care specifically for patients with renal and liver failure, most are concerned with maintaining the circulation and respiration in patients with potentially reversible illnesses such as acute asthma, sepsis, severe metabolic acidosis, drug overdosage and trauma.

SHOCK

Acute circulatory failure with inadequate cellular oxygenation is commonly referred to as shock. This can have a wide variety of causes (Table 3.1).
The body responds to shock in several different ways.

1. Increased sympathetic nervous system activity releases catecholamines from the adrenal medulla.
2. Renin release from the underperfused kidneys leads to an increase in angiotensin II levels. Angiotensin II is a very potent vasoconstrictor which also causes the adrenal cortex to release aldosterone, thereby retaining salt and water.
3. A variety of pituitary hormones (e.g. adrenocorticotrophic hormone, growth hormone, antidiuretic hormone), cortisol, glucagon and beta-endorphin are released into the circulation.

Table 3.1. Common causes of shock

Blood loss, e.g. gastrointestinal haemorrhage	Allergic (anaphylaxis)
	Cardiogenic (primary cardiac damage)
Fluid loss, e.g. severe burns	Cardiac tamponade (pericardial effusion)
Acute infection	Pulmonary embolus

All of these measures are intended to restore tissue perfusion. Where shock is caused by infection (septic shock) or tissue damage (e.g. crush injury) other changes occur. These include:

4. increased prostaglandin activity, especially prostacyclin, thromboxane and PGF_2
5. complement cascade activation
6. cytokine release
7. platelet activating factor release
8. release of lysosomal enzymes.

These mediators have a wide range of different, often opposing, activities; for example prostacyclin is a vasodilator that inhibits platelet aggregation while thromboxane is a vasoconstrictor and promotes platelet adhesion.

MICROCIRCULATORY CHANGES

The initial changes at the small arteriolar and capillary level depend on the type and degree of shock. Eventually local accumulation of metabolites (e.g. lactic acid) leads to vasodilatation with fluid loss into the interstitial spaces. This in turn makes the blood more coaguable and viscous, increasing the potential for intravascular coagulation. Paradoxically, because clotting factors are consumed so heavily within the microcirculation, the patient is often effectively anticoagulated. This condition is known as disseminated intravascular coagulopathy (DIC) or consumption coagulopathy (see p. 348).

Poor tissue perfusion leads to metabolic changes and anaerobic metabolism supervenes. All of the changes outlined eventually lead to multiple organ failure, which has a poor prognosis.

CLINICAL PRESENTATION AND TREATMENT

These depend on the cause. For example severe blood loss presents an entirely different picture from cardiac tamponade (pericardial effusion). Therefore it is important to establish a cause for shock although some general principles can be applied.

1. Adequate haemodynamic monitoring to ensure correct fluid balance, e.g. central venous pressure, direct arterial pressure (most frequently using the radial artery). Sometimes cardiac output and pulmonary artery occlusion (wedge) pressure, an indirect measurement of left atrial filling pressure, are also monitored. Correct volume restoration is very important in managing most forms of shock (Table 3.2).
2. Adequate oxygenation, which may require the patient to be ventilated. The balance between oxygen demand and delivery is critical. The oxygen requirements of the ventilatory muscles, including the diaphragm, for example, may be increased several fold in shock.
3. Analgesia and sedation.
4. Inotropic support and the use of vasoactive drugs to redistribute cardiac output.

Table 3.2. Fluids used to replace circulating volume in shock

SAGM blood*

Colloid solutions:
    Gelatin solutions, e.g. Gelofusine, Haemaccel
    Dextrans, e.g. Dextran 70 in saline 0.9%
    Hetastarch, e.g. Hespan, Elohes
    Human albumin solution 4% (HAS)
    Fresh frozen plasma (FFP)

Crystalloid solutions:
    Saline 0.9%
    Hartmann's solution

*SAGM blood = red cells suspended in an optimal preservative of Saline, Adenine, Glucose, Mannitol.

In most forms of shock, even where the heart was previously healthy, the myocardium is depressed. It is therefore important to monitor closely and adjust cardiac work by manipulating the factors affecting cardiac filling (pre-load) and impedance to ejection (afterload). In septic shock in particular, it is sometimes necessary to redirect the increased cardiac output from the vasodilated peripheral circulation to the major organs. It may also be necessary to stimulate cardiac output pharmacologically with inotropic drugs (Table 3.3).

Table 3.3. Inotropes and vasoactive drugs

Dobutamine	Vasodilating inotrope. Direct myocardial stimulant Ensure adequate circulating volume
Dopamine	At low doses: dopaminergic renal and splanchnic vasodilatation At high doses: beta-1 adrenergic stimulation and increasing alpha adrenergic vasoconstriction
Dopexamine	Dopamine analogue: 1/3 peripheral dopaminergic but 60 times more beta-2 and only 1/6 beta-1 stimulation. Significant vasodilator
Phosphodiesterase inhibitors, e.g. Enoximone, Milrinone	Increased myocardial and smooth muscle cAMP resulting in increased contractility and vasodilatation: 'inodilatation'
Noradrenaline	Alpha stimulant: vasoconstrictor redirecting cardiac output. Particularly useful in septic shock
Adrenaline	Beta stimulant and vasodilatation. Used in reversible myocardial depression

RESPIRATORY FAILURE

(See also p. 100.)

Type I. Occurs with damage to the lungs itself. This may be acute (e.g. pulmonary oedema) or chronic (e.g. pulmonary fibrosis). The PaO_2 is low and the $PaCO_2$ is low or normal.

Type II. Occurs with poor ventilation, as in chronic bronchitis and emphysema or neuromuscular disease. The PaO_2 is low but the $PaCO_2$ is high.

In patients suspected of developing ventilatory failure, blood gases and acid–base status need to be carefully monitored. These results and the clinical picture will determine the need for admission to an ITU and indicate the need for controlled ventilation. Sometimes specific ventilatory function tests are required.

Management
1. Seek the cause, e.g. acute exacerbation of chronic bronchitis, sepsis.
2. Achieve adequate oxygen delivery by supplementary oxygen administration with or without controlled ventilation (Table 3.4).

Table 3.4. Forms of ventilatory support

1. Controlled mandatory ventilation (CMV) by intermittent positive pressure ventilation (IPPV) through an endotracheal tube (ETT). A variety of functions may be adjustable, e.g. frequency, tidal volume, peak inflation pressure, ratio of inspiration and expiration times. This can be undertaken for several weeks.

2. CMV + positive end expiratory pressure (PEEP). During expiration a resistance of up to 20 cmH$_2$O is maintained which tends to increase functional residual capacity (FRC), enhancing oxygenation. There may be detrimental cardiovascular effects.

3. Synchronised intermittent mandatory ventilation (SIMV). The ventilator is programmed to deliver a predetermined number of mechanical breaths of specified tidal volume after a suitable pause in the patient's spontaneous ventilatory efforts. May help weaning from CMV.

4. Pressure support ventilation. Breaths initiated by the patient, sensed as a predetermined reduction in the ambient airway pressure, are assisted by a preset positive pressure supplement. This may assist weaning from CMV or SIMV.

5. Continuous positive airway pressure (CPAP). The patient breathes spontaneously through either an ETT or a tightly fitting face mask. There is a persistently positive airway pressure during both inspiration and expiration which increases FRC and reduces the work of breathing. It requires a large flow of gas to achieve the continuous positive pressure, especially during inspiration. It assists weaning from CMV or SIMV.

NB. Inspired oxygen concentration can always be independently adjusted.

ADULT RESPIRATORY DISTRESS SYNDROME (ARDS)

ARDS is sometimes referred to as shock lung. The pulmonary capillaries leak and result in hypoxia, reduced lung compliance and diffuse pulmonary infiltration radiographically. ARDS occurs as a non-specific reaction to a variety of problems that have a final common pathway of capillary cellular functional deficit. Common causes include sepsis, burns, blunt chest trauma, fat embolism and aspiration.

Cellular respiration can usually be maintained (Table 3.4) in the short term with increased inspired oxygen concentrations, CMV using minimised inflation pressures, adjusted inspiration : expiration ratios and PEEP.

A poor prognosis usually relates to the development of multiple organ failure rather than to the inability to maintain ventilation.

HYPERSENSITIVITY REACTIONS

ANAPHYLAXIS (TYPE I HYPERSENSITIVITY)

There is a marked allergic response occurring within 30 minutes of exposure, e.g. to a bee sting, pollen. It is now more commonly encountered in response to drugs, e.g. penicillin. Usually the patient has had a milder reaction to a previous exposure.

Symptoms and signs
There may be urticarial rashes with itching and paraesthesiae. Vasodilatation and increased capillary permeability result in hypotension and angioedema. Bronchospasm is also usually present. These patients are often shocked and profoundly unwell.

Treatment
Emergency administration of subcutaneous adrenaline (1 ml of 1:1000; 1 mg) given repeatedly (every 10–15 minutes) as indicated. Antihistamines are also given intravenously. Supportive measures such as intravenous fluids, oxygen or assisted ventilation may be required, as may tracheostomy for severe laryngeal swelling.

4

NEUROLOGY

Iain Ferguson

A good grounding in neuroanatomical and neurophysiological principles is essential to the understanding of how pathology disrupts normal function of thought, movement and sensation. However, it must be realised that the essence of neurology is a detailed clinical history complemented by physical examination.

Certain factors are important in the history, for example:

1. The age of the patient. A progressive, spastic paraparesis in a child is more likely to be caused by a tumour, whereas in the young adult multiple sclerosis is the more likely diagnosis.

2. Mode of onset. The dramatic onset of focal neurological symptoms may suggest a localised epileptic attack or ischaemic episode.

3. Duration of symptoms. A migraine rarely persists for longer than 48 hours, yet tension headache may last days or even weeks.

4. Family history. A tentative diagnosis of Huntington's chorea may be reinforced by establishing this disease in another relative.

5. Previous medical history. A subarachnoid haemorrhage in early life may predispose to hydrocephalus or syringomyelia.

Physical signs may range from a gross disturbance of gait, as in cerebellar ataxia, to a subtle, dissociated sensory impairment seen in spinal cord lesions. Such signs, and a detailed history, allow definition of the disease and its situation. Appropriate tests may then be applied to specific regions. Images of great clarity may be obtained using computed tomography (CT), magnetic resonance imaging (MRI) and Doppler ultrasound. Neurophysiological tests include electroencephalography (EEG) and nerve conduction studies with electromyography (EMG).

DISEASES OF THE CRANIAL NERVES

OLFACTORY (I) NERVE

Anosmia, or loss of the sense of smell, is commonly caused by nasal or sinus disease. Head injury may also cause anosmia. A subfrontal meningioma can cause anosmia although this is usually overlooked if visual failure and intellectual impairment are prominent features. Episodic disturbances of smell may be a feature of temporal lobe epileptic attacks (uncal fits).

OPTIC (II) NERVE

Disease here may affect colour vision, visual acuity, visual fields (Fig. 4.1) and optic disc appearance. Papilloedema, or swelling of the optic nerve head, has an identical appearance to papillitis but the latter is associated with a marked reduction of visual acuity. If left untreated, papilloedema will eventually result in reduction of acuity, concentric diminution of visual fields and finally blindness (Table 4.1).

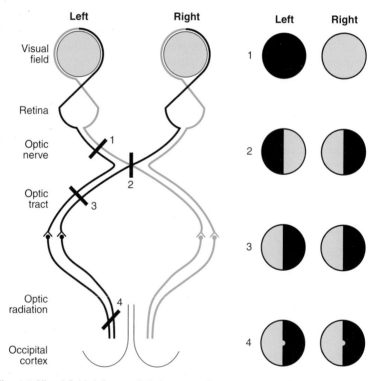

Fig. 4.1 Visual field defects and their causes. Common causes of lesion at site 1 = optic neuritis (MS), tumour, trauma, aneurysm; 2 = pituitary tumour, craniopharyngioma, aneurysm; 3 = tumour, stroke; 4 = stroke, tumour. The shaded area shows the visual defect. NB: Macular sparing at site 4.

Table 4.1. Causes of papilloedema

Raised intracranial pressure by tumour, abscess and meningitis due to failure of retinal venous drainage

Thrombosis of cerebral venous sinuses

Orbital tumour or pseudotumour

Malignant hypertension

Chronic hypercapnia and hypoxia

Benign intracranial hypertension

In papilloedema the blind spot is enlarged and this can be used as a sign to monitor treatment.

Optic neuritis

Painful eye movements caused by traction on the inflamed nerve, poor visual acuity, impaired colour vision, afferent pupillary defect and central scotoma are features of this condition. Optic neuritis can occur with multiple sclerosis (MS), syphilis, giant cell arteritis, tobacco and alcohol amblyopia, and methanol poisoning. Severe neuritis usually results in optic atrophy.

Optic atrophy

1. Primary. Leber's sex-linked recessive disease affecting males, Devic's disease (optico-myelopathy), multiple sclerosis and optic neuritis.

2. Secondary. Compression of the nerve by tumour or aneurysm, glaucoma, papilloedema, central retinal artery thrombosis, trauma, drugs and toxins, e.g. chloroquine, tobacco, quinine, and methyl alcohol.

The optic disc may appear pale in normal patients with myopia. Glaucoma causes enlargement of the optic cup.

Pupillary abnormalities

Large pupils occur in the young and smaller pupils in older healthy individuals. Irregular pupils may complicate chronic uveitis or follow iridectomy.

An Argyll Robertson pupil is small, irregular and unequal, unreactive to bright light, and reacts normally to accommodation. It occurs in neurosyphilis, diabetes mellitus and some autonomic neuropathies.

The myotonic or Holmes Adie pupil

This is benign and usually unilateral. Patients complain only of a mild blurring of vision. The pupil is dilated, and reacts sluggishly to light and accommodation. A brisk reaction may be obtained from dilute (2.5%) methacholine. Absent deep tendon reflexes may be present in the full syndrome.

Table 4.2. Site and causes of Horner's syndrome

Site of lesion in sympathetic pathway	Causes
Hypothalamus	Tumour
Brainstem	Stroke, trauma, tumour
Cervical cord	Syringomyelia, glioma, trauma
Cervical root-stellate ganglion	Pancoast tumour, cervical rib surgery, trauma
Carotid artery	Trauma, dissection or angiography
Cavernous sinus	Migrainous neuralgia
Retro-orbital	Aneurysm or tumour

Horner's syndrome

This is the result of a unilateral, rarely bilateral, sympathetic nerve lesion. The pupil is small (miosis) because of the unopposed action of the parasympathetic nerve. There is also a mild ptosis from weakness of Müller's muscle, and an apparent enophthalmos and lack of sweating in the upper and sometimes lower half of the face. The causes of Horner's syndrome are summarised in Table 4.2.

OCULO-MOTOR (III) TROCHLEAR (IV) ABDUCENS (VI) NERVES

Good ocular motility is essential to bring the full field system to bear on any new object. Horizontal eye movements are controlled by the pons. Failure of conjugate horizontal gaze may arise from a lesion in the medial longitudinal bundle, a fibre pathway that co-ordinates sixth and third nerve function. Nystagmus of the lateral rectus in the direction of gaze and weakness of the adducting eye (medial rectus) gives a clinical picture known as internuclear ophthalmoplegia. This is commonly caused by multiple sclerosis. Failure of vertical eye movement is seen in progressive supranuclear palsy and tumours of the midbrain periaqueductal region.

In a third nerve lesion there is weakness of all extraocular muscles except the lateral rectus and superior oblique. The nerve also supplies levator palpebrae superioris and the pupillo-constrictor fibres.

Features of a complete third nerve palsy are dilated pupil, marked ptosis and a downward and outward deviated eye.

Lesions of the third nerve nucleus in the midbrain are commonly vascular or tumour. In diabetes mellitus where there is microvascular damage, there is sparing of the peripherally lying pupillomotor fibres and so the pupil is unaffected. This is often called a 'medical' third nerve palsy. 'Surgical' third nerve palsy is commonly caused by a posterior communicating aneurysm or pituitary tumour and the pupil is affected. As the nerve leaves the dura it may be involved in an invasive basal process, such as tumour or sarcoid or tubercular granulomata.

A lone sixth nerve palsy is more common than isolated trochlear nerve lesions. More often, it occurs in association with third nerve palsy, when the lesion of the cavernous sinus is a tumour, granuloma or giant internal carotid aneurysm. Myasthenia gravis may present with ophthalmoplegia and a variable diplopia which is worse towards the end of the day. Thyroid eye disease causes ophthalmoplegia and proptosis.

TRIGEMINAL (V) NERVE

Facial sensation is appreciated via the three divisions (ophthalmic, maxillary and mandibular), supplying the skin of the face, cornea, sinuses, mucous membranes of nose, teeth, tympanic membranes, and sensation but not taste, to the anterior two-thirds of tongue. The motor division supplies the temporalis, masseter and pterygoid muscles. A brainstem lesion of the pons and medulla may cause numbness and tingling of the face. The pattern of sensory loss is sometimes in an 'onion skin' or concentric distribution. This is seen in syringobulbia, brainstem glioma or vascular disease. Trigeminal nerve trunk lesions occur from compression by an aneurysm of the internal carotid artery in the cavernous sinus or an acoustic neuroma in the cerebellopontine angle. Intrinsic nerve trunk disease may be caused by herpes zoster.

FACIAL (VII) NERVE

This nerve innervates muscles of facial expression and the chorda tympani with taste to the anterior two-thirds of the tongue. The nerve to stapedius muscle dampens bony ossicle movement which, if damaged, results in hyperacusis. Damage to parasympathetic fibres to the lacrimal gland may cause a dry eye.

Upper motor neurone facial palsy occurs with damage to the anterior frontal fibres controlling facial movements. It spares voluntary movements but affects emotional ones. The other type of upper motor neurone lesion damaging suprapontine fibres results in a lower half facial weakness with sparing of the upper half because of bilateral cortical innervation of the forehead muscles.

A lower motor neurone lesion will cause complete paralysis of half of the face because the final motor pathway is affected.

Bell's palsy is caused by swelling of the facial nerve in the facial canal (Fig. 4.2). Retroaural pain precedes palsy in 50% of patients. The facial muscles are stiff and weak; food collects in the mouth. Other features are loss of taste and excessive tears (crocodile). Early steroid therapy will aid recovery; however, 90% of patients recover spontaneously.

Causes of bilateral facial weakness include Guillain–Barré syndrome, myotonic and facioscapulohumeral dystrophy and myasthenia gravis.

Brainstem lesions more commonly cause unilateral facial weakness and are the result of cerebrovascular accident, multiple sclerosis, tumour, motor neurone disease or syringobulbia.

Blepharospasm (intermittent involuntary forceful closure of the eye) may also occur in Parkinson's disease, or as a more widespread oromandibular

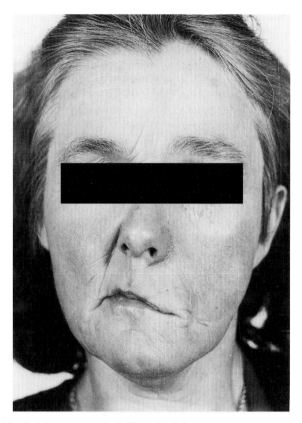

Fig. 4.2 The facial appearance in Bell's palsy (left side).

dyskinesia known as Meige's syndrome. Treatment is by intramuscular injection of small amounts of botulinus toxin.

Hemifacial spasm (clonic spasm of facial muscles involving the eye and mouth) is frequently distressing and also treated with botulinus toxin.

Facial myokymia, if restricted to the eyelids, is usually benign. When it involves facial muscles, producing a fine, rippling, 'bag of worms' appearance, it suggests pontine multiple sclerosis or glioma.

AUDITORY (VIII) NERVE

Sudden-onset lesions
1. Geniculate herpes zoster (Ramsay Hunt syndrome) causes vertigo, deafness, unilateral facial palsy and a vesicular rash in the external aural canal and hard palate.
2. Occlusion of the anterior inferior cerebellar artery will precipitate sudden unilateral deafness, more commonly in the elderly.
3. Mumps.
4. Head injury is a common cause of sudden deafness.

Gradual-onset lesions

1. An acoustic neuroma causes progressive deafness, with trigeminal and mild facial nerve involvement. There may also be unilateral cerebellar signs.
2. Other causes of deafness include bacterial meningitis, syphilis, sarcoidosis, Meniere's disease, streptomycin toxicity and brainstem multiple sclerosis.

GLOSSOPHARYNGEAL (IX) AND VAGUS (X) NERVES

The gag reflex, palatal and pharyngeal movement, and sensation and movement of the vocal cords are affected. Other features are bilateral vocal paralysis, a bovine cough, stridor and loss of explosive cough. These symptoms are collectively known as either a bulbar or pseudobulbar palsy (Table 4.3).

SPINAL ACCESSORY (XI) NERVE

This nerve supplies the trapezius and sternomastoid muscles. Unilateral lesions are rare. Causes of XIth nerve palsy include glomus tumour of the jugular foramen and surgical dissection of lymph glands in the neck and may result in weakness of shrugging of the shoulder with slight winging of the scapula.

An upper motor neurone lesion such as a stroke will cause weakness of the sternomastoid contralateral to the side of the hemiparesis.

HYPOGLOSSAL (XII) NERVE

The signs of XIIth nerve palsy are wasting and fasciculation, deviation of the tongue to the weak side, with difficulty in manipulating food. The causes are tumour and malignant meningitis, glomus tumour and skull base fracture. The lesion is unilateral.

Table 4.3. Bulbar and pseudobulbar palsy

Site of lesion	Clinical signs	Causes
Bulbar		
Lower motor neurone	Dysarthria—nasal, slow voice, dysphagia	Myasthenia gravis Motor neurone disease Muscular dystrophy (rare) Guillain–Barré syndrome
Pseudobulbar		
Upper motor neurone corticobulbar fibres —a supranuclear and nerve lesion	Dysarthria—jerky type, dysphagia, spastic rapid tongue movements, brisk jaw jerk, emotional lability	Stroke Multiple sclerosis Motor neurone disease

DISORDERS OF CONSCIOUSNESS

EPILEPSY

Epilepsy is defined as a continuing tendency to have seizures caused by a sudden excessive electrical discharge of cerebral neurones. Synchronous paroxysmal bursts of large numbers of neurones correlate with the EEG sharp and spike waves. These occur often in the inter-ictal period in patients with epilepsy and are extremely helpful in the diagnosis. Approximately 0.5% of the population will have a seizure. The highest incidence is in the first year of life, slowly declining between 10 and 50 years with another peak in the over 50s, usually caused by tumours, and vascular and degenerative diseases.

Ten to 20% of patients may not have epilepsy but rather syncope or pseudoseizures. A witness account is invaluable.

Aetiology

1. A birth history may suggest trauma, hypoxia, or metabolic insult.
2. A positive family history of epilepsy may be obtained.
3. Symptomatic disease may affect the cortex diffusely.
4. Medical conditions include alcohol excess, barbiturate withdrawal, uraemia, hypoparathyroidism, hypoxic encephalopathy, post-cardiac arrest, bacterial meningitis, viral encephalitis, subacute sclerosing panencephalitis and Creutzfeldt–Jakob disease.
5. Focal seizures are almost always an expression of intracranial localised pathology, such as trauma, tumours, abscess or stroke.
6. Trigger factors for seizure include alcohol, late nights, hypoglycaemia, drugs and flashing lights.

Classification of epilepsy

1. Generalised
   (a) tonic and/or clonic = 'grand mal'
   (b) absence = 'petit mal'
   (c) myoclonic
   (d) atonic
2. Partial (focal)
   (a) simple motor
   (b) simple sensory
   (c) complex partial with or without secondary generalisation (also known as psychomotor or temporal lobe epilepsy).

Symptoms and signs

Generalised seizures

These are characterised by clinical symptoms and EEG discharges which are bilaterally symmetrical with no focal onset.

Tonic/clonic or generalised attacks have an initial phase of widespread tonic muscular contractions, followed by rhythmical clonic jerks. Duration is 1–2 minutes with no aura. Consciousness is lost at onset and not recovered until minutes after the clonic phase. Lip or tongue biting and urinary incontinence occur frequently. The post-ictal confusion may last minutes or hours.

Absence and petit mal attacks are short-lived episodes of loss of consciousness (5–15 seconds) with only minimal motor manifestations. True petit mal appears only in childhood and is associated with an EEG pattern of 3 per second spike and wave abnormality.

Absence attacks must be differentiated from petit mal. They often occur in adults with complex partial epilepsy. Such patients may also have myoclonic jerking—brief sudden muscular contractions either affecting the whole body or localised to the hand or leg.

Tonic or akinetic seizures occur predominantly in childhood with repetitive short bursts (5–10 seconds) of tonic posturing or loss of tone, where the patient suddenly falls. This is often associated with mental retardation.

Partial or focal seizures
These are characterised by clinical symptoms and EEG changes localised to one region of the brain. The focus may move to other areas of the motor cortex resulting in a spreading movement or sensory disorder (Jacksonian seizure).

Sensory seizures may be simple from the primary sensory cortex, or more complex visual, auditory or even olfactory illusions or hallucinations. This often takes place at the aura or prodrome of an attack. Déja vu or entendu feelings of familiarity, or an epigastric sensation rising to the head may also occur.

Complex partial seizures arise from the temporal lobe, sometimes with automatisms such as lip smacking, grimacing and fugue-like states. Violent behaviour occasionally occurs but flailing of the arms is usually haphazard and poorly directed.

Investigations

The EEG may provide supportive evidence of the diagnosis (Fig. 4.3) but it can be normal in epilepsy and abnormal in non-epileptic individuals. A resting EEG or 24-hour ambulatory monitoring is useful in differentiating psychogenic from true seizures. The type and localisation of the epileptic discharge may be shown on EEG. MRI and/or CT are useful in determining the cause of epilepsy. Table 4.4 shows the differential diagnosis of epilepsy.

Treatment

Most recurrent seizures will improve with an appropriate anticonvulsant. Certain types of epilepsy respond to specific anticonvulsants.

1. Phenytoin and carbamazepine are most effective in partial and secondary generalised tonic/clonic epilepsy. The side-effects of phenytoin include hirsutism and gingival hyperplasia. Drug interactions occur. Phenytoin

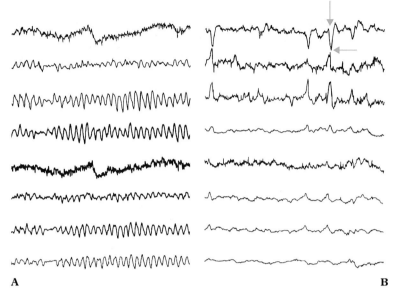

A   B

Fig. 4.3 (**A**) EEG from a normal subject. Left hemisphere leads show normal alpha rhythm. (**B**). A subject with spike focus and phase reversal in temporal leads from the left hemisphere. Both traces were recorded at a paper speed of 3 cm/s.

can reduce the efficacy of the oral contraceptive pill. The side-effects of carbamazepine include blurred vision, drowsiness, skin rash, ataxia and diplopia. Benign leukopenia in 30% of cases will settle with cessation of the drug. Aplastic anaemia and hepatitis are rare.

2. Sodium valproate is the drug of choice for primary generalised tonic/clonic seizures, myoclonic or absence seizures. Side-effects are nausea, vomiting, abdominal pain, tremor, hair loss and weight gain. Hepatotoxicity occurs rarely in children.
3. Ethosuximide is only of value for petit mal attacks.
4. Young patients with partial and secondary generalised fits often respond well to carbamazepine.

Second-line newer drugs, such as lamotriginè, gabapentin, vigabatrin and topirimate, may need to be considered.

Special problems relating to epilepsy

Pregnancy. All drugs can be teratogenic. Carbamazepine is the preferred drug.

Driving. If the patient has had even one witnessed seizure, and has an abnormal EEG, they should not drive until seizure-free for one year.

Social implications. Most patients lead a normal life, but some care has to be taken with certain activities such as swimming and climbing.

Table 4.4. Diagnostic features of loss of consciousness in epilepsy, vasovagal syncope and hypoglycaemia

	Epilepsy	Vasovagal syncope	Hypoglycaemia
Early warning	Uncommon Sometimes vague epigastric sensation in partial complex seizures	Blurred vision, lightheadedness	Pallor or bradycardia before and during attack
Onset	Dramatic	Gradual Helped or prevented by lying flat	Slow
Signs	Eyes roll up, often open Limbs rigid Tonic muscle contractions, pallor, normal heart rate or tachycardia	Eyes closed Hypnotic, pale, bradycardia	Variety of involuntary movements, pale, bradycardia
Plantar reflexes	Plantars extensor	Plantars flexor	Reflexes lost
Corneal reflexes	Absent	Present	Lost
Sphincter control	Lost	Preserved	Lost
Recovery	Disorientated, unreal feeling, sleepy Headaches lasting for hours	Drained, cold, sweaty Rapid recovery within 5 minutes	May be slow if glucose is not given

Status epilepticus. This is defined as the failure to recover consciousness between serial seizures. Permanent brain damage will occur if patients are allowed to continue fitting for more than 1 hour. Mortality is 12%. Principles of treatment include maintaining an airway and inserting an intravenous line with glucose, vitamin B complex and specific anticonvulsant therapy.

NARCOLEPSY

This is a rare disorder of the reticular activating system, characterised by excessive daytime sleepiness often associated with cataplexy (sudden loss of muscular tone with collapse precipitated by emotion such as laughing or crying). Hypnagogic hallucinations and sleep paralysis may also occur.

COMA

There is relative or total absence of cerebral activity caused by disturbance of metabolism, blood supply or by direct injury.

Coma of sudden onset

Cardiac arrest is associated with apnoea and absence of pulse. The patient is limp, with moist, cool skin because of peripheral shut down. Eyes are slightly open, pupils in midposition and there is no eye movement on passive head rotation. Rapid return of cerebral perfusion will result in complete recovery without any neurological damage.

There are many syndromes of cerebral damage resulting from inadequate brain perfusion, varying from cortical blindness and language difficulties to the persistence of coma and limb paralysis. Sudden rupture of blood into the subarachnoid space from an intracranial aneurysm is suggested by a cry, headache and vomiting before loss of consciousness. Subhyaloid haemorrhages in the optic fundus may appear.

The diagnosis is made by CT scan of the brain and a lumbar puncture. Other cerebral insults that can result in sudden coma include occlusion of the basilar artery and pontine haemorrhage.

Coma occurring over minutes or hours

This is often of the metabolic type caused by hyperglycaemia with or without ketosis, hypoglycaemia, drug overdose or hypoxia. Ruptured arteriovenous malformation, meningitis, encephalitis, cerebellar haemorrhage, hypertensive encephalopathy, metabolic, renal and hepatic failure are other causes.

Slow evolution of coma with lateralising signs

This is often associated with head injury. If there is a rapid rise in pressure from swelling or blood clot, then the temporal lobe will herniate downwards and compress the brainstem (Fig. 4.4).

Cerebellar infarction with swelling, may produce a brainstem compression syndrome with coma. There is little chance of recovery from a coma with pupillary and eye movement changes.

Investigations and treatment (see Tables 4.5 and 4.6)
Some patients fail to recover after a general anaesthetic. This may be from anoxia. A dramatic rise in temperature, pulse and respiration rate, and metabolic acidosis during anaesthesia, suggest malignant hyperpyrexia which is an inherited autosomal dominant trait. Sensitivity to succinylcholine or halothane in patients with muscle disease may be a problem. This is treated with intravenous dantrolene.

Special coma syndromes

The locked-in syndrome is caused by damage to the ventral pons, resulting in paralysis of all four limbs and lower cranial nerves. The patient is fully aware. Communication may be possible only with vertical eye movements.

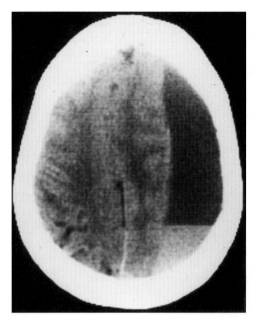

Fig. 4.4 Chronic subdural haematoma. Unenhanced CT scan shows a collection of altered blood with a fluid level from sedimentation of blood breakdown products.

Table 4.5. Assessment of the comatose patient

1. Inspect for signs of trauma to scalp and body
2. Endotracheal intubation if cyanosed
3. Smell for alcohol and acetone on the breath
4. Remove vomitus from throat
5. Suction and maintain clear airway
6. Insert intravenous line, check calcium, sugar and creatinine levels, osmolality, prothrombin time, APTT, drug screen, haemoglobin, white cell count
7. Infusion of intravenous glucose 50% and 50 mg thiamine to treat possible Wernicke's encephalopathy
8. Look for signs of drug abuse
9. Assess level of coma on Glasgow Coma Scale (see Table 4.6)
10. Observe the eye position and movement—horizontal roving eyes suggest intact brainstem, therefore a bihemisphere problem; check oculocephalic reflex only if a neck fracture has been excluded
11. Insert urinary catheter
12. If brain CT scan is negative then perform lumbar puncture providing there is no evidence of papilloedema: look for features of meningitis, encephalitis and haemorrhage. Centrifuge sample of cerebrospinal fluid (CSF) and look for xanthochromia
13. If brain CT scan shows mass lesion, refer to neurosurgeons.

Table 4.6. Glasgow Coma Scale

	Score
1. *Eye opening*	
Spontaneous	4
To speech	3
To pain	2
Nil	1
2. *Verbal response*	
Orientated	5
Confused conversation	4
Inappropriate words	3
Incomprehensible sounds	2
Nil	1
3. *Best motor response*	
Obeys command	6
Localises to pain	5
Withdraws to pain	4
Abnormal flexion to pain	3
Extension response	2
Nil	1
15 = fully conscious 3 = Severe brain damage	

This scale is widely accepted as a method for quantifying level of coma.

A chronic vegetative state occurs where there is no higher function. The patient has a normal sleep–wake cycle and the eyes are often open.

Brainstem death occurs where there is artificial ventilatory support in a patient whose heart continues to beat, yet the brain is irreversibly damaged. The cause of death must be known and hypothermia, metabolic disturbance such as hypoglycaemia, or drug effect, e.g. barbiturate, excluded.

To establish brainstem death, apnoea should persist after prior ventilation with oxygen, when the patient is taken off the ventilator. Oxygen is given via a tracheal cannula and the $PaCO_2$ must rise to stimulate the brainstem. The patient should be unresponsive except for spinal reflexes. All brainstem reflexes should be absent, including pupil response to light, oculo-cephalic, oculo-vestibular, corneal and gag reflexes.

MOVEMENT DISORDERS

PARKINSON'S DISEASE (PARALYSIS AGITANS)

The cause is unknown; 1% of the population aged over 60 is affected. Parkinson's disease (PD) results from degeneration, with neuronal loss, of the pigmented nuclei of the brainstem. Intracytoplasmic hyaline inclusions (Lewy bodies) are found in the remaining neurones. Chemical changes in the nigro-striatal system are responsible for the clinical features of PD, which emerges when 80% of the total dopaminergic cells are lost.

Symptoms and signs

The cardinal features are tremor at rest, rigidity and akinesia. Other signs include disturbance of posture and abnormal autonomic function. There is slow loss of agility, lack of facial expression, increased blinking, tilted trunk posture and hesitant rise from a chair. Generalised poverty of movement and problems with fine movements such as dressing occur.

Rigidity is cogwheel and often unilateral. Body posture is flexed, with the centre of gravity thrown forward. Gait is small and shuffling (festinant).

As the disease progresses, freezing occurs. Other problems include dysarthria, dysphagia and drooling of saliva. Autonomic features include thermal paraesthesiae, increased sweating and flushing, and postural hypoension with inadequate bladder emptying. The skin is often greasy and eczematous. 60% of patients will eventually develop dementia.

Differential diagnosis

A Parkinsonian syndrome occurs in patients on dopamine blocking drugs such as chlorpromazine.

The arteriosclerotic extrapyramidal syndrome is characterised by a 'marche a petit pas' and pyramidal signs often with a pseudobulbar palsy.

Benign essential postural tremor is of a faster frequency and does not have the other associated features.

Treatment

Benzhexol and orphenadrine suppress excess cholinergic activity in the striatal neurones. They help tremor but are limited by side-effects of dry mouth, constipation, prostatism and difficulty focusing.

Leva-dopa (L-dopa) with a dopa decarboxylase inhibitor, e.g. Sinemet-Plus or Madopar, represent the most effective medication. The duration of action of L-dopa may be up to 8–10 hours initially, but tends to diminish with time.

Dopamine agonists such as bromocriptine, lysuride and pergolide.

Subcutaneous apomorphine is only used in selected patients with severe unpredictable swings in motor performance.

The central nervous system side-effects of L-dopa and the dopamine agonists include abnormal movements of various types with 'on–off' effects and psychiatric problems. After many years, a range of involuntary movements may emerge: tics, chorea, dystonia and even ballismus. Treatment is by reducing the dose of L-dopa and adding a small amount of a dopamine agonist.

Psychiatric effects occur in 50% of patients who have had the disease for 5 years or more. These may take the form of vivid dreams, progressing to frank hallucinations. The psychosis may have a strong paranoid element. Treatment consists of reducing the dose of L-dopa or dopamine agonist. Drugs such as phenothiazines may exacerbate PD. Sudden cessation of anti-Parkinsonian drugs should be avoided because this can precipitate an acute confusional state and rigidity. Postural instability with frequent falls, freezing and swallowing problems are very difficult to manage.

Brain implantation with human fetal mesencephalic cells is still an experimental procedure. Surgical pallidotomy offers relief from distressing dyskinesias and may also help tremor, bradykinesia and rigidity.

Prognosis

PD patients are living longer—15 to 20 years from the time of diagnosis is not unusual—but the degree of disability by then is marked.

CHOREA

Chorea is characterised by non-rhythmical involuntary jerking movements affecting different areas of the body in an irregular, unpredictable fashion. It may affect the distal limbs, the face, swallowing, articulation or breathing.

Causes

1. In the young. Sydenham's chorea (St Vitus dance or rheumatic chorea) from *Streptococcus* group A infection, pregnancy and the contraceptive pill.

2. In the elderly. Huntington's disease, benign hereditary and senile chorea.

3. Systemic diseases. Systemic lupus erythematosus (SLE), thyrotoxicosis, hypoparathyroidism, patients with Parkinson's disease on L-dopa.

Vascular hemichorea, or hemiballismus, caused by infarction in the basal ganglia subthalamic nucleus, is treated with haloperidol or tetrabenazine.

Huntington's chorea is an autosomal dominant condition with complete penetrance and a very low mutation rate. Prevalence is 5–10 per 100 000. The onset of chorea, behavioural abnormality and dementia in the fourth and fifth decade is followed by a progressive course and death within 15–20 years. The pathological features are thinning of the head of the caudate nucleus from neuronal loss and gliosis. This is seen on MRI or CT scan as a flattening of the frontal horns of the lateral ventricles. The gene for Huntington's chorea is related to a DNA segment on the short arm of chromosome 4.

Treatment is with dopamine blockers, such as tetrabenazine, haloperidol or pimozide, to control movements.

ESSENTIAL TREMOR

There is regular rhythmical oscillation of segments of the limb and trunk whilst maintaining posture or moving parts of the body. It is a type of action tremor most noticeable when the arms are outstretched. It is often familial and is helped by alcohol. The most common cause of tremor is anxiety, but it is also seen with alcohol abuse and thyrotoxicosis. The incidence of Parkinson's disease is increased in patients with essential tremor. Treatment is with propranolol, clonazepam and sometimes prednisolone.

MYOCLONUS

Sudden involuntary contraction of muscle groups results in movement of the corresponding joint. Nocturnal myoclonus is a normal phenomenon associated with sudden jerking of the whole body during the hypnagogic state. Epileptic myoclonus, or epilepsia partialis continua, is often precipitated by sensory stimuli and occurs with a spike focus on the EEG. It is commonly the result of stroke, tumour or cerebral abscess. Other causes of myoclonus include post-cardiac arrest cerebral hypoxia, Creutzfeldt-Jakob disease, benign essential myoclonus and subacute sclerosing panencephalitis (SSPE). It also occurs as a complication of hepatic, renal and respiratory failure. Treatment is with clonazepam or sodium valproate.

DYSTONIA

Dystonia can be either focal or segmental and consists of muscle agonist and antagonist contracting in a slow fashion to distort limb posture, e.g. spasmodic torticollis. Patients on L-dopa or dopamine agonist treatment often develop dystonia affecting one foot or one arm.

The rare primary idiopathic dystonia musculorum deformans is a progressive disease requiring large doses of anticholinergics, phenothiazines, L-dopa and benzodiazepines.

Wilson's disease, an inherited disorder of copper metabolism, is characterised by stiff dystonic posturing and a fixed smile. If treated early it will respond to penicillamine.

Spasmodic torticollis and other dystonias may be treated with local injections of botulinus toxin into the affected muscles.

Writer's cramp is believed to be a form of focal dystonia.

ATHETOSIS

Slow, sinuous writhing movement occurs along the long axis of the limbs, as an L-dopa side-effect, but also in cerebral palsy.

TICS OR HABIT SPASMS

These are common, repetitive semi-purposive movements, which patients can suppress, and are often associated with stress. They can take the form of some purposeful action, such as winking or shrugging of the shoulder. An extreme form occurs in the Gilles de la Tourette syndrome.

PAIN SYNDROMES

At a peripheral level, unmyelinated C fibres are responsible for diffuse, long-lasting slow pain. A-delta fibre discharges result in well localised, brief, fast pain. Pain may be distributed to the dermatomes, in which case it is well localised and often associated with paraesthesiae. Pain may also radiate to the myotomes or sclerotomes (skeletal or ligamentous structures) where it tends to be less well localised. Dermatome pain is of a pricking, burning, nature. Deep pain is a diffuse dull ache and bears no relationship to skeletal or visceral structures, making diagnosis problematical. Disease of visceral or skeletal structures is referred to the skin supplied by the same spinal segments, e.g. cardiac pain. Central nervous system sources of pain are exemplified by thalamic pain after stroke. This is characterised by dysaesthesiae or pain on touching skin.

MIGRAINE

Fifty per cent of men and 30% of women will suffer such headaches at some time in their lives. Pain is caused by dilatation of the arteries in the distribution of the external carotid arteries. During the prodrome the blood flow is reduced by vasoconstriction and increased during the headache phase. This dilatation has been linked to increased levels of 5-hydroxytryptamine (5-HT) and other vasoactive substances in the serum. Migraine usually begins in the second to third decade, sometimes the fifth, and a positive family history is common.

Symptoms

Headaches begin suddenly, reaching a peak in minutes or hours. The pain is described as throbbing, pulsing or pounding. A typical migraine begins early in the day and often at weekends. Diuresis and euphoria are common. Common migraine is defined as unilateral headache with nausea and vomiting. Classical migraine has focal neurological features. The aura, e.g. a hemianopia, usually lasts 15 minutes. Flashing lights, shimmering, fortification spectra or teichopsia, bright moving lights, may be followed by a blind spot or hemianopia. Trigger factors include:

1. foods containing tyramine or other vasoactive substances, e.g. alcohol, cheese, caffeine, yoghurt
2. hormone fluctuations prior to and during menstruation, pregnancy and puerperium, and the contraceptive pill
3. vasodilator drugs including nifedipine, and glyceryl trinitrate
4. relaxing after a period of intense activity.

A variant of migraine is cluster headaches (migrainous neuralgia) and is characterised by localised pain around the eye, conjunctival injection, lacrimation and a Horner's syndrome. Other types of migraine include facial, ophthalmoplegic and basilar syndromes.

Treatment

The acute attack usually only requires simple analgesics and an anti-emetic. If these fail then a combination of ergotamine and caffeine may be required. This is best limited to younger patients without vascular disease. Prophylaxis takes the form of cyclizine, beta-blockers, clonidine or pizotifen. The anti-serotonin drug methysergide may be required in resistant cases. Sumatriptan, a selective 5-HT agonist which causes a selective vaso-constriction within the carotid arterial circulation, is used to treat acute migraine attacks.

GIANT CELL (TEMPORAL) ARTERITIS

This condition tends to afflict those over 60 and is rare under the age of 55 years.

Diffuse steady headache, sometimes spreading from the temples over the face, is typical. The scalp is often tender because of the inflamed superficial temporal and occipital vessels. General symptoms of fatigue, malaise and proximal stiffness (from polymyalgia rheumatica) may occur.

Although the erythrocyte sedimentation rate (ESR) is usually raised it may be normal in the early phase of the illness in 15% of cases. Patients may complain of a painful tongue, which may develop ischaemic ulcers or even gangrene. Jaw claudication from masseter ischaemia is secondary to external carotid artery involvement.

The most important complication is sudden loss of vision caused by occlusion of the ophthalmic artery. Vertebrobasilar and, rarely, carotid arteries may be affected before they enter the dura, resulting in focal ischaemic syndromes.

Diagnosis is confirmed by biopsy of the superficial temporal artery. Arteritic changes are often focal and segmental, so a negative biopsy does not exclude the diagnosis. The dramatic response to steroids is diagnostic. Patients may have to remain on steroids for 12–18 months.

TENSION HEADACHES

The pain is a constant tight pressure and may radiate into the neck and shoulders. It often builds up gradually and may continue for days. Headache lasting longer than 6 months is unlikely to be caused by serious intracranial disease. Alcohol and exercise alleviate tension headache whereas they exacerbate migraine. Cervical headache may be associated with spondylosis. Emotional factors can influence tension headaches. Physiotherapy, soft collar, muscle relaxants and antidepressants may alleviate the pain.

TRIGEMINAL NEURALGIA OR TIC DOULOUREUX

The pain is usually in the distribution of the maxillary and/or mandibular divisions. In idiopathic tic, degenerative or fibrotic changes in the Gasserian ganglia have been reported. Secondary causes of neuralgia include multiple sclerosis and compression of the nerve by tumour or anomalous blood vessel.

The onset of idiopathic trigeminal neuralgia is usually in mid to late life and is unusual under the age of 35.

Symptoms and signs

The symptom is a paroxysmal pain (like an electric shock) from a trigger zone, radiating out into the trigeminal divisions. It is often precipitated by cold wind, washing the face, shaving or eating. Paroxysms last for 1–2 minutes. There is no objective loss of sensation during or after an attack, although the patient may complain of hyperaesthesia. The frequency of attacks varies from many times a day to several times a month. The patient may be undernourished from a lack of eating or from fear of precipitating an attack.

Differential diagnosis

Facial pain involves disease of the temporomandibular joint, maxillary sinusitis, teeth, glaucoma, or nasopharyngeal disease. Atypical facial pain where no organic cause is found can be difficult to treat. Antidepressants and carbamazepine are usually employed.

Treatment

Simple analgesics are ineffective. Opiates will work but are addictive. Intravenous phenytoin will abort an attack. Oral carbamazepine is usually effective, but may cause sedation in the elderly. Surgery, including alcohol injection of the infraorbital nerve, can be effective. Radiofrequency thermo-coagulation of trigeminal nerve rootlets is often used, as is decompression by separating anomalous vessels from nerve roots via a small posterior fossa approach.

Prognosis

Remission of months or years in trigeminal neuralgia is very common.

LIMB PAIN

Causalgia. Severe limb pain and intense burning secondary to partial injury is often associated with varying degrees of sympathetic nervous system disturbance. It is similar to reflex sympathetic dystrophy secondary to minor limb trauma, also known as Sudeck's atrophy, where there are skin changes and reduced sweating.

Phantom limb pain as seen in amputees and caused by central mechanisms.

Radicular pain may be caused by herpes zoster, a tumour or irradiation.

Plexus pain is seen in brachial neuralgia, tumour and trauma.

Peripheral nerve pain is seen in amyloidosis, diabetes and entrapment mononeuropathy.

CERVICAL RADICULAR PAIN SYNDROMES

C5/6 level disease involving the C6 root produces pain in the trapezius ridge, shoulder, anterior arm, radial forearm and thumb.

C6/7 disc level involving the C7 root causes pain in the shoulder blade, pectoral region, posterolateral upper arm, dorsal forearm, elbow, index and middle finger.

Other causes of upper limb pain include polymyalgia rheumatica, fibromyalgia, viral myalgia, cellulitis, ischaemia, superficial venous thrombosis, collagen vascular disease and paraproteinaemia from vasospastic disease.

LOW BACK PAIN

Lumbar disc disease may cause pain by several mechanisms. These include a torn tendon at muscle attachment to vertebrae, stretching of the periosteum, a bulging disc against annulus fibrosis, inflammation around the disc (discitis), compression of nerve roots from bulging of the annulus or frank herniation of disc material, and a root compressed by osteophytes, intervertebral joints and facets. Abdominal or pelvic disease may also be referred to the back. Ninety-five per cent of lumbosacral disc lesions occur at L4/5 and L5/S1 level.

Symptoms

The clinical features of lumbar root lesions are shown in Table 4.7. The mode of onset and type of pain may give a clue to the aetiology of back pain.

1. Pain of gradual onset suggests tumour.
2. Pain of sudden onset suggests mechanical stress.
3. Intermittent pain associated with walking suggests spondylitic radiculopathy with narrow spinal canal.
3. Discomfort at rest with continuous irritation suggests inflammation of the pain-sensitive periosteum.

   The quality of bone pain is a referred discomfort, often a deep aching, whereas root pain is often very intense and sharp, and distally distributed to the dermatomes.

Differential diagnosis

Other causes of low back pain include lumbosacral or sacroiliac sprain, fractured lumbar vertebra, metastatic bone disease, infection of bone,

Table 4.7. Clinical features of lumbar root lesions

Root	Site of pain	Sensory loss	Weakness	Tendon reflex affected
L3	Anterior thigh	Anterior thigh	Hip flexion, adduction Quadriceps	Knee jerk
L4*	Anterior thigh	Anterior thigh	Quadriceps Tibialis anterior	Knee jerk
L5*	Lateral thigh	Lateral lower leg and dorsum of foot	Hip abduction Hamstrings Foot eversion	—
S1*	Posterior thigh	Lateral foot	Eversion of foot	Ankle jerk
S2	Posterior thigh	Rear calf	Small foot muscles	—

*Most commonly affected roots

spondylolisthesis (slip forward of vertebra), spondylosis and ankylosing spondylitis.

Investigations

These include plain X-ray of the lumbosacral spine. Spinal CT and MRI are very helpful, showing the soft tissue and bone. Contrast myelography shows indentation of the thecal sac by a mass lesion.

Treatment

Narcotics may be necessary for acute pain relief. Anti-inflammatory and anti-depressant drugs are used for chronic pain, as are physiotherapy, massage, traction and bedrest. Surgery is considered if medical treatment fails.

STROKE

Cerebrovascular disease is the third most common cause of death in Western society and a major cause of disability. Stroke is defined as the rapid onset of neurological deficit which may build up over minutes, hours or even days.

Pathology

1. reversible ischaemia
2. infarction—major vessel occlusion, either embolism or thrombosis
3. infarction with secondary haemorrhage
4. haemorrhage (15% of cases).

Aetiology of infarction

1. local thrombosis
2. emboli from the great vessels or heart
3. poor perfusion pressure
4. abnormal platelets or coagulation
5. vasospasm
6. arteritis.

Risk factors

1. Hypertension—persistently raised blood pressure, diastolic greater than 100 mmHg.
2. A family history of stroke, hypertension and coronary artery disease.
3. Cardiac disease, particularly valvular, with or without atrial fibrillation.
4. Transient cerebral ischaemic attacks.
5. Raised haematocrit, greater than 0.5.
6. Smoking, lack of exercise, high serum cholesterol levels, excess alcohol.
7. Oral contraceptive pill.

Symptoms and signs

The temporal syndrome

1. Transient cerebral ischaemic attack (TIA) lasts less than 24 hours.
2. Minor stroke lasts longer than 24 hours but less than 1 week.
3. Major stroke lasts longer than 1 week.

The anatomical syndrome

Carotid territory features include amaurosis fugax and language problems. Vertebrobasilar territory features include dizziness, dysarthria, double vision, dysphagia, hemianopia, clumsiness and loss of consciousness.

Specific arterial occlusive syndromes

Common carotid. Occlusion often fails to produce a deficit because of the good anastomosis between the two carotids, and vertebrobasilar systems.

Internal carotid. Stenosis with eventual thrombosis leads to a gradual stuttering onset with TIAs preceding the major event in several cases. Embolism is usually dramatic and calamitous. Features are those of unilateral hemisphere dysfunction:

1. contralateral hemiparesis
2. contralateral sensory loss
3. aphasia (dominant hemisphere)
4. homonymous hemianopia is infrequent and usually takes the form of temporary neglect of opposite visual fields.

Middle cerebral artery. This is the artery most likely to be affected by embolism. Damage is to the ipsilateral internal capsule and basal ganglia. Features include:

1. contralateral hemiplegia
2. contralateral hemianaesthesia
3. contralateral hemianopia
4. aphasia if dominant hemisphere is affected.

Anterior cerebral artery (Fig. 4.5). Features include:

1. contralateral numb weak leg
2. akinetic mutism and abulia (reduced rate and complexity of language and motor response) in bilateral disease.

Posterior cerebral artery. Contralateral homonymous hemianopia.

Vertebrobasilar arteries. Occlusion produces a wide spectrum of syndromes that depend on the site of thrombosis. If of sudden onset, usually embolic, occlusion results in quadraplegia and ocular dysfunctions. The lateral medullary syndrome is from occlusion of the basilar or posterior inferior cerebellar artery. Findings include:

1. vertigo, vomiting, nystagmus
2. dysphagia
3. hoarseness
4. ipsilateral loss of pain and temperature in the face, palate and vocal cord paralysis, Horner's syndrome and limb ataxia

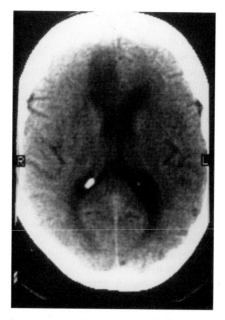

Fig. 4.5 Infarction in territory of right anterior cerebral artery—a low-density area in front of the right frontal horn involving grey and white matter. There is no compression of the ventricle.

5. contralateral pain and temperature loss in the limbs and trunk (there are *no* motor limb signs)
6. crossed hemiplegias occur with brainstem lesions when a cranial nerve nucleus and pyramidal tract are affected.

Investigations

These include haemoglobin, packed cell volume, ESR or viscosity, blood sugar, serum cholesterol (controversial because it is not known whether lowering blood cholesterol will reduce the incidence of stroke), serological tests for syphilis. In a patient with stroke a CT brain scan may:

1. be normal
2. show a low-density large lesion caused by a major vessel occlusion, or small lacunar infarctions (lacunes are 3–5 mm cystic lesions)
3. show patchy enhancing lesions thought to be caused by luxury perfusion
4. show evidence of haemorrhage.

Doppler carotid artery studies represent a non-invasive technique to show stenotic lesions. Carotid arteriography may be necessary to define stenotic lesions more accurately.

Treatment

TIAs, if untreated, lead to stroke in 22–50% of cases within 5 years. Treatment is with aspirin (300 mg/24 hours). If this fails then anticoagulants should be considered. Carotid endarterectomy may be effective when there is ≥ 70% carotid artery stenosis.

Anticoagulants may be of value for stroke in evolution and as prophylaxis in valvular heart disease, especially where there is atrial fibrillation. Surgery to evacuate a cerebellar haemorrhage may be beneficial.

Rehabilitation involves the physiotherapist, and the occupational and speech therapist. The role of thrombolysis in stroke of less than 6 hours' duration is under evaluation.

Prognosis

Forty to 50% of patients die within 3 weeks. The highest mortality occurs in cerebral haemorrhage (70–80%). Mortality is lower in infarction—20%. Adverse factors for long-term outlook include aphasia and incontinence; 50% of surviving patients will be left with a substantial neurological deficit.

SUBARACHNOID HAEMORRHAGE

Bleeding into the subarachnoid space is usually from a ruptured berry aneurysm (Fig. 4.6) or arteriovenous malformation. Saccular berry aneurysms are caused by a congenital defect in the supporting tissue of the arterial wall and are usually located at the division of a major intracranial artery.

A transient sudden increase in blood pressure often precedes rupture.

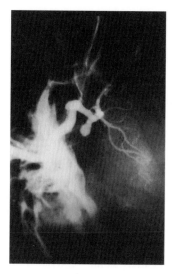

Fig. 4.6 Angiogram shows a berry aneurysm of the basilar artery.

The volume of blood released varies from a few millilitres to a massive haemorrhage which can be fatal in seconds. The consequences of rupture are:

1. direct brain injury
2. susceptibility to re-rupture
3. secondary hydrocephalus from blockage of CSF circulation
4. vasospasm.

Symptoms and signs

Symptoms include sudden onset of severe occipital headache, unconsciousness in 50% of patients, vomiting, epileptic fits and lumbar pain in the case of spinal subarachnoid haemorrhage. Neck stiffness, positive Kernig's sign, papilloedema, subhyaloid retinal haemorrhages, focal neurological signs, and cranial nerve palsies result.

Investigations

A CT scan may show subarachnoid blood in sylvian and interhemispheric fissures and occasionally in the ventricular system. If the CT scan is negative then lumbar puncture may be necessary. This should show a uniformly blood-stained CSF. Xanthochromia may persist for up to 14–20 days. Lymphocytes may be present in small numbers in the late phase.

Differential diagnosis

Other causes are encephalitis, meningitis, migraine and cervical spondylosis.

Treatment

The risk of re-rupture remains high at 1–2% per day for the first 3–4 weeks. Blood pressure should be well controlled. Intravenous nimodipine reduces the morbidity from vasospasm.

Surgery involves clipping the neck of the aneurysm and the best results are obtained in middle cerebral and posterior communicating aneurysms.

Prognosis

1. Thirty per cent of patients will die in the first 24 hours.
2. Thirty per cent will survive 8 weeks and 20% of these will re-bleed, usually within the first 3 weeks.
3. Fifty per cent of the survivors at 1 year will go back to work.
4. Persistent disability results from hemiplegia, cranial nerve palsies and epilepsy.

Arteriovenous malformations (AVM) comprise arteries and veins of mixed size but not capillaries. There is usually an arteriovenous (AV) fistula. The AVM may rupture, or cause epilepsy or headache. It is often detected incidentally on a CT brain scan. A proportion of patients will have a skull bruit. Treatment takes the form of catheter embolisation, surgery or radiotherapy.

DISEASES OF THE SPINAL CORD

The cord terminates at the L1 vertebra but lower lumbar sacral roots continue in the canal until they reach their point of exit.

In lesions of the spinal cord, the level of damage should be assessed so that appropriate radiology can be accurately directed. However, it is not always possible to determine the exact site of the cord lesion from symptoms and signs. It is often necessary during myelography to run the contrast medium the full length of the cord from conus to foramen magnum.

ACUTE SPINAL CORD LESION (MYELOPATHY)

Compressive lesions must be looked for immediately. Failure to do this and to treat surgically may result in permanent cord damage. Causes include:

1. Trauma.

2. Extradural compression from:
   (a) disc herniation, cervical and thoracic spine
   (b) metastatic tumour from primary prostate, lung, breast and also myeloma
   (c) osteomyelitis, tuberculosis.

Less common causes such as epidural abscess, haematoma and tumour may not be associated with bony X-ray changes.

Damage to the cord occurs by means of compression of its blood supply with subsequent ischaemia.

Other causes of acute myelopathy include:

1. transverse myelitis caused by viral infections, syphilis and HIV
2. multiple sclerosis
3. Devic's disease (neuromyelitis optica)
4. systemic cancer—necrotising non-metastatic myelopathy
5. vascular disease, haematomyelia or anterior spinal artery thrombosis.

Symptoms and signs

Symptoms include a painful back from bone disease, segmental root pain, progressive difficulty in walking, a numb tingling sensation in the legs and difficulty in passing urine.

The signs are sensory level below the point of lesion, enlarged bladder with overflow incontinence, and proximal hip flexion weakness leading to flaccid paralysis; spasticity emerges later with brisk reflexes and extensor plantars.

Investigations

1. Chest X-ray.
2. Rectal examination.
3. Lumbar puncture. CSF protein level may be very high, with xanthochromia, particularly if there is a complete block.
4. MRI and CT scanning.

Management of established complete paraplegia

1. Medical or surgical treatment of the cause.
2. Bladder function, with indwelling catheter using aseptic technique. Infections are treated with antibiotics.
3. Bowel care: enema, manual evacuation.
4. Regular turning to avoid pressure scores. A Ripple mattress should be used.
5. Avoidance of contractures with physiotherapy and regular passive exercises.
6. Later, transfer to a special paraplegic unit for rehabilitation.

CHRONIC SPINAL CORD DISEASE

This is slowly progressive, occurring over months or even years. Common causes include cervical spondylosis from osteoarthritic and degenerative changes in the neck, with osteophytes, disc protrusion posteriorly, resulting in local bony overgrowth. There may be progressive difficulty in walking, bilateral tingling, numbness in the hands, and neck stiffness (absence of local pain is common). Bladder dysfunction is rare.

Spastic paraparesis, brisk deep tendon reflexes and extensor plantar responses are seen. The sensory level may involve the dorsal column, or spinothalamic function, and is not always an accurate guide to the level of the lesion.

Investigations

Plain neck X-ray, CT scan with myelogram, MRI scan.

MOTOR NEURONE DISEASE

This is a condition of unknown aetiology where there is degeneration of the corticospinal tracts, anterior horn cells and bulbar motor nuclei. It affects patients aged 30–60 and has a male to female ratio of 2.5 : 1.

The symptoms and signs of the disease are summarised in Table 4.8 and a combination of syndromes is common. Widespread fasciculations beyond the focal weak muscles is a common picture.

Investigations

Investigations are directed to exclude other diseases. Nerve conduction studies and concentric needle EMG may show widespread features of denervation.

Differential diagnosis

1. cervical spondylitic myelopathy
2. pure motor neuropathy as in paraproteinaemia
3. foramen magnum or cord tumour
4. a pseudobulbar palsy may be secondary to vascular disease.

Management

There is no cure. Extension of life expectancy by 6–9 months may occur with the drug riluzole. Dysphagia may be treated by sucking ice or taking neostigmine 15 mg before meals. Feeding is by gastrostomy in cachectic patients. Physiotherapy, speech and swallowing therapy, suction machines and foot drop orthotic splints are needed. In the UK, Motor Neurone Disease Association care assistants will provide support.

Death almost invariably occurs within 3 years. Inhalation pneumonia is common because of the weak cough reflex.

SPINAL CORD TUMOURS

These may be caused by lesions arising from the nerve roots, the covering of the spinal cord, extradural fat, vascular networks and sympathetic chain of the vertebral column itself.

Benign encapsulated tumours (meningiomas and neurofibromas) account

Table 4.8. Symptoms and signs of motor neurone disease

Clinical syndrome (location of pathology)	Symptoms	Signs
Progressive muscular atrophy (PMA) (anterior horn cell)	Weakness, wasting fasciculations	Often asymmetrical proximal or distal wasting Preservation of deep tendon reflexes
Amytrophic lateral sclerosis (ALS) (corticospinal tracts)	Spastic gait, weak legs, cramps	No sensory signs Spastic quadraparesis Brisk reflexes, plantars extensor Bladder function preserved until very late
Bulbar palsy (motor lower cranial nerve nuclei)	Dysphagia, dysarthria, Dysphonia, weak cough, risk of inhalation	Nasal speech, nasal regurgitation, and a wasted fasciculating tongue
Pseudobulbar palsy (bilateral corticobulbar tracts)	Dysarthria, spastic tongue, dysphagia, emotional lability	Spastic tongue, increased jaw jerk

for the majority of all spinal cord primary tumours. Intramedullary tumours are more common in children and extramedullary tumours in adults. Tumours of the spinal cord are much less frequent than intracranial tumours, with a ratio of 1 : 4. Extramedullary tumours can cause symptoms by involving nerve roots and compression of the spinal cord, including occlusion of spinal blood vessels. Intramedullary tumours such as a glioma may extend the whole length of the spinal cord early in the disease (Fig. 4.7).

SUBACUTE COMBINED DEGENERATION OF THE CORD

Deficiency of vitamin B_{12} (cyanocobalomin) is the cause. Neurological lesions may result from inactivity of the B_{12} dependent enzyme methionine synthetase. This occurs in pernicious anaemia (PA), post-gastrectomy and some malabsorption syndromes. PA is often seen in association with other auto-immune diseases. The pathology is in the white more than the grey matter, although peripheral nerves are involved. There is loss of the myelin sheath and, to a lesser extent, the axons.

Neurological symptoms may appear early in the disease and even antedate the onset of anaemia (see p. 316).

FRIEDREICH'S ATAXIA

This most common of the spinocerebellar degenerations is an inherited disorder (autosomal recessive) causing degeneration of cells in the posterior

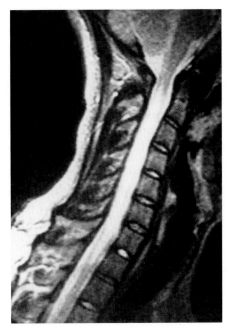

Fig. 4.7 Astrocytoma of the spinal cord. A sagittal MRI scan (T2 weighted) of the cervical spine showing a high signal from within the cord extending from C2 to C7.

root ganglia, with secondary change in the peripheral nerves and posterior column of the spinal cord and cerebellum.

Development is in childhood, although the disease can present for the first time in adults. The signs are difficulty in walking, cerebellar dysarthria, ataxic weak limbs, absent deep tendon reflexes and extensor plantar responses. Posterior column function is affected with Rhombergism. There may also be club foot, scoliosis and cardiac involvement.

The ECG is usually abnormal with widespread T wave inversion. There is no treatment and the mean age of death is 35 years, from heart failure.

SYRINGOMYELIA

This is caused by an irregular cavitation in the central grey part of the spinal cord and brainstem. In the early stage of what is mainly a slowly progressive disease, there is disruption of the central decussating pain and temperature fibres. The process then extends to the anterior horn cells, and eventually disrupts the corticospinal fibres. Dorsal column function abnormality is a late feature.

The disorder is occasionally associated with craniocervical junction anomalies. These include cerebellar tonsilar herniation and adhesions at the foramen magnum. They cause interruption of the free flow of CSF in and out of the fourth ventricle to the subarachnoid space. CSF is then forced downwards into the central cord.

Symptoms and signs

In the early stages patients may experience painless burns and sudden-onset pain in the back, chest or arms. The sensory signs are often dissociated anaesthesia with pain and temperature being affected, and sparing of dorsal column function. The hands may be weak and the reflexes are usually depressed or absent in the upper limbs. A Horner's syndrome and nystagmus may be present and some patients have a short neck with kyphosis.

Late in the disease, patients exhibit severe wasting of the hands, with difficulty in walking from spastic paraparesis. There is increasing sensory loss, and the skin of the hands takes on a red, shiny, dystrophic appearance. Charcot joints may develop, particularly involving the shoulders and elbows. Patients may develop a bulbar palsy (syringobulbia).

Differential diagnosis

Tumour of the cord, haematomyelia and cervical spondylitic myelopathy.

The diagnosis is made on an MRI scan (Fig. 4.8) of the cord, or CT myelogram.

Treatment is by craniocervical junction decompression. Most patients will do moderately well, although a small number of patients will experience slow progression despite surgery.

MULTIPLE SCLEROSIS (MS)

MS is the most common disorder of the central nervous system to affect the young in the Western World. Lesions are confined to the central nervous system white matter, with preservation of axons compared with loss of myelin. The multiplicity of lesions and their sclerotic appearance (plaques) are evident on gross pathological specimens. The MRI scan (Fig. 4.9) shows well-established periventricular high signal abnormalities. Lesions also occur in the brainstem, cerebellum and spinal cord.

A susceptibility to the disease may be acquired during childhood. Disease prevalence is 5 : 100 000 in Africa and Asia, whereas in northern Europe it is 80 : 100 000. If migration from one zone to another takes place before the age of 10 then individual susceptibility is determined by the new region, otherwise the patient takes with him or her the susceptibility of the home country. Altered host reaction to an agent (?virus) not yet identified is a possible factor, set against a background of genetic and immune abnormality. MS is more frequent in identical twins and amongst members of the immediate family.

An immunological basis for MS is supported by the finding of a raised CSF IgG with oligoclonal banding. Immunological studies show collection of T cells and macrophages in the perivenous white matter near the plaques.

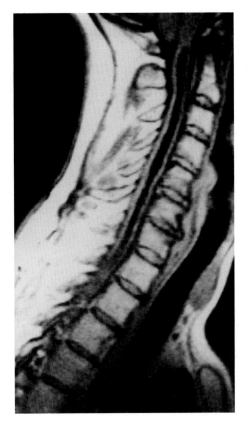

Fig. 4.8 Syringomyelia shown on an MRI scan (T1 weighted) showing cystic dilatation of the cervical cord.

The course of the disease is more severe in women with onset in the midthirties. Those patients whose disease begins with pure optic neuritis or pure sensory symptoms have a better prognosis than those with other syndromes. The average onset is between the second and fourth decades.

Symptoms and signs

These are listed in Table 4.9.

Relapses and remissions are very common in MS. The acute episodes may develop over several hours of days and resolve gradually over weeks.

The diagnosis of MS depends on demonstrating scattered lesions throughout the central nervous system. In some cases, usually the elderly, MS runs a chronic progressive course, with no remission, and it is essential to exclude other disease such as spinal cord compression.

Although there is considerable individual variation, most patients will

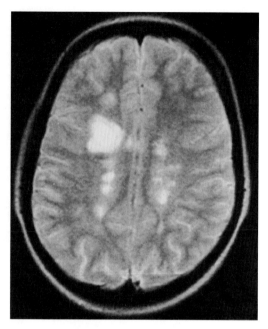

Fig. 4.9 Multiple sclerosis. Several high signal areas in a periventricular distribution within the white matter of the cerebral hemispheres are shown on the MRI scan (T2 weighted).

Table 4.9. Symptoms and signs in multiple sclerosis (in order of frequency)

Symptoms	Signs
Muscle weakness	Spasticity
Ocular disturbance	Hyperreflexia
Urinary disturbance	Extensor plantars
Gait ataxia	Absent abdominal reflexes
Paraesthesiae	Intention tremor
Dysarthria	Optic atrophy
Mental disturbance	Nystagmus
Pain	Impaired vibration sense
Vertigo	Impaired position sense
Dysphagia	Impaired pain appreciation
Convulsions	Facial weakness
Hearing loss	Impairment of touch
Tinnitus	Impairment of temperature

experience progressive deterioration, often punctuated with acute relapses. This results in a progressively increasing difficulty in walking, a spastic ataxic gait, failing vision and urinary difficulty.

Investigations

Although the diagnosis is commonly made on clinical grounds, laboratory support, particularly in the early stages, can be invaluable.

The CSF lymphocyte count is usually less than 20 cells per mm^3. The IgG total protein ratio is raised at greater than 15%. Oligoclonal banding in the CSF is the most sensitive test.

Electrophysiology—visual evoked potentials (VERs) are used to check the integrity of the visual pathway. This test is abnormal in all patients with a previous attack of optic neuritis, even if the visual acuity has returned to normal.

MRI scanning (Fig. 4.9) shows multiple lesions. T2 weighted images will show established pathology, and gadolinium enhances areas thought to relate to an acute breakdown in the blood–brain barrier associated with a new lesion.

Differential diagnosis

1. Visual loss—consider optic nerve compression, vascular or toxic disease.
2. Paraplegia—think of other causes of cord compression.
3. Ataxia—consider tumour and vascular disease.

Treatment

There is no cure for MS.

1. An acute relapse may be shortened by an intensive course of i.v. methylprednisolone 500 mg per 24 hours for 5 days.
2. Dietary regimens have been studied, but appear to confer no long-term benefit. Nevertheless many patients claim benefit from linoleic acid or sunflower seed oil, and take a low animal fat or gluten-free diet.
3. Immunosuppressive drugs such as azathioprine and cyclophosphamide confer no long-term benefit.
4. Trials of beta interferon and co-polymer I have indicated a modest reduction in the number of relapses in the relapsing–remitting type of disease.

Symptomatic management

1. Infections are controlled with antibiotics.
2. For bladder dysfunction anticholinergic drugs (propantheline and oxybutynin) may reduce urinary urgency and frequency but can precipitate acute retention. A Conveen sheath for males may help incontinence. Intermittent self-catheterisation is usually followed by a permanent indwelling catheter or a suprapubic catheter. A small number of patients

are managed with an ileal bladder, with the ureters transplanted into an ileal loop.

3. Baclofen, diazepam and dantrolene reduce muscular spasms but with higher doses, the limbs may become hypotonic, resulting in patients collapsing if they use their spasticity to maintain the upright posture. Some patients use a self-administered intrathecal baclofen pump.

4. If the immobile patient is left for periods without passive exercises, then tendon contractures appear that may have to be treated surgically.

5. Support services are required, including physiotherapy and occupational therapy.

Most patients remain active in the early stages of the disease. Thereafter they are managed at home and occasionally admitted for respite care. The average duration of the disease is 20 years from time of diagnosis. Some patients are still ambulant 20 years or more after onset.

CEREBRAL INFECTIONS

BACTERIAL MENINGITIS

Bacterial meningitis is due to inflammation of the meninges. Any cerebral cortex changes occur as the result of vascular occlusion. Meningitis in children is usually caused by blood-borne organisms spreading from paranasal sinuses, middle ear, mastoid or respiratory infections. Organisms may enter the skull from a fracture. Neonates are often infected with *Haemophilus influenzae* which is rare after the age of 6 years. Adults are usually affected by the meningococcus, with its haemorrhagic skin rash, or *Streptococcus pneumoniae*.

Symptoms and signs

These comprise fever, headache, fits, confusion and alteration of conscious level. There is a rapid onset over 24 hours. The patient is sick, irritable, with neck stiffness, photophobia and limited straight leg raising.

Diagnosis

Confirmed by CSF cell count and culture. If there are papilloedema and focal neurological signs, a CT brain scan is required to exclude an abscess. CSF usually contains 1000 white cells per ml and most are polymorphs. There is increased protein and a low glucose. Organisms may be hard to find in the partially antibiotic-treated patient.

Chronic meningitis with cranial nerve signs, hydrocephalus and a moderate CSF lymphocytic pleocytosis raises the possibility of tuberculous meningitis. Confirmation of this diagnosis may be difficult but is aided by a positive history of tuberculosis contact, TB on the chest X-ray, or a positive Heaf test.

Treatment

In bacterial meningitis, intravenous antibiotics are given as soon as possible, e.g. ampicillin, chloramphenicol, benzyl penicillin, cefatoxime. When sensitivity of the organism is known, a specific antibiotic is used and continued for 14–21 days. Serial CSF examinations may help to monitor difficult cases.

Prognosis

The mortality is 8–10%. Long-term complications include deafness, epilepsy and mental retardation.

NEUROSYPHILIS

This is a rare condition. Most deaths occur from cardiovascular or neurological complications caused by the spirochaete *Treponema pallidum*. The early stages of primary infection may be followed years later by meningovascular involvement. Gummata in the brain occasionally occur and will mimic a space-occupying lesion. Tabes dorsalis and general paralysis of the insane may develop years later.

Tabes dorsalis

Tabes is due to degeneration of posterior roots of spinal nerves and posterior column of the spinal cord.

Symptoms and signs

These include lightning pain (rectal and bladder 'crises'), painless urinary retention, impotence, falling in the dark because of the loss of proprioception, Argyll Robertson pupils, bilateral ptosis, optic atrophy, high stepping, stamping gait, Romberg's test positive and patchy sensory loss to the face in a cuirasse distribution. Charcot joints develop with absent deep pain and joint position sense.

General paralysis of the insane (GPI)

GPI is caused by progressive inflammation of the brain parenchyma by the spirochaete.

Symptoms and signs

Lack of judgement, personality deterioration, grandiose ideas. Cognitive impairment, Argyll Robertson pupils, tremor of tongue (rare), limb tremor, increased reflexes with extensor plantars are also present.

Investigations

CSF and blood, VDRL, *Treponema pallidum* haemagglutination assay (TPHA), fluorescent treponemal antibody test (FTA). Lymphocytic pleocytosis is seen in most cases. The IgG/total protein ratio is raised.

Treatment

Three weeks of intramuscular penicillin. Response to treatment is measured by the number of cells and amount of protein in the CSF.

INTRACRANIAL ABSCESS

CT brain scanning has improved early diagnosis but the mortality is still 30%. Local spread of infection occurs from middle ear, mastoid, sinuses or local bone infection. Blood spread is often from a remote site such as chronic pulmonary or cyanotic congenital heart disease. Abscesses develop in areas of focal ischaemia or necrosis in grey or white matter, cerebral cortex and cerebellum. Beginning as a cerebritis with a necrotic centre, it slowly enlarges with capsule formation. If untreated, the abscess slowly expands or ruptures.

Symptoms and signs

The local infection site may be apparent, e.g. mastoid. Focal neurological symptoms may be seen. Headaches and papilloedema point to raised intracranial pressure. Focal signs are:

1. Dominant hemisphere—dysphagia, hemiparesis
2. Temporal lobe—dysphasia, quadrantanopia and epilepsy
3. Frontal lobe—disinhibition, epilepsy
4. Cerebellum—nystagmus and ataxia.

Investigations

CT and MRI scans are useful. EEG will show a focal abnormality. Lumbar puncture should be avoided because of the risk of coning.

Blood cultures, especially in haematogenous spread, are required, as are chest, skull, middle ear and mastoid X-rays.

Complications

Pus may rupture into a ventricle. Epilepsy is often difficult to control.

Differential diagnosis

Other intracranial masses and meningitis.

Treatment

Surgical drainage with instillation of antibiotics, and intravenous antibiotics, usually broad spectrum with cover for gram-negative bacteria and anaerobes.

INTRACRANIAL THROMBOPHLEBITIS

This may occur in the presence of infection but is now more common in a non-infective form. It is also seen in women on the contraceptive pill and in patients with an increased tendency to thrombosis (thrombophilia, see p. 350).

1. Cavernous sinus thrombosis may result from spread of infection from the

face or nose. It is characterised by orbital oedema and proptosis, leading to chemosis and ophthalmoplegia.
2. Thrombosis of the lateral sinus may be caused by spread of infection from the middle ear and lead to raised intracranial pressure.
3. Superior sagittal sinus thrombosis is characterised by headaches, monoparesis or hemiparesis and fits.

Investigations
1. CT brain scans may show a contrast-enhancing venous sinus.
2. MRI scans may show a venous filling failure.
3. Intravenous digital subtraction angiography shows a failure to fill affected venous sinuses.
4. CSF may show raised pressure and protein, but no cells.

Treatment is with antibiotics. Anticoagulants may be indicated. Although many patients make a good recovery, morbidity and mortality are significant.

VIRAL DISEASE OF THE CENTRAL NERVOUS SYSTEM

1. Neurotropic viruses attack certain nerve cells, e.g. poliomyelitis affects the anterior horn cell and herpes zoster the dorsal root ganglion.
2. Viruses cause inflammation of the meninges.
3. Viruses cause acute demyelinating disease with inflammation. This affects the white matter, causing an encephalitis and myelitis.
4. 'Slow' viruses are unconventional agents or 'prions'. They cause a spongiform encephalopathy, the rare Creutzfeldt–Jakob disease. This condition is transmitted in a specific way, either by the use of contaminated instrumentation or by injection or implantation of affected tissue, e.g. corneal transplant. The disease usually presents after a very long incubation period. The suggested link with bovine spongiform encephalopathy (BSE) is controversial.

Acute aseptic viral meningitis

This is a self-limiting illness with meningeal irritation and CSF pleocytosis. Most cases are viral but *Leptospira* and *Mycoplasma pneumoniae* have been reported. Non-infectious agents, such as contrast dye and fluid from CSF cysts, can cause a similar picture. The most common viruses involved are enteroviruses, coxsackie, Epstein–Barr, herpes simplex, polio, HIV and lymphocytic choriomeningitis. This condition is usually seen in children and young adults and is uncommon over the age of 50.

Symptoms and signs
These include fever, neck stiffness and headache. The CSF is clear, with a raised lymphocyte count, raised protein and sterile culture.
The duration of the illness is 1–2 weeks. The prognosis is excellent.

Differential diagnosis
Partially treated bacterial meningitis, with a low CSF cell count, epidural or

subdural abscess, tuberculous meningitis, neurosyphilis, fungal (crypto-coccal) infection, neurosarcoidosis, carcinomatous meningitis and leukaemia.

ENCEPHALITIS

Encephalitis is defined as inflammation of the surface of the brain. Encepha-litis must be distinguished from metabolic or toxic causes of stupor, fits and confusional states. Common viruses causing encephalitis include mumps, measles, varicella and influenza. Herpes simplex encephalitis is often a fatal condition characterised by haemorrhagic necrosis of the temporal lobe.

Symptoms and signs
These include headache, drowsiness, confusion, odd behaviour, focal neuro-logical signs, coma, fits and papilloedema.

Investigations
A CT brain scan shows a swollen low-density temporal lobe in herpes simplex encephalitis. The EEG is helpful, showing focal slow wave abnormality.

Specific features of herpes simplex encephalitis (HSE)

1. It is abrupt in onset.
2. There is a rapid progression but great variability in the clinical picture.
3. Seventy-five per cent have fever, personality change, headache or dysphasia.
4. Thirty per cent have fits, autonomic dysfunction, ataxia, hemiparesis.
5. The EEG is abnormal in 80%, characterised by high-voltage complexes of a periodic nature over the temporal lobe.
6. A brain biopsy of the temporal lobe is diagnostic.

Treatment
Intravenous acyclovir, if given rapidly, can improve the survival rate to 80%. If untreated, the mortality from HSE is 70%. Intravenous dexamethasone may reduce cerebral oedema.

Acute disseminated post-infectious encephalomyelitis

There is perivascular cerebral infiltration and patchy demyelination of the white matter of brain and spinal cord; this differs from acute viral encephalitis in which there is grey matter involvement and no demyelination. There are 100 cases per 100 000 population. It may complicate measles, influenza, rubella and Epstein–Barr virus infection and rarely follows vaccination for influenza, rubella, smallpox and rabies. There are encephalitic and myelitic forms and the CSF findings are the same as those in acute viral encephalitis. Early vaccination reduces the risk of this condition. Steroids may reduce complications. Mild cases may recover but morbidity and mortality are significant.

HERPES ZOSTER (SHINGLES)

There is acute inflammation of the dorsal root ganglia, with a painful vesicular eruption in the involved dermatome. Motor root involvement occurs in 15% of cases. The risk increases with advancing years. It may complicate trauma, surgery or deep X-ray therapy, and there is an increased incidence in patients with systemic illness such as pneumonia.

Symptoms and signs
1. The skin is hypersensitive and associated with painful paraesthesiae.
2. When it affects the ophthalmic division, it may produce corneal ulceration, scarring and blindness.
3. Geniculate herpes (Ramsay Hunt syndrome) is characterised by vertigo, pain in the ear, and facial palsy with a vesicular rash on the tongue, palate and external auditory canal.

Treatment
1. Herpes zoster infection is treated with aciclovir.
2. Topical preparations are available.
3. Idoxyuridine in solution can also be applied to the skin. The pain of post-herpetic neuralgia may be severe enough to warrant pethidine.

OTHER INFECTIOUS DISEASES AFFECTING THE NERVOUS SYSTEM

Poliomyelitis

Though effective vaccination has made this disease rare, it still occurs in the Third World and sporadically elsewhere. There are three types of polio virus and the incubation period is 3–21 days.

Symptoms and signs
An initial febrile illness with sore throat and headache that may be very mild. The major illness is accompanied by signs of meningism with muscle pains and flaccid paralysis of the limbs. Bulbar involvement causes dysphagia, dysphonia and instability of the blood pressure. Respiratory paralysis may be a result of diaphragmatic, intercostal or bulbar involvement.

The paralysed limbs are hypotonic, areflexic and quite characteristic of an anterior horn (lower motor neurone) lesion. There is no sensory involvement. Paralysis, though rare, is more likely if vigorous exercise has been taken at the time of the initial illness.

Investigations
1. The diagnosis is principally a clinical one.
2. Lumbar puncture shows a CSF with increased numbers of cells (early on polymorphs, then lymphocytes) together with increased protein levels.
3. The virus can be isolated from throat swabs but more successfully from the stools.

Treatment

Treatment includes analgesia for muscle pain and respiratory support if there is a reduction in regular measurements of vital capacity. Recovery from paralysis may take up to 6 months and the patient may be left with one or more wasted, weak and hypotonic limbs, as well as possibly needing long-term respiratory support. Intensive physiotherapy is required for muscle weakness.

Prophylaxis is with three doses of oral live polio vaccine. In children it is given in a sugar lump with a 6–8 week interval between the doses. A reinforcing dose is given at school entry. HIV-positive subjects may excrete the virus for longer than normal subjects and household contacts should be warned.

Tetanus

Tetanus results from infection of a wound, often trivial, with *Clostridium tetani*, a commensal in the human gastrointestinal tract also found commonly in soil. Farm and agricultural workers are especially at risk. The tetanus spores can remain dormant for years and only germinate when conditions are correct, i.e. anaerobic. Tetanus neonatorum occurs in neonates when the umbilical stump is infected.

Pathology

The organism stays locally at the site of infection but produces a neurotoxin which attacks motor nerve endings and the anterior horn cells of the spinal cord. It also attacks sympathetic nerve fibres.

Symptoms and sings

After a variable incubation period there is:

Trismus. Spasm of the masseter muscles (lockjaw) spreads to affect other facial and neck muscles (risus sardonicus). Eventually muscle spasm may affect the trunk and back, which is arched.

Violent spasms. In severe cases there may be generalised spasms occurring every few minutes. These can be provoked by disturbance or noise.

Exhaustion. The severe spasms or convulsions may exhaust the patient.

Pneumonia. Involvement of the respiratory muscles together with the convulsions leads to inhalation pneumonia.

Local tetanus. Sometimes tetanus remains localised to the area around the wound site.

Treatment

Local. An obviously infected wound should be opened and drained. Surgery should be delayed for at least 1 hour following the administration of antitoxin.

Antitoxin. Either human or equine antitoxin should be given as soon as the diagnosis is suspected (diagnosis is usually made on clinical grounds alone).

Antibiotics. Large doses of intravenous penicillin are required immediately.

Supportive. Minor spasms may be relieved by diazepam. In more severe cases curarisation and artificial ventilation are required.

Prevention. Tetanus is preventable and everyone should be immunised with toxoid vaccines. The initial course should be maintained by booster injections at 5 yearly intervals. Boosters should also be given following at-risk wounds when a long-acting penicillin is also given.

Prognosis
The neonatal form of tetanus is almost always fatal, while the local form has a good prognosis. The rate of onset and severity of convulsions determines the outcome in others. Overall mortality is 40–50%.

Botulism

This is caused by poisoning with an enterotoxin derived from *Clostridium botulinum* found in contaminated and often tinned meat or fish.

Symptoms and signs
After nausea, vomiting and diarrhoea, which develop 10–40 hours after ingestion of the contaminated food, the hallmark of the disease is the presence of severe autonomic (hypotension and dryness of the mouth and throat) and bulbar (diplopia, dysphagia and nasal regurgitation) palsy. Respiratory and limb weaknesses also occur.

Treatment
This is supportive only, and mortality, if there is bulbar involvement, is high.

INTRACRANIAL TUMOURS

Tumours of the brain may cause symptoms of a focal nature depending on their location. Raised intracranial pressure forces the brain downwards. Herniation of the medial temporal lobe occurs through the tentorium, and so the brainstem becomes compressed against the opposite free edge of the tentorium. The cerebellar tonsils are forced downwards between the foramen magnum and the medulla. Vital brainstem functions such as respiration, conscious level, blood pressure, heart rate and circulation are then impaired. Patients are treated by acute medical and surgical decompression.

The behaviour of a tumour depends on several factors:

1. histology, speed of growth and tendency to bleed
2. local invasion
3. oedema surrounding the tumour mass
4. obstruction to CSF flow leading to hydrocephalus in the posterior fossa fourth ventricular tumour

5. location: tumour on the parasagittal cortex on one side will produce weakness of the opposite leg
6. raised intracranial pressure.

PRIMARY BRAIN TUMOURS

Most primary brain tumours are malignant and do not respond to treatment. Death for most patients occurs within 2 years. In adults the primary brain tumour arises from supporting tissues not from neurones. Of primary tumours, 50% are glial in origin, 30% arise from the meninges and 20% from pituitary or ependymal tissue. Glial tumours include astrocytoma and oligodendroglioma. A glioblastoma is a poorly differentiated, highly malignant tumour (Fig. 4.10). Assessing the degree of malignancy is important. This depends on the number of mitotic figures and amount of vascular hyperplasia, necrosis, cellularity and haemorrhage. The pilocytic astrocytoma and the radiosensitive reticulum sarcoma are relatively benign tumours. Glioblastoma and oligodendrogliomas are prone to haemorrhage and may therefore be mistaken for a stroke.

Ependymomas represent 5% of primary brain tumours and develop at any site along the ependymal lining of the walls of the ventricles, even in the aqueduct and spinal cord. They spread via the ventricles and subarachnoid space in 20% of cases.

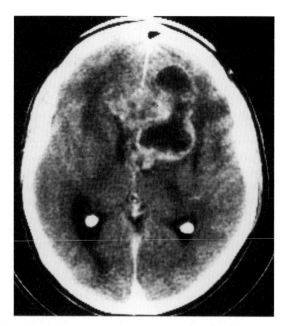

Fig. 4.10 Malignant glioma. Contrast-enhanced CT scan shows irregular enhancement with surrounding oedema involving the left frontal lobe and extending into the right hemisphere across genu of the corpus callosum.

Investigations

The diagnosis is usually confirmed by CT or MRI. Biopsy is recommended in most cases of single tumour to determine histology.

Differential diagnosis

This includes brain abscess, infarction and encephalitis.

Treatment

Treatment is surgical and by irradiation. Chemotherapy is disappointing. Dexamethasone reduces brain oedema. Primary brain lymphoma is rare but is increasing with HIV and the use of immunosuppressives. This type of tumour metastasises to the dura and is treated by radiotherapy.

CNS METASTASES

1. These represent 20% of all brain tumours (Fig. 4.11).
2. 80% are solitary with an identifiable primary; 15% are late manifestations after the primary has been successfully treated and 5% are solitary lesions with no known source.
3. The mode of spread is often haematogenous via microtumour emboli.
4. Deposits occur in proportion to the size and blood flow of various regions of the brain.
5. Lung and breast adenocarcinomas and malignant melanoma have a

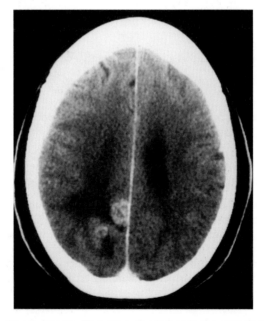

Fig. 4.11 Malignant deposits. Two enhancing lesions in the upper hemisphere and a cystic lesion with an enhancing ring in the right thalamus.

high microembolic release rate, and are prone to vascular endothelial penetration into brain tissue.

6. A biopsy may be necessary for a single lesion, and often yields an adeno-carcinoma but no indication of the primary site.

Treatment

1. Radiotherapy.
2. Intrathecal radiolabelled monoclonal antibodies for targeting radiotherapy to the tumour tissue represents an important development. This is useful in carcinomatous meningitis but less successful with solid tumours.
3. Methotrexate and cytarabine are usually of value in meningeal metastases.

MENINGIOMAS

Fifteen per cent of intracranial tumours are meningiomas. Common sites include cerebral convexity, sphenoid wing, parasagittal regions, olfactory groove, posterior fossa tentorium, cerebellopontine angle, and occasionally the sellar region.

Symptoms and signs

Patients may present with seizures from the indentation of healthy cerebral cortex. Focal sensory hallucinations are often mistaken for transient cerebral ischaemic attacks. Focal motor or dysphasic episodes are often a presenting feature in a slow-growing benign tumour.

Sometimes there are no symptoms until the tumour is very large, when it presents with raised intracranial pressure or a progressive hemiparesis.

Investigations

A CT brain scan shows a dense mass with a uniform pattern of enhancement after contrast.

Treatment

Treatment is by surgical removal if possible (sometimes the tumour is too large to remove). Recurrence is common but slow growth is measured in years.

TUMOURS IN THE SELLAR REGION (Fig. 4.12)

Acidophilic adenomas present with acromegaly, and basophilic adenomas with Cushing's disease. Microadenomas and prolactinomas are prolactin-secreting tumours which cause less obvious physical changes.

Infertility, galactorrhoea and amenorrhoea may be present. A tiny lesion, prolactinoma is sometimes difficult to detect on a CT scan even with high resolution and contrast. MRI scanning is more accurate. Serum prolactin levels are helpful.

Treatment

Treatment is with either oral bromocriptine 2.5 mg twice daily or surgical

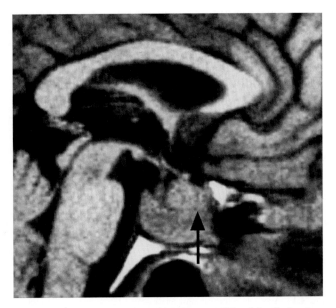

Fig. 4.12 Pituitary adenoma. Mid-sagittal MRI scan (TI weighted) showing normal midline structures. The pituitary gland is grossly expanded up into the suprasellar cistern.

removal, particularly if there are signs of compression of optic nerves. Radiotherapy may be necessary.

Chromophobe adenoma

This tumour may present as a mass with no endocrinopathy or with hypopituitarism and diabetes insipidus. CT appearances are of a high-density lesion with contrast enhancement. Fifty per cent of cases are referred because of visual failure. This is often of very gradual onset and patients are unaware of the deficit. Routine skull X-ray may show a large sella turcica.

Treatment is by surgical removal.

ACOUSTIC NEUROMAS (Fig. 4.13)

Representing 8% of all intracranial tumours, acoustic neuromas are generally unilateral but bilateral in 5%. Tumours arise from Schwann cells that envelop axons of the vestibular branch of the eighth nerve.

Symptoms and signs

Presentation is often of very gradual onset. There is progressive unilateral deafness, numbness of the ipsilateral face and an absent corneal reflex.

Mild seventh nerve weakness, brainstem compression with ataxia, weak legs and upper motor neurone signs occur. Papilloedema is a late feature.

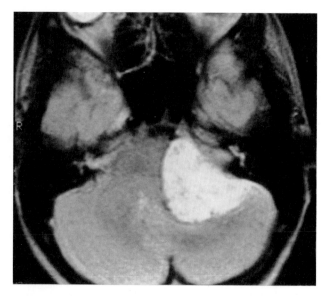

Fig. 4.13 Acoustic neuroma. An MRI scan (T2 weighted) through level of the internal auditory meati. The large high signal area in the cerebellopontine angle is a tumour.

Investigation and treatment

Brainstem auditory evoked potential monitoring is sensitive. MRI scanning is more sensitive than CT, especially for intracanalicular tumours.

Treatment is by surgical removal. Intraoperative brainstem auditory evoked potential monitoring is used to detect excessive traction on the brainstem. This has reduced morbidity to less than 3%. Care must be taken to preserve facial nerve function.

NERVE ROOT AND PLEXUS DISEASE

The peripheral nervous system is that part of the nervous system lying outside or distal to the pia arachnoid membrane. Disease of these fibres is characterised by weakness, wasting, pain, and sensory and reflex loss. Anterior horn cell diseases, including syringomyelia and motor neurone disease, also produce lower motor neurone signs. Motor and sensory nerve conduction velocities may distinguish between segmental demyelination and axonal disease. Identification of slowing of nerve conduction across two points of the nerve may point to a source of entrapment, e.g. in carpal tunnel syndrome. Concentric needle EMG is of value in nerve and muscle disease. Nerve biopsy, usually sural or superficial radial, may be of value in identifying some causes of peripheral nerve disease.

CERVICAL ROOT LESIONS

Symptoms and sings (Table 4.10)
These may manifest with pain in the arm, shoulder and neck, often in a radicular distribution or in the myotomes, with numbness and paraesthesiae in the dermatomes. Wasting and weakness occurs in a radicular distribution.

Causes are most commonly cervical spondylosis, but also the Pancoast lung tumour affecting the T1 root, herpes zoster and Guillain–Barré syndrome.

BRACHIAL PLEXUS DISEASE

The brachial plexus consists of three trunks—upper, middle and lower— comprising C5/6/7/8 T1 nerve roots. The plexus is liable to damage by trauma, tumour invasion and compression by a fibrous band or cervical rib.

1. Lower plexus. C8/T1 (medial cord) may be damaged by hyperextension

Table 4.10. Clinical features of cervical root lesions

	Segmental root
Pain	
Shoulder	C5
Lateral forearm, thumb and index finger	C6
Posterior arm	C7
Medial forearm	C8
Medial arm and hand	T1
Weak muscles	
Spinati, deltoid, rhomboid, biceps	C5
Biceps, brachioradialis, pronator, supinator, extensor carpi radialis	C6
Sternal head of pectoralis major, triceps, wrist extensors	C7
Finger flexors	C8
Intrinsic hand muscles	T1
Sensory loss to lateral upper arm	
Lateral forearm, thumb and index finger	C5 and C6
Middle finger, posterior forearm	C6 and C7
Medial forearm, little finger	C8
Inner aspect of upper arm	T1
Deep tendon reflexes affected	
Biceps	C5
Brachioradialis	C6
Triceps	C7
Finger flexors	C8
Interossei	T1

of the arm, with or without traction. A birth injury is called Klumpke's paralysis. Acquired lesions include dislocation of the shoulder, thoracic outlet syndrome (cervical rib or fibrous band) and tumour invasion. These result in paralysis of the small muscles of the hand, and painful paraesthesiae of the medial part of the forearm and hand.

2. Middle plexus. C5/6/7/8 (lateral cord) is often damaged in a motorcycle accident, with violent downward pulling on the arm which may result in paralysis of biceps, flexors of the wrist and fingers, together with sensory loss to the lateral aspects of the forearm and hand.

3. Upper plexus. C5/6/7 (posterior cord) damage causes a Duchenne-Erb's paralysis, an unusual paralysis of deltoid, triceps, brachioradialis and extensor muscles of wrist and fingers. The patient has a 'waiter tip' posture.

NEURALGIC AMYOTROPHY

This is an acute syndrome of excruciating pain in the shoulder or arm, which when resolved is followed by rapid-onset focal weakness and wasting, not always of a specific root or peripheral nerve type.

It often follows infection, inoculation, trauma or surgery and is the result of acute inflammation of the nerve roots, plexus or its branches. Patients slowly recover, but weakness may persist for months.

THORACIC OUTLET SYNDROME

This is produced by pressure on the medial cord of the brachial plexus, often by a cervical rib or fibrous band. Features include pain in the inner aspect of the arm, after carrying heavy weights, and weakness of the small muscles of the hand and sensory loss in a C8/T1 distribution. There may be a supraclavicular bruit and thrill and obliteration of the radial pulse on arm hyperabduction.

A chest X-ray may show a cervical rib but not a fibrous band or thickened scalenus anticus muscle. A subclavian arteriogram may show kinking or compression of the subclavian artery. Differential diagnosis includes carpal tunnel syndrome and cervical spondylitic radiculopathy.

Treatment is surgical.

CAUDA EQUINA LESIONS

Common causes include fracture dislocation of the vertebra, tumour, arteriovenous malformation and prolapsed intervertebral disc. Posterolateral protrusion affects one root only; central disc lesions may affect several roots.

Symptoms and signs

There is neurogenic claudication, i.e. pain and foot drop worsening on walking.

Reduction in straight leg raising, weak muscles, depressed deep tendon reflexes and sensory impairment depend on which roots are involved. There is urinary retention with bladder distension and incontinence, loss of anal reflex, impotence, and numb legs and buttocks.

Investigations and treatment

Plain X-rays of lumbar sacral spine, CT radiculogram and an MRI scan are useful.

Early surgical decompression is mandatory if bladder function is involved. Single nerve root disease with pain and paraesthesiae may respond to traction. Bedrest on hard boards may help. Surgery may be required if there is wasting and weakness, or central disc protrusion.

PERIPHERAL NEUROPATHY

The following types are recognised:

1. acute Guillain—Barré syndrome
2. subacute or chronic distal neuropathy, which can be motor, sensory, autonomic or mixed
3. mononeuropathies
   (a) entrapment type
   (b) non-compressive mononeuritis multiplex as seen in diabetes mellitus, polyarteritis nodosa, carcinoma and amyloidosis.

Pathology

1. Acute infective allergic process e.g. Guillain–Barré syndrome.
2. Occlusion of the vasa nervorum with focal infarction of the nerve, e.g. polyarteritis nodosa.
3. Amyloid infiltration.
4. Segmental demyelination, such as in diabetes and diphtheria.
5. Peripheral dying back phenomenon, as in hereditary neuropathy.

ACUTE GUILLAIN–BARRÉ SYNDROME (GBS)

This acute demyelinating neuropathy accounts for 40% of all adult neuropathies. It is multifocal and proximal, and appears to be caused by an immune response directed against a component of myelin in the peripheral nerve. The decreased suppressive T cell response in GBS is consistent with a cell-mediated immune response. There may also be humoral antigen, although the basis for this is unknown. It is the rationale behind plasma exchange treatment. A non-specific viral infection precedes the onset of neurological symptoms by 2–4 weeks in 50% of cases.

Symptoms and signs

Weakness spreads upwards from the legs. Involvement is diffuse, symmetrical, and usually reaches maximal effect within 4 weeks. There is mild distal paraesthesiae, back muscular pain in 50% of cases and dysphagia.

Areflexia, proximal weakness, and later total paralysis are seen. Asymmetrical facial weakness occurs in 50% of cases. Other cranial nerve motor weakness gives rise to dysphagia, dysarthria and a weak cough.

Respiratory weakness occurs and is sometimes not easily detected because of facial involvement. Serial lung function measurements are essential.

Autonomic signs appear in 70% of cases. Sympathetic features include orthostatic hypotension even when sitting, transient bladder paralysis and tachycardia. Parasympathetic features are generalised warmth, bradycardia and the inappropriate ADH syndrome.

Investigations
There is a raised CSF protein yet no increase in the number of white cells. Nerve conduction studies may be normal or show slow conduction velocity and block with increase in distal latency.

Treatment and prognosis
All patients should be admitted to hospital because respiratory failure may occur at any stage during the illness. Some patients need artificial ventilation.

The major causes of a 13% mortality are pulmonary embolism, autonomic dysfunction and overwhelming infection.

The illness is usually complete within 3–6 months but intravenous gamma-globulin or plasmapheresis within the first 2 weeks may accelerate recovery. Five per cent are left with some disability and 10% experience relapses.

SUBACUTE AND CHRONIC NEUROPATHIES

The picture is motor, sensory, autonomic or mixed. In most cases the feet are more severely affected than the hands. Although in 50–60% no cause can be identified, it does occur with diabetes mellitus, toxins (N-hexane), drugs (amiodarone) and alcohol, carcinoma (often occult) or vasculitis (SLE or polyarteritis), vitamin deficiency, e.g. B_{12}, and hereditary Charcot-Marie-Tooth disease.

Symptoms and signs
There is slowly progressive sensory loss, with numbness and tingling in the feet and hands. The fingers are clumsy and the feet often catch the ground.

Wasting of distal muscles occurs with areflexia (sensory neuropathies may have intact deep tendon reflexes). A glove and stocking distribution of sensory loss is found.

Perforating skin ulcers, neuropathic joints and foot deformities occur.

Investigations
1. Drug, alcohol, occupational, social and family history.
2. Blood sugar, vitamin B_{12} level, porphyrins, paraproteins.
3. Chest X-ray.
4. Nerve conduction studies, EMGs.
5. CSF. If CSF protein is high, there may be inflammatory demyelinating neuropathy which can respond to steroids or plasma exchange.

Treatment
1. Depends on underlying cause.

2. Vitamin B_{12} injections, tight control of diabetes, removal of tumour.
3. Symptomatic treatment: below-the-knee orthotic splints.

Prognosis
Toxic neuropathies will improve when the cause is removed. Hereditary neuropathies will slowly progress but rarely shorten lifespan.

ENTRAPMENT MONONEUROPATHY

Incomplete injury to the peripheral nerve where the nerve is macroscopically intact is common in compressive neuropathy. In initial stages the patient may only complain of numbness and paraesthesia, but when the syndrome is well developed a fixed sensory loss and muscle atrophy may be present and treatment is unlikely to result in complete recovery. Early diagnosis is therefore important.

Features of upper and lower limb peripheral nerve lesions are shown in Tables 4.11 and 4.12.

CARPAL TUNNEL SYNDROME

This is caused by compression of the median nerve at the wrist. Features include tingling, numbness and pain in the tips of the thumb, index and middle fingers which may waken the patient at night. Less commonly there will be weakness of the abductor pollicis brevis.

The syndrome is most common in females in their fifties. There is an increased frequency of the syndrome with hypothyroidism, acromegaly, the contraceptive pill, pregnancy and rheumatoid arthritis.

Table 4.11. Peripheral nerve lesions—arm

Nerve	Weakness	Sensory loss
Axillary/circumflex	Deltoid	Patchy over deltoid
Long thoracic	Serratus anterior—winged scapula	None
Musculocutaneous	Biceps (and absent jerk)	Lateral forearm
Radial spiral groove of humerus (upper arm)	Brachio-radialis (and absent tendon jerk) wrist extensors, finger extensors, supinator and forearm plus triceps muscle (and absent tendon jerk) for a high lesion	Back of hand at base of thumb
Median at wrist	Thenar eminence (abductor pollicis brevis)	Radial 3½ fingers
Ulnar at elbow	Flexor digitorum profundus (4/5, fingers), lumbricals (4/5), interossei, and hypothenar eminence.	Ulnar 1½ fingers

Table 4.12. Peripheral nerve lesions—leg

Nerve	Weakness	Sensory loss	Affected tendon reflex
Femoral	Quadriceps— iliopsoas (in a proximal lesion)	Anterior thigh, medial shin	Knee jerk
Lateral cutaneous nerve of thigh	None	Anterior and lateral thigh	None
Obturator (rare)	Adductors of hip	Medial thigh	—
Common peroneal (lateral popliteal)	Dorsiflexors and eversion of foot = foot drop	Lateral shin, dorsum of foot	None
Posterior tibial	Plantar flexion of foot	Sole of foot	Ankle jerk
Sciatic	Hip extension abduction and knee flexion	Lateral shin, sole, rear of calf	Ankle jerk

There is reduced pinprick and light touch in the tips of the radial 2½ fingers and thumb with later wasting and weakness of the thenar muscles.

Treatment
Immediate relief of pain may be achieved by injecting steroids into the carpal tunnel and by wearing a night splint. Definitive treatment is section of the transverse carpal ligament.

ULNAR NERVE COMPRESSION

Repetitive minor injuries (often not reported by the patient) to the medial epicondyl region may result in localised slowing of ulnar nerve conduction across the elbow. This will ultimately result in progressive wasting of all small muscles of the hand except the thenar group. Sensory loss involves the fifth and ulnar half of the fourth finger.

Treatment consists of transposition of the ulnar nerve from the cubital tunnel to the anterior aspect of the arm.

LATERAL CUTANEOUS NERVE OF THE THIGH

This may be compressed by the inguinal ligament, usually in overweight people, producing the syndrome of meralgia paraesthetica. There is burning pain experienced over the anterolateral aspect of the thigh. Weight loss is required and, sometimes, local steroid injection or, rarely, section of the nerve.

COMMON PERONEAL NERVE

It may be compressed at the head of the fibula from too tight a plaster cast.

Sitting cross-legged for long periods may also result in weakness of dorsiflexion and eversion of the foot. The pattern of sensory loss involves the lateral aspect of the leg, dorsum, and lateral aspect of the foot.

POSTERIOR TIBIAL NERVE

Entrapment at the transverse intertarsal ligament in the ankle produces pain and paraesthesiae in the toes and ball of the foot. These symptoms are often worse on walking. Treatment is by avoiding the precipitating cause, weight loss or surgical release of the transverse intertarsal ligament.

DISEASE OF THE NEUROMUSCULAR JUNCTION

MYASTHENIA GRAVIS

Myasthenia gravis (MG) is an autoimmune disease characterised by fluctuating fatigueable weakness caused by a defect in neuromuscular transmission. It is often associated with other autoimmune disease, such as pernicious anaemia, hypothyroidism and rheumatoid arthritis. Although the cause is unknown, an autoimmune response may be centred on the thymus with production of antibodies directed against striated muscle acetylcholine receptors. The antiacetylcholine antibody is positive in 95% of patients. The condition is associated with thymic hyperplasia in 70% of cases, thymic tumour in 15% and atrophy in the remainder.

Penicillamine may induce a temporary autoimmune myasthenia, with high antibody titres.

Symptoms and signs
The disease affects mainly adults. The purely ocular form is seen in 20% of patients and is more benign, with lower titres of antiacetylcholine receptor antibodies. Transient neonatal MG affects the offspring in 11% of affected mothers. It is a temporary condition, disappearing within 4–6 weeks of birth.

There is diplopia, dysarthria, dysphagia, weakness of mastication and of the facial and proximal limb muscles.

Diagnosis is by a positive intravenous edrophonium chloride 'tensilon' test or repetitive nerve stimulation studies demonstrating a decremental muscle response.

Treatment
Treatment is with the long-acting anticholinesterase drug, pyridostigmine. The shorter-acting neostigmine can aid swallowing. Alternate-day prednisolone and immunosuppressive drugs such as azathioprine and cyclophosphamide may be required in severely affected patients.

Thymectomy is of benefit, particularly in young females, and is mandatory in all patients with thymoma.

Intravenous gammaglobulin and plasmapheresis may be particularly helpful.

MUSCLE DISEASES

Features of the inherited dystrophies are shown in Table 4.13. Muscle diseases are often classified by the affected muscle group, e.g. facioscapulo-humeral dystrophy. Metabolic disorders of muscles are rare and include McArdle's disease (myophosphorylase deficiency), periodic paralysis (hypo-normo- or hyperkalaemic), glycogen storage disorders, lipid myopathies and mitochondrial defects. Myotonia or a failure of muscle relaxation may accompany certain disorders, such as dystrophia myotonica.

DUCHENNE MUSCULAR DYSTROPHY (DMD)

This is an inherited sex-linked recessive disorder affecting males. The female offspring are carriers. There is a milder variant (Becker's muscular dystrophy). Prenatal diagnosis has been greatly improved by the availability of DNA markers for the DMD gene. The disease has the following features:

1. The onset of DMD is often before 4 and always under 10 years.
2. Walking is delayed in half the patients, and they present with clumsiness and frequent falls.
3. Signs include a waddling gait, and positive Gower's sign, characterised

Table 4.13. Inherited muscular dystrophy

Type	Inheritance	Onset	Progress	Muscles affected	Serum CPK level
Duchenne (DMD) and the milder Becker's form	Sex-linked recessive; males affected, 30% spontaneous mutation rate	Early childhood < 4 years	Rapid In wheel-chair by age 10, dead by age 20	Pelvic, pectoral girdle, myocardium	Very high, 10–20 000 iu/l
Limb girdle	Autosomal recessive	Variable Age 20–30 years	Variable slow progression	Pelvic, pectoral girdle	Slightly elevated, may be high
Facioscapulo-humeral	Autosomal dominant	Variable Age 10–20 years	Variable, severe within 20 years of onset	Facial, scapular, humeral, pelvic girdle	Elevated or normal
Dystrophia myotonica (myotonia congenita, rare, no wasting)	Autosomal dominant	Variable Age 20–60 years	Most patients unable to walk 20 years after onset	Facial, sternomastoid, distal limbs	Normal

by the patient climbing up his own legs from a seated position on the floor.

4. Proximal limb weakness and pseudohypertrophy of the calves are common.

5. Cranial nerve muscles and bladder function are spared.

6. When confined to a wheelchair, these boys often develop kyphoscoliosis and hip and knee contractures. Reduced lung function then follows.

7. Most patients die before the age of 20 years.

8. The ECG is abnormal in 60% but clinical cardiac involvement is rare.

Investigations

The serum creatine phosphokinase (CPK) is very high. Concentric needle EMGs show a myopathic pattern. Muscle biopsy shows a typical pattern with increased internal nuclei and variation of fibre size in the early stages, leading to fibrosis and fat replacement in severely affected muscles.

Treatment

There is no cure but treatment is with passive muscle stretching and spinal supports. It is important to keep weight down. Genetic counselling is essential.

5

ENDOCRINOLOGY

Roger Corrall

THE PITUITARY

ANTERIOR PITUITARY

Control of anterior pituitary function is via hypothalamic hormones released into the hypophyseal portal system. The activity of hypothalamic and pituitary cells is affected by circulating levels of the relevant hormone by negative and sometimes positive feedback. Many of the hypothalamic hormones, or synthetic analogues, are used in clinical practice.

POSTERIOR PITUITARY

Hormones are synthesised in hypothalamic neurones and are transferred along axons to the posterior lobe where they are secreted into the circulation (neurosecretion).

PITUITARY TUMOURS

Endocrinologically active tumours of the anterior pituitary may be derived from any of the hormone-secreting cells and are classified according to the hormone(s) secreted.

Effects of pituitary tumours

Pituitary tumours may cause endocrine and local pressure effects. The most common pressure effects are headaches and visual field defects, the latter from upward extension of the tumour affecting the optic chiasma, classically causing a bitemporal hemianopia.

The bony margin of the pituitary fossa can be seen on skull radiology but this gives no indication of pituitary anatomy. This can be demonstrated by either a CT or, better, MRI scan, which shows suprasellar extensions and may outline microadenomas.

HYPERSECRETION

Prolactin: hyperprolactinaemia

Hyperprolactinaemia is common. It is much more frequent in women than in men and causes 10–15% of all secondary amenorrhoea in gynaecological clinics. The main causes are pregnancy, prolactinomas, hypothalamus/pituitary stalk lesions, primary hypothyroidism, chronic renal failure and the use of dopamine antagonists such as phenothiazines.

Symptoms and signs

Amenorrhoea, infertility, oestrogen deficiency and galactorrhoea are seen in women. Rarely, impotence is seen in men.

Investigations

Diagnosis is by detection of a raised serum prolactin on at least two occasions. Pregnancy must be excluded, a drug history taken and serum thyroid function tests performed. Many prolactinomas are too small to be seen on plain X-ray of the skull (microadenoma) but are detected on a CT or MRI scan.

Differential diagnosis

The normal serum prolactin level is up to approximately 700 mU/l. Even higher levels in normally menstruating women are unlikely to be significant. Levels above 5000 mU/l usually indicate a prolactinoma. In women with a lesser degree of hyperprolactinaemia, a prolactinoma must be distinguished from a lesion affecting the hypothalamus or pituitary stalk, e.g. other tumour that induces hyperprolactinaemia by depleting the pituitary of dopamine, the inhibitory controller of prolactin secretion.

Treatment

Dopamine agonist treatment, usually with bromocriptine, is very effective, reduces prolactin levels to normal and relieves symptoms. During a subsequent pregnancy there is a risk of prolactinoma enlarging, rarely causing a visual field defect. A major long-term indication for treatment is prevention of osteoporosis, by restoration of ovarian function, which necessitates contraception. Because dopamine agonist treatment also reduces the size of prolactinomas, they can usually be treated with long-term bromocriptine, and surgery or pituitary irradiation is not often needed.

Growth hormone (GH): acromegaly/gigantism

This is uncommon, with physical and biochemical changes arising from excessive GH secretion, almost always from an anterior pituitary tumour.

Symptoms and signs (see Table 5.1, Fig. 5.1)

Investigations

Diagnosis is predominantly clinical and is confirmed biochemically by measuring serum GH levels during an oral glucose tolerance test when,

Table 5.1. Symptoms and signs of acromegaly

Symptoms	Signs
Change in facial appearance	Acromegalic facies
Enlargement of hands and feet	Large extremities
Paraesthesiae of hands	Carpal tunnel syndrome
Sweating	Greasy, sweaty skin
Headaches	Prognathism (protrusion lower jaw)
Joint pains	Osteoarthrosis
Diabetes mellitus	Hypertension
Gigantism in children (before fusion epiphyses)	

because of the suppressive effect of hyperglycaemia, the level normally falls to < 5 mU/l. In acromegaly, owing to autonomous secretion of GH by the underlying tumour, normal suppression is not seen and GH levels may even rise paradoxically. A CT or MRI scan of the pituitary demonstrates the tumour. The classical syndrome is readily recognised, but may be overlooked because of its slow progression; comparison with old photographs is invaluable.

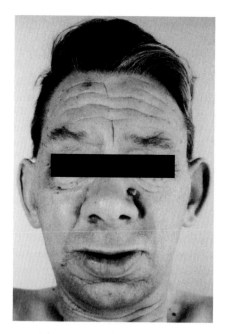

Fig. 5.1 Facial features of acromegaly showing soft-tissue enlargement and coarse skin.

Treatment

This is usually surgical, using the trans-sphenoidal route, when relatively small tumours may be excised, leaving normal pituitary function intact. Otherwise subsequent ablative treatment with pituitary irradiation may be required. Medical treatment with bromocriptine can also be used in a minority sensitive to dopamine agonists. In addition there is now an analogue of somatostatin available, given by subcutaneous injection, which reduces GH levels.

Adrenocorticotrophic hormone (ACTH): Cushing's syndrome
(See p. 179)

Follicle stimulating hormone/luteinising hormone (FSH/LH): Sexual precocity

Sexual precocity occurs when changes of puberty are seen in girls and boys before the ages of 8 and 9 respectively. It may arise from an organic lesion, such as a pinealoma affecting the hypothalamus, or, more often in girls than boys, as a functional disorder.

Symptoms and signs
The precocious puberty commonly causes associated psychological problems.

The signs are those of precocious puberty and disordered growth. The premature secretion of gonadal steroids results in early excessive growth but ultimate shortness from fusion of the epiphyses.

Investigations
Serum gonadotrophin levels are raised and a CT or MRI scan of the hypothalamus/pituitary may detect an underlying tumour.

Differential diagnosis
The condition must be distinguished from sexual precocity caused by congenital adrenal hyperplasia and gonadal hormone secreting tumours.

Treatment
Treatment is of the underlying condition, if possible, or by subcutaneous injection of an LHRH analogue that inhibits FSH and LH secretion. Resolution of the endocrine syndrome and reduction in the excessive rate of growth results.

Vasopressin: Syndrome of inappropriate antidiuretic hormone secretion

Although tumours of the posterior pituitary do not occur, inappropriate secretion of vasopressin is common and found in many conditions such as primary hypothyroidism, pneumonia and head injury. In addition, some malignant tumours, in particular small cell carcinomas of the bronchus, secrete vasopressin ectopically. Inappropriate secretion of vasopressin results in water retention and, eventually, the syndrome of water intoxication, the clinical features of which depend upon the severity and rapidity of onset.

Symptoms and signs
The patient may have headaches and progress to fits, drowsiness and, ultimately, coma and death. Peripheral oedema is not seen.

Investigations
Diagnosis is based on finding hyponatraemia with normal or low levels of serum urea and creatinine. Urine osmolality is inappropriately high compared with plasma.

Differential diagnosis
The serum biochemical findings must be distinguished from those of depletional hyponatraemia, resulting from sodium deficiency, in which hyponatraemia is associated with impairment of renal function because of the depletion of extracellular fluid volume.

Treatment
Treatment is with fluid restriction to 500–1000 ml per 24 hours when the serum sodium level gradually rises. Rarely, emergency treatment is needed, for instance because of fits, in which case hypertonic saline (3 or 5%) is given. This may precipitate heart failure, and too rapid correction can also cause the rare, but fatal, neurological condition of central pontine myelinolysis.

HYPOSECRETION

Non-selective

Non-selective hypopituitarism is usually caused by a pituitary tumour or its treatment. Other causes include pituitary infarction, which occurs particularly post-partum (Sheehan's syndrome), and granulomas.

Symptoms and signs
These depend on the extent of pituitary hormone deficiency. Thus, deficiency of GH in a child results in shortness, of gonadotrophins in hypogonadism, of ACTH in glucocorticoid deficiency, of thyroid stimulating hormone (TSH) in (secondary) hypothyroidism and of vasopressin in diabetes insipidus.

Investigations
Serum GH levels during a stimulation test, serum gonadotrophins, thyroid function tests and serum cortisol, usually also during a stimulation test, may need to be measured. A CT or MRI scan of the pituitary is usually indicated.

Differential diagnosis
Secretion of gonadotrophins and GH is almost always impaired before that of TSH and ACTH. Thus, preservation of normal gonadotrophin secretion as indicated by persistent menstruation or the normal post-menopausal

elevation of gonadotrophins in a woman, and normal potency and serum testosterone in a man, virtually excludes significant hypopituitarism.

Treatment

Treatment depends upon the age of the patient and extent of hypopituitarism. Patients with panhypopituitarism require full replacement therapy with thyroxine, glucocorticoids, GH (for children and some adults) and desmopressin for diabetes insipidus. Thyroxine should not usually be given without glucocorticoid as TSH and ACTH deficiency commonly occur together and thyroxine treatment alone may precipitate an adrenal crisis. Men are treated with androgens and women, at least until the age of 50, with oestrogens, both for their immediate effects and the long-term prevention of osteoporosis. Infertility can be treated with injections of gonadotrophins.

Growth hormone: Shortness

This may occur as an isolated idiopathic defect or from an organic lesion such as a craniopharyngioma.

Symptoms and signs

The child is markedly short, usually more than 2.5 standard deviations below the mean, and is usually chubby as GH has a lipolytic effect.

Investigations

Subnormal GH levels are found during one or more stimulation tests, of which the most definitive is insulin-induced hypoglycaemia.

Differential diagnosis

See section on Growth (p. 191).

Treatment

Growth can be restored with subcutaneous injections of human GH which is manufactured by recombinant DNA technology. This has replaced material extracted from human pituitaries, which has been responsible for cases of Creutzfeldt–Jakob disease.

ACTH

ACTH deficiency occurs rarely as an isolated defect, and more commonly from long-term treatment with glucocorticoids or ACTH.

FSH/LH: HYPOGONADOTROPHIC HYPOGONADISM

Gonadotrophin deficiency occurs as a manifestation of hypopituitarism, e.g. secondary to craniopharyngioma, or as an isolated hypothalamic defect. The latter is more common in boys than in girls and may be associated with other congenital disorders, including anosmia in Kallmann's syndrome.

Investigations
Serum gonadotrophin levels are measured and a skull X-ray and CT or MRI scan may be performed.

Differential diagnosis
Isolated gonadotrophin deficiency must be distinguished from constitutional delayed puberty; this may only be possible after a period of follow-up.

Treatment
Treatment is with androgens or oestrogens but, when inducing puberty, it is very important that the dosage is kept low to avoid premature maturation and fusion of the epiphyses and shortening of ultimate height.

Vasopressin: Diabetes insipidus

Diabetes insipidus is caused either by a lesion of the posterior pituitary and pituitary stalk leading to vasopressin deficiency (cranial diabetes insipidus), or by resistance to the action of vasopressin on the renal tubules (nephrogenic diabetes insipidus) as in hypercalcaemia, hypokalaemia, the action of certain drugs, e.g. lithium, and in a rare sex-linked congenital abnormality. The deficiency of, or resistance to, vasopressin results in failure to concentrate urine.

Symptoms and signs
Thirst is the predominant symptom, with polyuria of > 3 litres per 24 hours. If the subject is unable to maintain an adequate fluid intake (e.g. after a head injury) there is the risk of rapid and profound water depletion.

There are usually no signs unless the patient becomes fluid depleted.

Investigations
Urine volume should be measured and plasma electrolytes and serum calcium levels determined. To confirm the diagnosis, a fluid deprivation test should be performed in which fluid intake is stopped, usually for up to 8 hours, and bodyweight, plasma and urine osmolality serially measured.

Differential diagnosis
Polyuria needs to be distinguished from frequency of micturition. The most difficult differential diagnosis is from compulsive water drinking, which is not uncommon and does not necessarily indicate a serious underlying psychiatric disorder.

Treatment
Treatment is with desmopressin, a synthetic long-acting analogue of vasopressin. It is given intranasally, usually twice daily.

THE THYROID

The thyroid gland synthesises thyroxine (T4) and tri-iodothyronine (T3), and also calcitonin in the C cells. Control of thyroid hormone production is by TSH, the secretion of which is stimulated by TRH from the hypothalamus. Circulating levels of thyroid hormones exert a negative feedback effect upon the hypothalamus and anterior pituitary.

Synthesis of the thyroid hormones begins with the trapping of iodide from blood and ends with the release of T4 and T3 into thyroid capillaries. Over 99% of T4 and T3 circulate bound to plasma proteins, particularly thyroxine binding globulin (TBG), and it is the free concentrations that determine the thyroid state of the individual.

HYPERFUNCTION: THYROTOXICOSIS, HYPERTHYROIDISM

Thyrotoxicosis has a prevalence in the UK of 1.1% for established cases and 1.6% with the inclusion of possible cases. It is commonly due to Graves' disease, an autoimmune condition in which thyroid overactivity is caused by circulating thyroid-stimulating immunoglobulins that bind to and activate the TSH receptor. Graves' disease occurs in association with other organ-specific autoimmune diseases such as Addison's disease, diabetes mellitus and pernicious anaemia.

Autonomous oversecretion by one or more thyroid nodules, associated with suppression of the activity of the rest of the gland, underlies thyrotoxicosis of the elderly. Transient thyrotoxicosis occurs in thyroiditis—either autoimmune or subacute viral (de Quervain's)—caused by the release of preformed thyroid hormone from the inflamed gland.

Symptoms and signs

The effects of excessive thyroid hormone secretion are listed in Table 5.2

Table 5.2. Symptoms and signs of excessive thyroid hormone secretion

	Symptoms	Signs
General	Loss of weight (despite good appetite) Heat intolerance Increased sweating	Evidence of weight loss Warm, moist skin
Cardiovascular system	Shortness of breath Palpitations	Tachycardia Peripheral vasodilatation Increased pulse pressure Atrial fibrillation } Particularly in Cardiac failure } the elderly
Muscles	Weakness	Muscle weakness and wasting (thyrotoxic myopathy)
Nervous system	Anxiety state Irritability	Fine tremor Brisk tendon jerks
Gastrointestinal system	Diarrhoea	
Eyes	Staring appearance	Lid retraction, lid lag

Usually, but not always, a goitre which is diffuse in Graves' disease and nodular in the elderly is palpable.

Ophthalmopathy

Ophthalmopathy (Fig. 5.2) is characteristic of patients with Graves' disease and is also autommune in origin. It is not necessarily associated with thyrotoxicosis and can occur in patients who are euthyroid and, rarely, hypothyroid. The external ocular muscles are grossly hypertrophied and the orbital contents increased from oedema, fat, connective tissue, inflammatory cells and mucopolysaccharide deposition. It comprises one or more of the following features:

1. *Exophthalmos (protrusion)*. This is occasionally unilateral and then may be confused with an intraorbital tumour.
2. *Impaired eye movement (ophthalmoplegia)*. Upward gaze is affected most often from tethering of the inferior recti.
3. *Periorbital oedema*.
4. *Oedema of the conjunctiva (chemosis)*.

Rarely, the eye involvement causes visual impairment from corneal ulceration (with severe exophthalmos) or from pressure on the optic nerve.

Pretibial myxoedema. This occurs in up to 5% of patients with Graves' disease. It is an infiltration with a mucopolysaccharide which characteristially affects the front of the shins, sometimes asymmetrically, causing redness, thickening and puckering of the skin.

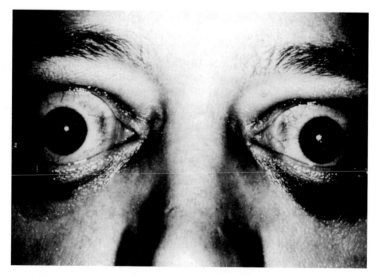

Fig. 5.2 Eye appearances in Graves' disease showing marked exophthalmos and lid retraction.

Investigations

There is raised serum free T3 and suppressed serum TSH.

Differential diagnosis

The diagnosis of thyrotoxicosis is essentially clinical. However, particularly in the elderly, the clinical features may be occult with non-specific symptoms such as weight loss and cardiac arrhythmias. The condition may be difficult to distinguish from an anxiety state and, indeed, the two conditions may coexist.

Treatment

Medical. Antithyroid drugs block the synthesis of thyroid hormone and will relieve the symptoms while they are taken. Persistent thyrotoxicosis is likely to be caused by inadequate dosage or lack of compliance with drug taking.

Carbimazole is the most commonly used drug. It is given in an initial dosage of 10–20 mg 12 hourly until the patient is euthyroid, which usually takes 4–8 weeks. On attaining a euthyroid state, T4 may be added (100–200 µg daily) and adjusted in accordance with thyroid function tests. Carbimazole is usually well tolerated, but may cause rashes and/or scalp hair loss, in which case propylthiouracil can be substituted. Both drugs very rarely cause agranulocytosis which appears to be an idiosyncrasy. Treatment is maintained for 12–18 months. However, relapse occurs in 50% and cannot be predicted. The best results are seen in young women with small goitres.

Non-selective beta-blockers are sometimes also used in the initial treatment of thyrotoxicosis as they relieve some of the symptoms, such as anxiety and palpitations, although they have no effect upon thyroid hormone secretion.

Radioiodine. The radioisotope ^{131}I, administered in a drink of water, is very effective and will cure the condition in approximately 75% of patients after a single dose. If thyrotoxicosis persists, one or more further doses are given as necessary, after an interval of at least 3 months. The treatment must not be given to pregnant mothers as ^{131}I crosses the placenta, and is best avoided in children. Its use was formerly restricted to those over the age of 40 to avoid unnecessary radiation of the gonads in childbearing years, but it is now considered a first-line treatment for all adults. The main disadvantage of ^{131}I therapy is the high incidence of subsequent hypothyroidism: 15% in the first year and 3% per year thereafter. It is essential therefore that patients are aware of this risk.

Surgery. Surgery is by partial thyroidectomy, which relieves the condition in more than 90% of patients and has a low incidence of relapse. There is a small risk of serious complications, such as damage to the recurrent laryngeal nerve and hypoparathyroidism. Hypothyroidism also occurs but the incidence is probably lower than that with radioiodine. It is essential that patients are euthyroid prior to surgery; initial treatment with antithyroid drugs is required.

The advantages and disadvantages of each form of treatment must be discussed with the patient. Radioiodine is being used more as first-line treatment for adults, but it is common in young adults to use antithyroid drugs first, and then either radioiodine or surgery if there is subsequent relapse.

Ophthalmopathy

The symptoms and signs of ophthalmopathy are difficult to treat but, fortunately, gradual improvement may occur after months or years.

Associated thyrotoxicosis should be treated and hypothyroidism avoided as this can worsen the condition. Watering and discomfort may respond to hypromellose eyedrops and diuretics. Active symptomatic thyroid eye disease may require orbital radiotherapy and immunosuppression. Rarely, operative orbital decompression is merited for threatened optic nerve function. Surgery to external ocular muscles may be indicated for severe diplopia.

Thyrotoxic crisis

Rapid clinical deterioration of thyrotoxicosis occurs with florid clinical signs, e.g. marked tachycardia, tremor, pyrexia. There is usually some precipitating event such as infection, surgery or intercurrent illness.

This is a rare medical emergency with a significant mortality. Urgent treatment is with beta-blockers, carbimazole and potassium iodide.

HYPOFUNCTION: HYPOTHYROIDISM, MYXOEDEMA

Hypothyroidism, like thyrotoxicosis, is common. Causes of the condition are shown in Table 5.3.

Primary hypothyroidism is the most common type. Globally the major cause is iodine deficiency, but in industrialised countries it is autoimmune thyroiditis and secondary to the treatment of thyrotoxicosis.

Symptoms and signs

Hypothyroidism can cause many different clinical features (Table 5.4) and thus presents in several different ways. In addition, there may be a goitre depending upon the cause. Hypothyroidism induces (secondary) hyperlipoproteinaemia with an increased incidence of ischaemic heart disease.

Table 5.3. Causes of hypothyroidism

Primary	Iodine deficiency
	Autoimmune thyroiditis (Hashimoto's disease)
	'Idiopathic atrophy' (end stage of autoimmune destruction)
	Iatrogenic: antithyroid drugs, radioiodine, surgery
	Drugs (e.g. lithium, amiodarone)
	Congenital enzyme defect
	Failure of development (cretinism)
Secondary (pituitary disease causing TSH deficiency)	
	Hypopituitarism
	Isolated TSH deficiency (rare)

Table 5.4. Symptoms and signs of hypothyroidism

	Symptoms	Signs
General	Cold intolerance Weight gain	Dry, coarse skin and hair Pallor
From myxoedematous infiltration of tissues	Change in appearance Hoarseness of voice Paraesthesiae of hands	Puffiness of face and extremities Involvement of larynx Carpal tunnel syndrome
Cardiovascular system	Angina of effort	Bradycardia Evidence of IHD Pericardial effusion
Muscles	Generalised aches	Stiff swollen muscles
Nervous system	'Slowing up' Poor memory Unsteadiness Sometimes frank psychosis	Slowness of speech and thought Delayed relaxation tendon jerks Cerebellar ataxia 'Myxoedema madness'
Gastrointestinal system	Constipation	Abdominal distension Paralytic ileus (rare) Ascites (rare)
Children	Retardation of growth	Shortness
Infants	Mental deficiency (if treatment delayed)	Cretinism

Investigations

The biochemical hallmark of primary hypothyroidism is a raised serum TSH, absence of which excludes the diagnosis. A raised serum TSH and normal serum T4 indicates subclinical hypothyroidism and an increased risk of developing frank hypothyroidism. In secondary hypothyroidism a low serum T4 is usually associated with a low or paradoxically normal TSH level.

Differential diagnosis

Typically the onset is gradual and the changes may be missed by those who see the patient frequently. The diagnosis must be considered in patients presenting with such diverse symptoms as weight gain, angina and rheumatic pains.

Treatment

Treatment is with T4, which is cheap and stable. In middle-aged and elderly patients it is important to begin with a small dose of 25–50 µg per 24 hours to avoid exacerbating, or precipitating, underlying ischaemic heart disease. The usual maintenance dose varies within 50–200 µg per 24 hours and is determined not only clinically but by levels of serum TSH which should be neither suppressed, which indicates overtreatment, nor elevated, indicating undertreatment.

Table 5.5. Causes of goitre

Bilateral	Unilateral
Iodine deficiency	Solitary palpable nodule in a multinodular goitre
Multinodular goitre (MNG)	
Graves' disease	Thyroid adenoma
Autoimmune thyroiditis (Hashimoto's)	Thyroid carcinoma
Subacute thyroiditis (de Quervain's)	
Goitrogen induced	
Congenital enzyme defect	

GOITRE

The term goitre is used for any swelling of the thyroid gland, the causes of which (Table 5.5) overlap with those of primary hypothyroidism.

Symptoms and signs

The patient usually becomes aware of a goitre because of the cosmetic appearance. True pressure effects, such as difficulty in swallowing and shortness of breath, are very unusual with benign goitres unless they are retrosternal.

Goitres vary in size, consistency and nature of their surface. Classically they are bilateral neck swellings which rise on swallowing.

Investigations

Measurement of thyroid autoantibodies and thyroid ultrasound may be indicated in addition to thyroid function tests.

Differential diagnosis

The most important distinction to be made is between a benign goitre (generally bilateral), for whatever reason, and thyroid carcinoma (generally unilateral).

Treatment

With small goitres, no treatment other than reassurance may be required. Autoimmune goitres often respond to T4 therapy but multinodular goitres do so rarely. Surgery may be required for large goitres that do not respond to medical treatment.

THYROID CARCINOMA

Carcinomas of the thyroid are rare. In the young they are usually differentiated, either papillary (most often) or follicular, whereas in the elderly they are often undifferentiated (anaplastic). Differentiated thyroid carcinomas may arise from exposure of the neck to ionising radiation, especially in childhood.

An additional type of malignant tumour is medullary thyroid carcinoma, arising from parafollicular (C) cells. This may occur sporadically or as part of the syndrome of multiple endocrine adenomatosis.

Symptoms and signs

The presentation is usually with a goitre. There may be pressure effects such as dysphagia, shortness of breath and hoarseness, from recurrent laryngeal nerve involvement.

The goitre is typically a hard, apparently single, thyroid nodule of recent onset, or there may rarely have been rapid increase in size of an existing goitre. There may be pressure effects, such as stridor, and enlarged cervical lymph glands.

Investigations

Thyroid carcinomas characteristically do not take up radioisotope ('cold' nodule) and on ultrasound are either solid or, if cystic, are > 4 cm in diameter. Diagnosis is by fine-needle aspiration cytology. Raised levels of serum calcitonin are found in medullary thyroid carcinomas.

Differential diagnosis

The possibility of a carcinoma has to be considered in anyone with a goitre.

Treatment

Initial treatment for differentiated carcinomas is surgical. Subsequently T4 is given long term, as many are sensitive to TSH suppression, together with therapeutic doses of radioiodine for residual tumour and/or functioning metastases. Medullary thyroid carcinomas are also treated surgically. Anaplastic carcinomas are rapidly fatal but may respond temporarily to irradiation.

Prognosis

The prognosis for differentiated carcinomas is good, with a 10-year survival of papillary carcinomas of > 80%.

ADRENALS

ADRENAL CORTEX

Three main groups of steroid hormones are secreted by the adrenal cortex: glucocorticoids and mineralocorticoids, the most important in man being cortisol (hydrocortisone) and aldosterone respectively, and androgens. All are derived from cholesterol by a series of enzyme steps (Fig. 5.3).

HYPERFUNCTION

Glucocorticoids: Cushing's syndrome

Cushing's syndrome is rare but of particular importance since it is part of

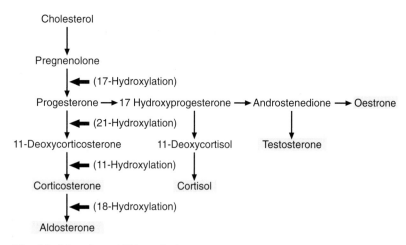

Fig. 5.3 Adrenal steroid biosynthesis.

Table 5.6. Causes of Cushing's syndrome

Type	Relative incidence (%)	Comments
Pituitary dependent	65	Underlying lesion usually a pituitary (micro) adenoma. Most common in young to middle aged women
Adrenal tumour		
Benign	10	
Malignant	10	
Ectopic ACTH secretion	15	Particularly small cell bronchial carcinoma, thymic and pancreatic tumours, bronchial carcinoid

the differential diagnosis of common conditions such as obesity and hypertension, and because high-dose glucocorticoid treatment causes the same clinical features. Causes of Cushing's syndrome are shown in Table 5.6.

Symptoms and signs (Table 5.7, Fig. 5.4)
These depend upon the duration of the condition. Patients with ectopic ACTH secretion from a malignant tumour may die before typical features can be detected, but their very high cortisol levels commonly cause mental confusion and weakness, the latter from potassium deficiency.

Investigations
These are used initially to establish the diagnosis and then, if confirmed, to determine the cause (Table 5.8). The overnight dexamethasone suppression

Table 5.7. Symptoms and signs of Cushing's syndrome

Effect of glucocorticoid	Symptoms and signs
Protein catabolic	Muscle wasting, weakness, proximal myopathy Thinning of skin, easy bruising, striae (particularly abdominal) Osteoporosis In children: stunting of growth
Anti-insulin	Clinical features of diabetes mellitus
Others	Redistribution of body fat with central obesity, 'buffalo hump'. Round (moon), red face Hypertension Psychiatric disorders, especially depression Hirsutism, oligo/amenorrhoea Pigmentation (in types with increased ACTH secretion)

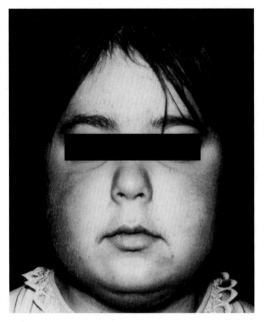

Fig. 5.4 Facial appearance in Cushing's syndrome classically described as a 'moon-face'.

test is a particularly useful screening procedure, normal suppression of the serum cortisol virtually excluding the diagnosis.

Differential diagnosis
Patients with depression may have steroid abnormalities similar to those

Table 5.8. Investigation of Cushing's syndrome

Test	Procedure	Typical findings
To establish diagnosis		
Overnight dexamethasone suppression	2300 h: 1 mg dexamethasone 0900 h: serum cortisol	Failure to show normal suppression
Low-dose dexamethasone	0.5 mg dexamethasone 6-hourly for 2 days	Failure to show normal suppression of serum/24 h urinary cortisol
Urinary free cortisol	24 h urine	Elevated levels
To determine cause		
Plasma ACTH	0900 h/2200 h— MN blood samples	Levels *high* in pituitary-dependent CS. Levels *very high* with ectopic ACTH secretion Levels *suppressed* in adrenal tumour
High-dose dexamethasone	2.0 mg dexamethasone 6-hourly for 2 days	Suppression of serum/24 h urinary free cortisol, in pituitary-dependent CS Other types show little or no suppression
Abdominal/skull MRI scan		May show adrenal/pituitary tumour
Screening tests for non-adrenal tumour	e.g. chest X-ray, LFTs	May show site/evidence of source of ectopic ACTH secretion

CS = Cushing's syndrome; LFTs = liver function tests; MN = Midnight

of Cushing's syndrome and alcoholics may develop a 'pseudo' Cushing's syndrome which remits on alcohol withdrawal.

Treatment
Treatment depends on the type of Cushing's syndrome. Patients with pituitary-dependent disease are usually treated by trans-sphenoidal pituitary surgery. If this fails, total adrenalectomy may be necessary but is a more serious surgical procedure and requires gluco- and mineralocorticoid replacement therapy. In addition, there is a risk of stimulating the growth of a pituitary adenoma, the patient commonly developing skin pigmentation (Nelson's syndrome) from the very high ACTH levels.

Adrenal tumours are treated by surgery, as may occasional ectopic ACTH-secreting tumours as appropriate. Preoperatively, or when it is not possible to relieve the condition, medical treatment with drugs, such as metyrapone, that block cortisol synthesis may be used.

Mineralocorticoids: Primary aldosteronism

Primary aldosteronism is most commonly caused by an adrenal tumour (almost always benign) or by bilateral hyperplasia. The excessive aldosterone secretion results in hypertension, from sodium retention, and hypokalaemia, from potassium loss in urine. It is an uncommon cause of raised blood pressure.

Symptoms and signs
The main clinical feature is hypertension. In addition, the patient may have symptoms of potassium deficiency, such as polyuria, polydipsia and muscle weakness. Peripheral oedema does not occur.

Investigations
Serum potassium is low, serum bicarbonate elevated and serum sodium is in the upper part of the normal range. The diagnosis is established by finding an elevated plasma aldosterone level and suppressed plasma renin activity. A CT scan may show an adrenal adenoma.

Differential diagnosis
The condition should be suspected in someone with hypertension and hypokalaemia, but the latter is more often the result of thiazide diuretic treatment of hypertension.

Treatment
Treatment is either by surgical excision of an adrenal tumour or medically with spironolactone or amiloride, which blocks the actions of aldosterone on the renal tubules.

Androgens: Congenital adrenal hyperplasia (CAH)

CAH is caused by a congenital, and sometimes familial, defect of one of the enzymes of cortisol synthesis, most commonly 21-hydroxylase. Although the main defect is of glucocorticoid secretion, there may be associated severe mineralocorticoid deficiency which results in a salt-losing state in newborn infants. Because of the glucocorticoid deficiency, there is stimulation of ACTH secretion which causes excessive adrenal androgen production.

Symptoms and signs
CAH may be recognised at birth because of masculinisation of the genitals of a female baby or, soon afterwards, from an acute salt-losing syndrome. The enzyme defect may be partial and the condition only recognised because of precocious puberty in boys and late-onset hirsutism in women.

Investigations
Urinary and plasma steroid levels are abnormal with high levels of glucocorticoid precursors and adrenal androgens.

Differential diagnosis

The condition must be distinguished from other causes of masculinisation of a female infant and, later, from other causes of male precocious puberty and hirsutism in women.

Treatment

Treatment is with glucocorticoids and fludrocortisone, an orally active mineralocorticoid, in the salt-losing form. In infants and children the glucocorticoid dose must be monitored carefully to avoid stunting of growth.

HYPOFUNCTION

Primary: Addison's disease

Addison's disease is uncommon. The destruction of the adrenal cortices was formerly most often due to tuberculosis, but is now usually the result of autoimmune destruction. Adrenal hypofunction may present acutely during a septicaemic illness, such as meningococcal infection, from bilateral adrenal infarction or haemorrhage.

Symptoms and signs

Acute adrenocortical deficiency causes a shock-like syndrome. Otherwise, the condition develops insidiously over several weeks or months with non-specific symptoms such as anorexia, weakness and weight loss.

The cardinal physical sign is brown pigmentation of the skin, particularly affecting exposed areas, scars and creases, and of the mucous membranes of the mouth and conjunctiva. This arises from excessive secretion of pituitary ACTH. Hypotension, with a further fall on standing, is also seen.

Investigations

The initial diagnosis is essentially clinical. In addition, serum biochemistry typically shows low serum sodium and raised serum potassium, urea and creatinine levels. If Addison's disease is strongly suspected, treatment should be started immediately to avoid an adrenal crisis and the diagnosis later confirmed by an adrenocortical stimulation test with tetracosactrin (Synacthen), a synthetic derivative of ACTH.

Treatment

Treatment of acute adrenocortical deficiency is with i.v. saline and cortisol 300–400 mg per 24 hours which, at this high dosage, also has adequate mineralocorticoid effect. Chronic replacement therapy is with 20–30 mg hydrocortisone per 24 hours in two divided doses, or an equivalent dose of an alternative glucocorticoid (see below), together with fludrocortisone, an orally active mineralocorticoid, 50–300 µg per 24 hours. The patient must double or treble the glucocorticoid dosage in the event of an intercurrent illness or accident.

Secondary

Isolated glucocorticoid deficiency occurs from ACTH deficiency either rarely as an isolated hormonal defect or because of long-term glucocorticoid or ACTH treatment. Mineralocorticoid treatment is not necessary since aldosterone secretion is intact.

Glucocorticoid therapy

Many glucocorticoids are available (e.g. cortisol, prednisolone, betamethasone, dexamethasone, triamcinolone). Replacement therapy for glucocorticoid deficiency, whether primary adrenocortical or secondary to ACTH deficiency, must be distinguished from pharmacological therapy when glucocorticoid is given for a variety of non-endocrine conditions such as rheumatoid arthritis or asthma. Occasionally ACTH rather than glucocorticoid is used. The higher the glucocorticoid/ACTH dose, and the longer it has to be given, the greater the risk of side-effects, which are the same as the clinical features of Cushing's syndrome (Table 5.7); in addition, there is a risk of adrenocortical suppression.

ADRENAL MEDULLA

Hyperfunction

Phaeochromocytoma

These tumours of the adrenal medulla, and similar tissue found around the aorta, are known as phaeochromocytomas. They are rare and may be unilateral or bilateral. The latter may be associated with conditions such as neurofibromatosis or medullary thyroid carcinoma. The tumours secrete adrenaline and noradrenaline sometimes intermittently. Hypertension is the major clinical feature (see p. 38).

THE GONADS

FEMALES

The ovaries contain oocytes and secrete oestrogens, progesterone and androgens. The predominant circulating oestrogen during reproductive years is oestradiol whilst, after the menopause, it is oestrone.

Delayed puberty

Delayed puberty results from disorders of the hypothalamus, anterior pituitary and ovary (Table 5.9).

Symptoms and signs

Disorders of the hypothalamus or pituitary are not necessarily associated with failure of development of secondary sexual characteristics, as there may

Table 5.9. Causes of delayed puberty

Hypothalamic–pituitary disorders	Primary gonadal disorders
Constitutional	Chromosomal abnormalities
	Gonadal dysgenesis (girls)
Isolated gonadotrophin deficiency (Kallmann's syndrome)	Klinefelter's syndrome (boys)
Chronic disease, e.g. chronic renal disease, coeliac disease	Surgical excision Cytotoxic chemotherapy
Low bodyweight Anorexia nervosa (in extreme cases)	
Hypothalamic/pituitary disease, e.g. tumours, granulomas, post-irradiation	
Primary hypothyroidism	
Hyperprolactinaemia (uncommon in children)	

be adequate gonadotrophin secretion to achieve this but failure of normal cyclical secretion resulting in amenorrhoea.

Investigations
Detection of elevated serum gonadotrophin levels indicates a primary ovarian disorder, whilst the levels are normal or low with hypothalamic/pituitary disease. X-ray of the left hand for bone age indicates skeletal development.

Differential diagnosis
This is sometimes evident on clinical examination, e.g. gonadal dysgenesis.

Treatment
Treatment depends upon the cause. If it is not possible to restore ovarian function, replacement therapy with oestrogen is needed. Small doses of ethinyl oestradiol (up to 10 µg per 24 hours) are given initially to avoid disproportionate maturation of the epiphyses and stunting of growth. Later it is convenient to give a combined oral contraceptive.

Gonadal dysgenesis (Turner's syndrome) (see p. 465)

Gonadal dysgenesis occurs in approximately 0.4 per 1000 female births. It is a disorder of sex chromosomes and a variety of different karyotypes are found, of which the most common is XO. The ovaries fail to develop and are present as undifferentiated (streak) gonads.

Symptoms and signs
Clinical features are absent ovarian function, shortness and associated abnormalities that include webbing of the neck, increased carrying angle of the forearm, short fourth and fifth metacarpals and skin naevi. Diagnosis may be made at birth from lymphoedema of the hands and feet.

Investigations
Serum gonadotrophin levels are elevated and the karyotype is abnormal.

Differential diagnosis
The diagnosis is essentially clinical, but the condition needs to be distinguished from other causes of shortness and absent pubertal development.

Treatment
Severe stunting of growth is now treated with injections of an anabolic steroid, sometimes together with human GH. Subsequently, oestrogen replacement therapy is given (as above), which eventually induces withdrawal menstrual bleeds and prevents the development of osteoporosis.

Amenorrhoea

Failure of development of periods is known as primary amenorrhoea and its causes overlap with those of delayed puberty discussed above. Development of amenorrhoea at any time after periods have become established is known as secondary amenorrhoea of which there are several causes (Table 5.10).

Symptoms and signs
In addition to the absence of periods there may be features of oestrogen deficiency (see below).

Investigations
Serum prolactin is measured to detect hyperprolactinaemia and serum FSH/LH levels to distinguish between a disorder of the hypothalamus/pituitary (the levels are normal or low), and, less commonly, of the ovary (the levels are elevated).

Table 5.10. Causes of secondary amenorrhoea (after exclusion of pregnancy)

Hypothalamic–pituitary	Ovarian	Endometrial
Functional defect of gonadotrophin secretion	Polycystic ovarian disease	Fibrosis
Emotional upset	Primary ovarian failure	Tuberculosis
Excessive physical exertion	Autoimmune oophoritis	
Intercurrent illness	Cytotoxic chemotherapy	
Low bodyweight	Pelvic irradiation	
Anorexia nervosa	Premature menopause	
Obesity	Surgical excision	
Hyperprolactinaemia		
Organic defect of gonadotrophin secretion		
Pituitary tumour		
Granuloma affecting the hypothalamus		

Treatment

Treatment is of the cause, if possible. Otherwise treatment may be indicated for absence of periods, associated infertility or oestrogen deficiency. Cyclical oestrogen therapy, most commonly with a preparation of the combined oral contraceptive, induces withdrawal bleeds unless there is a uterine disorder.

Oestrogen deficiency

This is inevitable at the time of the menopause and may occur in association with amenorrhoea in younger women, depending upon the cause.

Symptoms and signs

Oestrogen deficiency causes hot flushes, sweats and dyspareunia, the latter from dryness of the vagina. It results in excessive loss of bone mineral content with a risk of osteoporosis.

Investigations

Serum oestradiol levels are low.

Treatment

Treatment is with oestrogen replacement therapy. However, this must be given in combination with a progestogen since unopposed oestrogen causes endometrial hyperplasia and a risk of carcinoma. In younger women it is convenient to use a preparation of the combined oral contraceptive.

Hirsutism

Excessive body hair is a common symptom in women and often causes great distress. It must be assessed in relation to the patient's country of origin since there are large racial variations. It is most often caused by idiopathic hirsutism and polycystic ovarian disease, but is occasionally seen with other conditions such as adult congenital adrenal hyperplasia (CAH) and virilising syndromes, e.g. androgen-secreting tumours of the adrenals and ovaries.

Symptoms and signs

The excessive hair may affect the face, arms, legs, trunk and abdomen, the latter in the male type distribution. Disturbances of the menstrual cycle may occur and, rarely, there is frank virilisation with amenorrhorea, increased muscularity, marked loss of scalp hair and enlargement of the clitoris.

Investigations

Serum testosterone and plasma/urinary adrenal androgen levels are measured. An ultrasound of the ovaries may show polycystic ovarian disease.

Differential diagnosis

Women with clinical virilisation require full investigation to detect the cause.

Treatment

Patients with CAH are treated with glucocorticoid. Adrenal or ovarian tumours require surgical excision. Otherwise, if various cosmetic measures are not effective, oestrogen treatment, with a preparation of the combined oral contraceptive, may be helpful. In women with severe hirsutism, the anti-androgen cyproterone acetate may help. It is given cyclically with ethinyl-oestradiol to ensure contraception.

MALES

Spermatogenesis occurs within the seminiferous tubules of the testes, whilst testosterone is secreted by the interstitial (Leydig) cells. Testosterone is converted peripherally to dihydrotestosterone which, in some tissues, is the active form of the hormone.

Delayed puberty

Causes of delayed puberty are shown in Table 5.9. It is more often constitutional in boys than girls.

Symptoms and signs

Clinical features are those of lack of pubertal development of the genitalia and body hair, together with those of the underlying condition. Measurement of testicular size is particularly important, and enlargement is a clear sign that puberty is developing.

Investigations

Measurement of serum gonadotrophin levels and determination of the bone age and karyotype may be indicated.

Differential diagnosis

It is often difficult to distinguish functional delayed puberty from hypo-gonadotrophic hypogonadism except after a period of follow-up.

Treatment

Any treatment with androgens must be undertaken cautiously for fear of causing disproportionate maturation of the epiphyses and stunting of growth. It is given either by monthly low-dose intramuscular injection of testosterone ester or of human chorionic gonadotrophin (HCG), once or twice weekly.

Klinefelter's syndrome (see p. 465)

Klinefelter's syndrome is caused by a chromosomal abnormality which affects approximately 1 in 550 male births. Failure of normal development of the seminiferous tubules, which are hyalinised, and varying degrees of deficiency of interstitial cell function are seen. The most frequent chromosomal abnormality is an XXY karyotype.

Symptoms and signs

It commonly presents with delayed puberty and gynaecomastia associated with very small (pea-sized) testes. However, if there is normal androgen secretion, it may not be recognised until adult life because of infertility.

Investigations

Serum gonadotrophins are invariably raised and plasma testosterone often reduced. Karyotype typically is 47 XXY. Semen examination shows azoospermia.

Differential diagnosis

Klinefelter's syndrome must be distinguished in children from other causes of delayed puberty and gynaecomastia and must be considered in the investigation of infertility in adults.

Treatment

Gynaecomastia, if embarrassing, may need surgery. Androgen deficiency requires replacement therapy. The infertility is, unfortunately, untreatable.

Adult hypogonadism

The onset of hypogonadism in men is relatively rare and may have a hypo-thalamic/pituitary cause, such as pituitary tumour, or a primary testicular cause, such as mumps orchitis.

Symptoms and signs

The testes are small and there may be clinical features of androgen deficiency with soft smooth skin, loss of body hair and impotence, as well as infertility. Osteoporosis is a complication of long-standing hypogonadism.

Investigations

Measurement of serum gonadotrophin levels distinguishes a hypothalamic/pituitary lesion, when the levels are normal or low, from a primary testicular lesion when they are elevated.

Treatment

Treatment is of the cause, if possible. There are several different preparations of testosterone. Some can be taken orally, but testosterone esters, given intra-muscularly 3–4 weekly, are often more effective. Infertility due to pituitary hormone deficiency may be treated by injections of gonadotrophins.

Gynaecomastia

Gynaecomastia (enlargement of the breasts in males) occurs at puberty, probably from conversion of androgen to oestrogen, but usually resolves spontaneously over 1–2 years. In an adult it may signify serious disease (Table 5.11).

Table 5.11. Causes of gynaecomastia

Pubertal	Drugs
Klinefelter's syndrome	Androgens (transiently on
Post-pubertal	starting treatment)
Chronic renal failure	Anti-androgens
Cirrhosis of liver	Cimetidine
Hormone-producing tumours	Spironolactone
Adrenal cortex (oestrogens)	Digoxin
Carcinoma of bronchus (HCG)	Methyldopa
Germinal cell (HCG)	Oestrogens
Thyrotoxicosis	

Symptoms and signs

Although fat deposition in the breasts is often found in overweight men, true gynaecomastia consists of glandular tissue which can be felt as a bud under the areolae and may cause marked breast enlargement.

Investigations

There is usually no need for any investigations in boys with apparently pubertal gynaecomastia, unless there is clinical evidence of Klinefelter's syndrome. Similarly, mild gynaecomastia in the elderly does not necessarily need investigation. Otherwise, chest X-ray, liver function tests, serum testosterone, oestradiol, LH and HCG levels may be helpful.

Differential diagnosis

In adolescent boys the main differential diagnosis is between simple pubertal gynaecomastia and Klinefelter's syndrome.

Treatment

Medical treatment of pubertal gynaecomastia with an anti-oestrogen, such as tamoxifen, is sometimes effective but, if the condition is marked, surgery may be required. In adults, treatment is of the underlying condition.

GROWTH

The growth of an individual is determined by genetic and environmental factors, the latter including those in utero. Growth is assessed by comparison with growth charts derived from heights and weights of a large number of apparently normal girls and boys of different ages. In addition, parental height must be taken into account. Predictions of ultimate height can be made from bone age determined from an X-ray of the hand and wrist.

SHORTNESS

Shortness is usually considered to exist if the height is less than the third centile (below the mean). Shortness may be familial or constitutional, or the result of 'light for dates' birthweight, nutritional or emotional deprivation, skeletal or chromosomal disorders may result from chronic disease, such as bronchial asthma, diabetes mellitus, coeliac disease and chronic renal disease (Table 5.12).

Symptoms and signs
As well as shortness, there may be clinical features of the underlying condition. With food deprivation, comparison of weight and height centiles illustrates the thinness of the child.

Investigations
These include measurement of bone age, screening tests for chronic disease such as serum electrolytes, creatinine, ferritin and full blood count, blood glucose, thyroid function tests, stimulation tests of GH secretion, X-ray of the pituitary and determination of the karyotype.

Differential diagnosis
Although diagnosis may be apparent clinically, or made from results of initial investigations, the cause of shortness is sometimes difficult to establish, for instance with emotional deprivation or occult chronic disease such as coeliac disease.

Treatment
Treatment is of the underlying condition, if possible. When specific treatment is available, for instance with a gluten-free diet in coeliac disease, children

Table 5.12. Causes of shortness

Familial	Chromosomal disorders
Constitutional delayed puberty	Down syndrome
'Light for dates' birthweight	Gonadal dysgenesis
Food deprivation	Endocrine disorders
Emotional deprivation	GH deficiency
Skeletal abnormalities	Hypothyroidism
	Glucocorticoid excess
Chronic disease	Dysmorphic*
bronchial asthma	
chronic renal failure	
coeliac disease	
diabetes mellitus	

*Includes a variety of conditions often associated with unusual facies, skeletal abnormalities and a low IQ.

show 'catch up' growth to attain the height they would have achieved without the intercurrent disorder.

TALLNESS

Causes of excessive height are familial, Marfan's syndrome, homocystinuria and gigantism. Children with predicted excessive height from either of the two first causes are sometimes treated with large doses of gonadal steroid which, despite initial acceleration of growth, cause disproportionate maturation of the epiphyses and a reduction in ultimate height.

HYPOGLYCAEMIA

Hypoglycaemia is defined as a blood glucose level < 2.2 mmol/l. There are a variety of causes (Table 5.13), insulin treatment in diabetes being by far the most common.

Insulinomas are rare and may be part of the syndrome of multiple endocrine adenomatosis; they occur usually as a single adenoma and 10–20% are malignant. The mechanism(s) of hypoglycaemia with non-pancreatic tumours involves the secretion of insulin-like growth factors. Reactive hypoglycaemia without prior gastric surgery is rarely a convincing cause of symptoms.

Symptoms and signs

Hypoglycaemia produces a variety of symptoms and signs that originate in the nervous system (neuroglycopenia) or are from stimulation of the autonomic nervous system. These include hunger, shaking, anxiety, palpitations, sweating, poor concentration, slurred speech, fits, disorientation, drowsiness and ultimately unconsciousness, coma and death.

Table 5.13. Causes of hypoglycaemia

Endocrine disease	Drugs
Addison's disease	Alcohol
Hypopituitarism	Insulin
Hepatic disease	Sulphonylureas
Inborn errors of metabolism	Reactive (post-prandial)
Glycogen storage disease	especially after gastric surgery
Fructose intolerance	
Insulinoma	
Non-pancreatic tumour, particularly:	
Mesenchymal	
Hepatoma	
Adrenocortical carcinoma	

Investigations

It is first necessary to establish that the subject's symptoms are due to hypoglycaemia, and subsequently to establish its cause.

If an insulinoma is suspected, the serum insulin level must be measured at the time of hypoglycaemia, when it is inappropriately high.

Differential diagnosis

There may be particular difficulty in detecting hypoglycaemia caused by self-administration of insulin or a sulphonylurea (factitious hypoglycaemia).

Treatment

Individual episodes are treated with sugar by mouth or, if the patient is unable to swallow, with i.v. glucose. Otherwise, treatment of the underlying condition, if possible, is indicated, including resection of pancreatic insulinomata. The drug diazoxide reduces insulin secretion and is sometimes used in the medical management of hypoglycaemia.

CALCIUM AND BONE

The main bone-forming cells are the osteoblasts and those that resorb bone are the osteoclasts. The activity of the latter is stimulated by parathyroid hormone (PTH) and inhibited by calcitonin. Vitamin D, either taken in the diet or derived by the action of sunlight on the precursor 7-dehydrocholesterol in skin, is hydroxylated first in the liver and then the kidney to form the active compound 1,25-dihydroxycholecalciferol. Vitamin D promotes calcium absorption in the gut and normal mineralisation of bone. Approximately 50% of circulating calcium is bound to plasma proteins, in particular albumin, the level of which must be considered when assessing the total serum calcium.

HYPERCALCAEMIA

There are many causes of hypercalcaemia (Table 5.14) of which the most common in adults are primary hyperparathyroidism (see p. 197) and a tumour, usually malignant. Tumour-associated hypercalcaemia may be due to local cytokine production (haematological malignancy) or to local and systemic production of a PTH-related peptide (solid tumours).

Symptoms and signs

Mild hypercalcaemia (< 3.0 mmol/l) is often asymptomatic, but higher levels, especially of rapid onset, cause nausea, vomiting, polyuria, polydipsia, constipation, confusion and, eventually, coma and death.

Investigations

Once the presence of hypercalcaemia has been established, the most useful investigations in determining its cause are tests for an underlying malignancy, such as chest X-ray and serum immunoglobulins (myeloma), and measure-

Table 5.14. Causes of hypercalcaemia

Common	Rare
Hyperparathyroidism (primary or tertiary)	Acromegaly
	Addison's disease
Malignant tumours particularly carcinoma of breast, bronchus (squamous cell), renal tract, multiple myeloma	Familial hypocalciuric hypercalcaemia
	Immobilisation
	Milk-alkali syndrome
Sarcoidosis	Paget's disease of bone (on immobilisation)
Vitamin D overdose	Thiazide diuretics (? only in patients with primary hyperparathyroidism)
	Thyrotoxicosis

ment of serum PTH levels. Familial hypocalciuric hypercalcaemia is detected by measuring the calcium/creatinine clearance ratio and checking the serum calcium levels of first degree relatives.

Differential diagnosis

In most patients with tumour-associated hypercalcaemia, the tumour has already been diagnosed or is readily detected.

Treatment

Treatment is of the underlying condition, if possible. Acute treatment of symptomatic hypercalcaemia is with i.v. saline, often in large amounts, which may lower the calcium level sufficiently. Drug treatment is with a bisphosphonate. Glucocorticoids are specifically indicated for hypercalcaemia caused by vitamin D overdose and sarcoidosis.

HYPOCALCAEMIA

Hypocalcaemia is relatively uncommon. It occurs with hypoparathyroidism, in association with hyperphosphataemia causes of which include auto-immune destruction of the parathyroid glands and thyroid surgery. Other causes include vitamin D deficiency, magnesium deficiency, which reduces the secretion and effect of PTH, and acute pancreatitis.

Symptoms and signs

(See Table 5.15).

Investigations

Measurement of serum magnesium and PTH levels may be indicated.

Differential diagnosis

The cause of hypocalcaemia may be evident clinically, e.g. shortly after

Table 5.15. Symptoms and signs of hypocalcaemia

Symptoms	Signs
Muscle cramps, paraesthesia of extremities and lips	Overt
	Carpopedal spasm
Fits, psychiatric abnormality	Papilloedema*, cataracts*
In children:	Latent
Choking attacks from spasm of muscles of glottis (laryngismus stridulus)	Positive Trousseau's sign
	Positive Chvostek's sign

*After prolonged hypocalcaemia

thyroid surgery. Hypocalcaemia in patients presenting with fits is rare but should be considered.

Treatment

Hypoparathyroidism is treated with either 1-hydroxy or 1,25-dihydroxy-cholecalciferol. Other causes of hypocalcaemia are treated as appropriate. Acute hypocalcaemia, e.g. after thyroid surgery, requires immediate treatment with i.v. calcium until vitamin D has become effective.

OSTEOPOROSIS

Osteoporosis is thinning of bone from loss of mineral content, the bone itself being of normal architecture. Peak bone mineral content is established between the ages of 20 and 30 and thereafter is reduced in both men and women. Once bones have reached a critical degree of thinness, fractures occur, either spontaneously or with minor trauma, when the diagnosis of osteoporosis is made. The most important factor causing an accelerated decline is oestrogen deficiency at the menopause, or earlier if there is premature cessation of ovarian oestrogen production. Other risk factors include dietary deficiency of calcium, thyrotoxicosis, glucocorticoid treatment, smoking, alcohol and thinness.

Osteoporosis predisposes to vertebral fractures and fractures of long bones, particularly the neck of the femur and the wrist.

Symptoms and signs

Vertebral collapse causes back pain and ultimately kyphosis and loss of height.

Investigations

The diagnosis is radiological. Serum biochemistry is typically normal, other than a raised serum alkaline phosphatase for a few weeks following a fracture.

Differential diagnosis

The main differential diagnosis is from diffuse infiltration of the skeleton with a malignancy, particularly multiple myeloma.

Treatment

Every effort should be made to avoid the condition by attention to risk factors. Women with premature cessation of oestrogen secretion, for whatever reason, should receive oestrogen therapy, and women with a normal menopause should be considered for oestrogen replacement therapy. Bone density can be measured to help in the evaluation. Established osteoporosis is treated by either oestrogens or bisphosphonate.

PRIMARY HYPERPARATHYROIDISM

Primary hyperparathyroidism is usually from a single parathyroid adenoma, but sometimes from two or more adenomas, hyperplasia or, occasionally, carcinoma. It occurs particularly in middle-aged or elderly women and may cause renal calculi or, in the more severe form, bone disease (osteitis fibrosa cystica) and symptoms of hypercalcaemia. Nowadays the condition is commonly detected on routine screening of serum calcium.

Symptoms and signs

Patients with mild hypercalcaemia are usually asymptomatic but may have renal calculi. With more severe disease, patients may experience bone pain and deformities and symptoms of hypercalcaemia.

Investigations

In addition to serum calcium, serum electrolytes, urea and/or creatinine levels should be determined and X-ray of the abdomen for urinary tract calculi undertaken. The pathognomic radiological bone abnormality, seen only with severe hyperparathyroidism, is subperiosteal erosions of the phalanges.

Differential diagnosis

Other causes of hypercalcaemia (Table 5.14) need to be considered, but diagnosis depends upon the absence of clinical or laboratory evidence of a malignant tumour and a serum PTH level that is inappropriately high for the level of serum calcium.

Treatment

Treatment is by surgical excision of the underlying parathyroid tumour(s). However, particularly in elderly women, the condition is often benign and may be managed conservatively. Severe hypercalcaemia, bone disease, renal calculi and possibly osteoporosis are indications for surgery.

OSTEOMALACIA/RICKETS

Vitamin D deficiency causes osteomalacia in adults and rickets in children. Histologically there are widened osteoid seams and the bone is liable to deformity and fracture. Vitamin D deficiency may be dietary in origin and is rare nowadays in the UK except in the Asian population. It can also be caused by a malabsorption syndrome or by impaired production of 1,25-dihydroxycholecalciferol in renal disease.

Symptoms and signs

In children, vitamin D deficiency results in failure to thrive, bone pains and deformities. In adults, the condition is often subtle with non-specific aches and pains, sometimes with symptoms of a proximal myopathy.

Investigations

The serum calcium level is typically subnormal or in the lower half of the normal range, and the bone isoenzyme of serum alkaline phosphatase is elevated. Pseudofractures (Looser's zones) may be seen on X-rays.

Treatment

Dietary vitamin D deficiency responds to relatively small doses of vitamin D (ergocalciferol), e.g. 50 µg (2000 units) daily, without any risk of hyper-calcaemia. With malabsorption syndromes, once-monthly injections of vitamin D are given. In vitamin D resistant syndromes, it is best to use either 1-hydroxy or 1,25-dihydroxycholecalciferol as they act more rapidly than ergocalciferol and their duration of action is shorter, so any hypercalcaemia is less prolonged.

PAGET'S DISEASE

Paget's disease is a bone disorder of unknown aetiology with disturbed bone architecture caused by initial excessive osteoclastic and subsequent osteo-blastic activity. The bone is thickened and spongy with a greatly increased blood supply. The condition is very common in certain parts of the world, including the UK where it affects approximately 3.5% of those over the age of 40.

Symptoms and signs

In most subjects it is asymptomatic. It can, however, cause bone pain and deformity (Fig. 5.5). The skull, femur and tibia are commonly affected causing characteristic enlargement of the skull and bowing of the thigh and leg. The main complications are fractures, otosclerosis and neurological com-pression syndromes of the cranial nerves (especially the 8th) and the spinal cord. High output cardiac failure, hypercalcaemia on immobilisation and osteogenic sarcoma are rare complications.

Investigations

The serum calcium level is almost always normal but levels of the bone isoenzyme of serum alkaline phosphatase are raised, often grossly. The characteristic radiological changes include coarsening of the trabecular pattern with expansion and cortical thickening.

Differential diagnosis

It is often difficult to distinguish the pain of Paget's disease from other causes of pain affecting an elderly population, such as osteoarthritis.

Treatment

The usual indication for treatment is for bone pain. Courses of up to 6

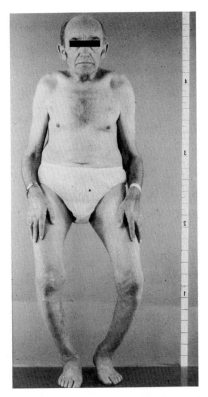

Fig. 5.5 A patient with Paget's disease with marked bone deformities.

months of one of the bisphosphonates are given by mouth or, less commonly, calcitonin given by subcutaneous injection 2–3 times weekly. If pain is not relieved within 4–6 weeks, its cause should be reviewed.

HYPERLIPOPROTEINAEMIA

The major clinical significance of hypercholesterolaemia and, to a lesser extent, of hypertriglyceridaemia is as risk factors for the development of atheroma affecting, in particular, the coronary arteries and causing ischaemic heart disease (IHD). In addition, they can cause skin and tendon xanthomata and severe hypertriglyceridaemia may induce acute pancreatitis.

HYPERCHOLESTEROLAEMIA (WHO Classification: Type IIa)

The predominant cholesterol-carrying lipoproteins are the low-density lipoproteins (LDL) and the concentration of both total LDL and cholesterol has been shown to be directly related to the risk of developing IHD. Familial hypercholesterolaemia (FH), a single gene defect inherited as an autosomal dominant, results in deficiency or abnormality of the LDL receptor and consequent hypercholesterolaemia. Those with homozygous FH have very high total serum cholesterol levels (>10 mmol/l) and develop IHD as children or young adults; the heterozygous form has an incidence of ~1 in 500 in the UK. However, in most people the hypercholesterolaemia is partly environmental (chiefly dietary) and partly genetic (via a polygenic mode of inheritance) in origin.

High-density lipoproteins (HDL) take up cholesterol from the periphery, returning it to the liver, and have a protective effect upon the development of IHD, the level of serum HDL cholesterol having an inverse relationship with risk of developing IHD.

In several diseases, such as hypothyroidism, biliary cirrhosis and the nephrotic system, hypercholesterolaemia exists as a secondary condition.

Symptoms and signs
Most often hypercholesterolaemia is only detected because of the development of arterial disease, usually IHD.

Investigations
Serum cholesterol can be measured on a random (i.e. not necessarily fasting) blood sample. The possibility of secondary hypercholesterolaemia should be considered. Serum HDL cholesterol should also be measured in asymptomatic subjects being considered for hypocholesterolaemic drug treatment.

Treatment
The mainstay of treatment is a reduction in dietary fat intake. Polyunsaturated fats (e.g. vegetable oils) and monounsaturated fats (e.g. olive oil) should be substituted for saturated (animal) fats. Other important dietary changes are reduction of calories in those who are overweight and an increase in fibre intake. A variety of hypocholesterolaemic drugs are available for those whose serum cholesterol levels remain too high despite dietary modifications (Table 5.16).

Every attempt should be made to reduce the total serum cholesterol level to < 6.0 mmol/l in subjects with established IHD (secondary prevention) and ideally to 5.2 mmol/l or less. Asymptomatic subjects with hypercholesterolaemia (primary prevention) should be given dietary advice. If their cholesterol levels remain > 6.5 mmol/l, serum HDL/LDL cholesterol levels should be determined and drugs considered for those whose total serum cholesterol levels are > 7.8 mmol/l. Other factors to be considered prior to drug therapy are age, sex and other IHD risk factors, e.g. hypertension, smoking, diabetes.

HYPERTRIGLYCERIDAEMIA (WHO classification: Type IV)

Hypertriglyceridaemia is caused by the elevation of VLDL and is commonly secondary to some other condition, particularly obesity and/or alcoholism.

Symptoms and signs
There may be clinical features of IHD. In addition, those with markedly

Table 5.16. Drugs used in the treatment of hyperlipoproteinaemia

Drug	Comments
Hypercholesterolaemia	
Anion exchange resin	Not absorbed
Cholestyramine	Binds cholesterol/bile salts in gut
Colestipol	Commonly cause GI symptoms
Statin	
Pravastatin	Inhibit HMG-Co A reductase
Simvastatin	May cause rise in hepatic transaminase and (rarely) myositis
Fibric acid derivative	
Bezafibrate	Complicated mechanism(s) of action
Fenofibrate	Potentiate oral anticoagulants
Gemfibrozil	(Rarely) causes myositis
Ciprofibrate	Avoid in gallbladder disease
Acipimox	Decrease release of non-esterified fatty acids
(nicotinic acid derivative)	(NEFA) from adipose tissue
	Side-effects common, especially flushing of face
Probucol	Reduces serum HDL
	Nevertheless can cause shrinkage of xanthomata
Hypertriglyceridaemia	
Fibric acid derivative	As above
Nicotinic acid	As above

elevated serum triglyceride levels (>10 mmol/l) are at risk of developing acute pancreatitis.

Investigations

Serum triglyceride levels should be measured on a *fasting* blood sample.

Treatment

Hypertriglyceridaemia often responds to treatment of underlying factor(s), e.g. reduction of weight and/or alcohol intake; drug treatment (Table 5.16) is needed far less often than with hypercholesterolaemia.

MIXED HYPERCHOLESTEROLAEMIA AND HYPERTRIGLYCERIDAEMIA (WHO classification: Type IIb)

This occurs commonly and is associated with an increased incidence of IHD. The clinical features, investigation and management are similar to those of hypercholesterolaemia and hypertriglyceridaemia considered above.

HYPERCHYLOMICRONAEMIA (WHO classification: Type I)

This is a rare condition of inherited deficiency of lipoprotein lipase. It does not predispose to arterial disease but is associated with skin lesions and a risk of acute pancreatitis. Treatment is with a low-fat diet.

INTERMEDIATE-DENSITY HYPERLIPOPROTEINAEMIA
(WHO classification: Type III)

This congenital abnormality results in raised levels of intermediate-density lipoprotein and there is a markedly increased risk of IHD. The condition responds to treatment with dietary modifications and a fibric acid derivative.

MIXED HYPERTRIGLYCERIDAEMIA AND
HYPERCHYLOMICRONAEMIA (WHO classification: Type V)

This is a relatively rare condition which may be an extreme form of hyper-triglyceridaemia. As with hypertriglyceridaemia, it is commonly associated with overweight and/or alcoholism and may respond to treatment of these; in addition, treatment with a fibric acid derivative is often necessary.

6

DIABETES
Roger Corrall

Diabetes mellitus is characterised by chronic elevation of blood glucose levels. There are two types of primary diabetes. Insulin-dependent diabetes mellitus (IDDM), formerly known as juvenile onset diabetes, is dependent on insulin treatment, has a tendency to ketosis and usually a relatively young age of onset. Non-insulin-dependent diabetes (NIDDM), formerly referred to as maturity onset diabetes, does not require treatment with insulin, is ketosis resistant and most cases are diagnosed beyond 40 years of age. These two varieties of diabetes are entirely separate disorders.

Diabetes may be secondary to other conditions, e.g. pancreatic and endocrine disease, the latter generally involving hypersecretion of insulin antagonists. It may also be drug induced, e.g. by thiazide diuretics.

NON-INSULIN-DEPENDENT DIABETES

In NIDDM, insulin secretion from the pancreatic islets in response to food is reduced in amount compared with non-diabetic individuals of comparable obesity and the early rapid phase of secretion is impaired. Secondly, NIDDM is associated with a state of insulin resistance, i.e. a reduced biological effect of circulating insulin on peripheral cells.

The causative mechanisms underlying NIDDM are incompletely understood. The condition runs in families and identical twin studies show an almost 100% concordance rate. Insulin resistance may also be associated with hypertension and atheroma and is linked with a low birth weight in affected individuals. Its effect is enhanced by concomitant obesity.

Symptoms

Many patients are asymptomatic and glycosuria is noted on routine medical examination. Patients may complain of thirst, polydipsia, polyuria and nocturia related to a glucose-induced osmotic diuresis. Tiredness and weight loss are common. Pruritus vulvae and balanitis are related to candidal infections of the genitalia. Visual disturbance is caused by a temporary lens malfunction. Pain and paraesthesiae in the limbs may be present, caused by a painful neuropathy. The clinical history is typically insidious over months or years.

Signs

Patients are frequently obese. Chronic diabetic complications such as neuropathy or retinopathy are sometimes seen at diagnosis in NIDDM.

Investigations

Although glycosuria arouses suspicion, the diagnosis of NIDDM must be confirmed by demonstrating raised blood glucose levels (Table 6.1). In a glucose tolerance test, circulating glucose levels are determined in the fasting state and 2 hours after ingestion of 75 g of glucose. In clinical practice, an abnormally raised fasting level or a blood glucose value taken more than 2 hours after a meal in excess of 10 mmol/l (plasma 11.1 mmol/l) confirms the diagnosis.

The condition of impaired glucose tolerance (see Table 6.1), where blood glucose levels fall outside strictly normal limits, is not associated with the specific microvascular complication of diabetes. It is, however, linked with a propensity to premature atheroma and may worsen to frank NIDDM.

Differential diagnosis

This includes other causes of polyuria, weight loss and general tiredness.

Treatment

The aim is to achieve as normal a state of metabolic control as possible without inducing any side-effects or toxicity. Newly diagnosed diabetic patients can generally be categorised on simple clinical criteria as NIDDM or IDDM. Those with NIDDM are treated initially with dietary modification and taught how to monitor their own control. If this is inadequate, they may need oral

Table 6.1. Diagnostic criteria for diabetes

| | Venous glucose (mmol/l) | |
	Blood	Plasma
Impaired glucose tolerance		
Fasting value	<6.7	<7.8
2 h value of glucose tolerance test	6.7–10	7.8–11.1
Diabetes mellitus		
Fasting value	>6.7	>7.8
2 h value of glucose tolerance test	>10.0	>11.1

hypoglycaemic drugs. These may prove successful, although failure may be seen at the beginning (primary failure) or after a period of satisfactory control (secondary failure). In these cases, insulin will be required.

Diet

Diet is the basis of all diabetic treatment. Appropriate diets, tailored to individual requirements, are based on the following principles:

1. Foods containing significant amounts of refined carbohydrates (monosaccharides and disaccharides, foods generally tasting sweet) are forbidden but those containing unrefined carbohydrates (starchy, non-sweet foodstuffs) are allowed.
2. High fibre foods are encouraged.
3. Animal fats (saturated) are reduced and replaced by vegetable oils (polyunsaturates and monounsaturates).

This simple diet alone is sufficient to achieve satisfactory control in many non-obese patients with NIDDM. Obese patients will need to reduce their overall calorie intake by limiting starchy and fatty foods.

Oral hypoglycaemic agents

Sulphonylureas. (Table 6.2) act primarily by increasing secretion from the pancreatic beta cells. They are started at a low dose, increasing until either satisfactory blood glucose control or a maximum tolerable dose is achieved.

Hypoglycaemia is the most common side-effect and often necessitates a reduction in dosage. Flushing after ingestion of alcohol is specific to chlorpropamide. Other side-effects, including skin rashes and marrow depression, are uncommon. Chlorpropamide should be avoided in the elderly and in those with impaired renal function.

Biguanides. Biguanides act primarily on peripheral cells to enhance insulin sensitivity and suppress hepatic gluconeogenesis. They are often the preferred option in obese patients. Metformin is given after food in two or three daily doses. The most common side-effects are gastrointestinal—predominantly

Table 6.2. Sulphonylurea drugs

Drug	Duration of action (h)	Site of elimination	Initial dose	Maximum dose
Tolbutamide	8	Liver > Kidney	500 mg	3 g
Chlorpropamide	36	Kidney >> Liver	100 mg	500 mg
Glibenclamide	12	Liver = Kidney	2.5 mg	20 mg
Gliclazide	18	Kidney > Liver	40 mg	320 mg
Glipizide	10	Kidney > Liver	2.5 mg	20 mg

diarrhoea, nausea and vomiting. These effects are lessened by increasing the dose gradually (at not less than weekly intervals) and by taking the medication after meals. The rare potentially fatal complication of lactic acidosis only occurs if the drug is given to patients with renal or hepatic failure, alcoholism and conditions associated with peripheral cell hypoxia.

Monitoring control

Diabetic control should be monitored both by the patient in the community and at visits to the outpatient clinic. In many centres, urine testing for glucose is still the preferred home method in NIDDM. It is best performed using quantitative reagent sticks such as Diastix. The normal renal threshold is 10 mmol/l and therefore positivity indicates that blood glucose levels are above the physiological range. In NIDDM, urine specimens tested in the fasting state and at least 2 hours after the main evening meal will suffice in monitoring control. With a normal renal threshold, such tests would generally be negative in a well-controlled diabetic.

There is an increasing tendency to assess control in NIDDM by blood glucose testing, the standard monitoring method for IDDM. In NIDDM, good control is associated with fasting levels lower than 7 mmol/l.

At clinic visits, a retrospective estimate of overall glycaemic control may be made using indices of blood protein glycosylation. Both haemoglobin in red cells and plasma proteins (fructosamine) combine chemically with glucose (glycosylation) in both normal and diabetic individuals. The level of glycosylation is increased in diabetes and its magnitude reflects prior metabolic control.

INSULIN-DEPENDENT DIABETES MELLITUS

IDDM is characterised by a virtually total destruction of the pancreatic beta cell mass with very low or zero plasma insulin levels despite hyperglycaemia. The onset usually occurs before 30 years of age. Beta cell destruction is confirmed histologically in the early stages with round cell infiltration characteristic of an autoimmune destructive process. Hyperketonaemia and ketonuria are often present at diagnosis, reflecting the absence of sufficient circulating insulin to suppress lipolysis and hepatic ketogenesis.

IDDM is a familial condition. There is an association of IDDM with the HLA haplotypes DR3 and DR4. When both are present, the relative risk of IDDM is increased 14 times. Identical twins have shown approximately 50% concordance for IDDM, indicating a strong genetic component but raising the possibility of environmental influences. Circulating islet cell antibodies are commonly present at diagnosis. They may be present for several years before the development of clinical diabetes, which manifests overtly when more than 90% of islet cells have been destroyed. It is possible that a viral infection may trigger the autoimmune destructive process in those genetically predisposed. Coxsackie B4, mumps and rubella are possible contenders.

Symptoms and signs

These are similar to those of NIDDM but the history is more acute, often no more than a few weeks. Rarely, patients may present in diabetic keto-acidosis. They often show evidence of weight loss and obesity is uncommon. Evidence of chronic diabetic complications is extremely rare at diagnosis in IDDM.

Investigations

The condition must be confirmed by blood glucose assay using the same criteria as in NIDDM. Ketonuria is commonly noted.

Treatment

Diet

This is based on the standard diabetic formula described above but quantitatively the starchy, carbohydrate component is more rigorously apportioned to particular meals in order to minimise variation in oral carbohydrate intake.

Insulin therapy

Insulin preparations. Insulin of bovine, porcine and human origin is used. Human insulin is made by genetic recombinant techniques and is very similar to porcine insulin. When injected subcutaneously, beef insulin is absorbed more slowly into the circulation than human or porcine varieties.

Each variety of insulin has a characteristic time of onset, peak effect and total duration of action and on this basis can be divided into three groups (Table 6.3). Neutral soluble insulin is unmodified insulin in solution at a neutral pH and appears clear. All other insulins have a cloudy appearance.

Table 6.3. Time actions of insulin preparations

Insulin	Time action (h)			Proprietary examples
	Onset	Peak	Total duration	
Short-acting				
Neutral soluble	0.25–1	2–4	5–8	Velosulin
Intermediate-acting				
Semilente	0.5–1	4–6	8–12	Semitard
Isophane	2–4	6–10	12–24	Insulatard
Long-acting				
Ultralente	3–4	14–20	24–36	Ultratard
Protamine zinc	3–4	14–20	24–36	

Premixed preparations are also available, such as lente insulin (30% semilente, 70% ultralente) and Mixtard 30 insulin (30% Velosulin, 70% Insulatard). The time actions of all insulins after injection are very variable. In practice, most clinical problems can be resolved using a combination of neutral soluble and isophane insulins.

Choice of insulin regimens. In the elderly, a single or two injections of isophane or a premixed formulation will often achieve acceptable control. In this age group, relatively high blood glucose levels may be acceptable in the absence of symptoms of poor diabetic control.

In younger patients, a greater flexibility and a desire for better diabetic control necessitate the use of multiple injection regimens. Two systems that have proved satisfactory are shown in Fig. 6.1. Both regimens are associated with four peak times of insulin action before the four main meals. In regimen

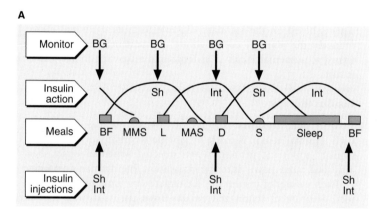

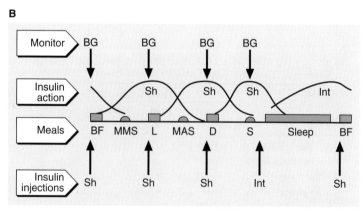

Fig. 6.1 Use of insulin injections in a twice daily **(A)** and four times daily regimen **(B)** BF = breakfast; MMS = mid-morning snack; L = lunch; MAS = mid-afternoon snack; D = dinner; S = supper; BG = blood glucose; Sh = short-acting insulin; Int = intermediate-acting insulin.

B, the short-acting insulin may be given from a cartridge-loaded pen device that may be carried in the pocket to facilitate injection.

Monitoring and adjustment of insulin dose. In some elderly patients, urinary glucose monitoring with reagent sticks may suffice. However, in the great majority of patients, direct home monitoring of blood glucose levels after digital puncture is preferred. Perfect control in a young insulin-dependent diabetic would be associated with preprandial blood glucose levels between 4 and 7 mmol/l with an absence of hypoglycaemic reactions. Lesser degrees of metabolic perfection are accepted in many patients, including the elderly, those with low IQ and those prone to hypoglycaemia.

Insulin dosage is adjusted to correspond to its peak time of action according to trends in blood glucose levels. In the absence of unprovoked hypoglycaemia or intercurrent illness, only infrequent and small changes are usually required. Clinic monitoring using glycosylated haemoglobin or fructosamine will give additional objective assessment of metabolic control.

Hypoglycaemia

Hypoglycaemia in IDDM is caused by a failure to match correctly food intake, exercise and insulin dosage. Subtle intellectual and psychomotor impairment—mild neuroglycopenia—is experienced as blood glucose levels fall below 3 mmol/l. At levels below 1 mmol/l, severe neuroglycopenia is experienced with confusion, disturbed behaviour, fits and ultimately coma. A generalised autonomic activation is triggered at blood glucose levels below 2 mmol/l which causes acute symptoms, including palpitations, sweating and tremor. Awareness of hypoglycaemia may be chronically reduced or lost in IDDM patients after many years of insulin treatment. Acute intensive insulin therapy may induce a reversible blunting of hypoglycaemic awareness.

To prevent hypoglycaemia, patients must learn to avoid missed or late meals, cover significant exertion with extra carbohydrate and avoid blood glucose profiles that are bordering on hypoglycaemia. Blood glucose guidelines may have to be relaxed in those with chronic hypoglycaemic unawareness. In conscious patients, hypoglycaemia is usually reversed by 20 g oral glucose. Unconscious patients may respond to glucose gel squirted into the mouth. Glucagon 1 mg s.c. or i.m. may be given by doctors or trained relatives or intravenous glucose (30 ml of 20% solution) may be required.

Intercurrent illness

This decreases insulin sensitivity in IDDM and thus tends to cause impairment of diabetic control. Urine should be tested for ketone concentration. Injections of insulin should never be omitted and insulin doses may need to be progressively increased depending on changes in blood glucose levels. If appetite is affected, carbohydrate exchanges should be maintained as liquid equivalents. Vomiting may require the administration of anti-emetics.

DIABETIC KETOACIDOSIS

Diabetic ketoacidosis (DKA) is a life-threatening complication of diabetes with an average mortality of 7%. The commonest causes are acute infection and management errors; it is also seen in new diabetics. DKA is the result of an absolute or relative insulin deficiency associated with an increase in catabolic hormones, particularly glucagon, cortisol and catecholamines. Unrestrained gluconeogenesis gives rise to hyperglycaemia with secondary water and electrolyte depletion. Increased hepatic ketogenesis causes raised levels of ketone bodies which are responsible for the acidosis and hyperventilation. Average adult deficits of fluid and electrolytes are listed in Table 6.4.

Symptoms and signs

There is polyuria with polydipsia, weight loss, weakness and drowsiness leading to coma. Abdominal pain may be present in the absence of pathology.

There may be evidence of salt and water depletion with tachycardia, hypotension, reduced skin turgor and low intraocular pressure. Hyperventilation may be marked with deep sighing breaths (Kussmaul's respiration). The odour of acetone on the breath is characteristic though not obvious to all.

Investigations

1. Urine shows heavy glycosuria and ketonuria.
2. A blood glucose reagent stick confirms significant hyperglycaemia (usually > 22 mmol/l) and centrifuged plasma reads ++ or +++ on Ketostix.
3. Plasma urea and electrolytes should be obtained: a depressed bicarbonate (< 5 mmol/l in severe cases) confirms the metabolic acidosis and arterial blood gases may show acidaemia with a depressed arterial pH value.
4. A full blood count commonly shows a neutrophil leukocytosis which in this context may not necessarily indicate acute infection.
5. Infection is sought with blood and urine culture and a chest X-ray.

Table 6.4. Average fluid and electrolyte deficits in diabetic ketoacidosis

Water	5–8 litres
Sodium	400–600 mmol
Potassium	300–1000 mmol
Calcium	50–100 mmol
Magnesium	25–50 mmol
Phosphate	50–100 mmol

Table 6.5. Treatment plan for diabetic ketoacidosis

Fluid and electrolytes

Volume:	Initially 3 litres in first 3 h then according to needs (total in first 24 h: 6–10 litres)
Fluids:	1. Isotonic saline (150 mmol/l) as basic replacement fluid
	2. Consider hypotonic saline (75 mmol/l) if plasma sodium > 150 mmol/l
	3. 5% Dextrose when blood glucose < 14 mmol/l
	4. Consider sodium bicarbonate (1.4%) if arterial pH < 7.0, 100 mmol/l over 45 min (with 20 mmol KCl) repeated if necessary
Insulin	By continuous i.v. infusion 5–10 u/h initially, 2–4 u/h when blood glucose falls below 14 mmol/l
Potassium	Monitor serum levels regularly, initially 2-hourly. Add the following amounts to each 1 litre of fluid:
	if plasma K^+ < 3.5 mmol/l, add 40 mmol KCl
	3.5–5.5 mmol/l, add 20 mmol KCl
	> 5.5 mmol/l, add no KCl

Treatment (see Table 6.5)

Infection should be treated energetically with appropriate antibiotics. Gastric aspiration is indicated in those with impaired consciousness. Cerebral oedema may rarely occur during treatment and is associated with deepening coma. Thrombo-embolic complications may develop.

Diabetic non-ketotic hyperosmolar coma

In non-ketotic hyperosmolar coma there is insidious development of marked hyperglycaemia (generally > 50 mmol/l) and salt and water depletion but without acidosis. A minor elevation of plasma ketone bodies may occur (up to 3 mmol/l, normal 0.05–0.5; DKA 5.0–50.0). Mortality is in excess of 30%. Precipitating factors include infections, administration of diuretics, steroids and phenytion and an over-enthusiastic ingestion of glucose-rich drinks.

Symptoms of polyuria, intense thirst and progressive clouding of consciousness are characteristic. Coma and severe dehydration are common. Patients are frequently moribund on admission to hospital but Kussmaul's respiration is not seen. Treatment involves rehydration, insulin therapy and electrolyte replacement in a manner similar to that used for DKA.

LONG-TERM COMPLICATIONS OF DIABETES

Diabetics, after many years, are prone to pathological changes in their blood vessels.

1. Premature and widespread atheroma in large and medium sized arteries, which is not specific to diabetes, may be responsible for complications such as myocardial infarction or peripheral limb ischaemia.
2. Microvascular changes, which are specific for diabetes and do not occur in the absence of long-standing hyperglycaemia, are a major pathogenetic factor in the development of three classical complications: retinopathy, neuropathy and nephropathy. The duration of diabetes and the quality of diabetic control are important determinants of these and constitute the basis for advocating good metabolic control from an early stage in young patients with IDDM. Immaculate diabetic control with intensive insulin treatment reduces the development of microvascular disease.

Diabetic eye disease

Diabetic retinopathy remains the most common cause of new blind registrations in those aged under 65. Background retinopathy, the earliest stage on ophthalmoscopy, is characterised by normal visual acuity and minor retinal changes sited maximally at the posterior pole of the eye. This may remain static for many years or develop into either maculopathy (commonest in NIDDM) or proliferative retinopathy (commonest in IDDM). In maculopathy, more advanced changes develop at the posterior pole with oedema and impaired visual acuity. Early treatment with retinal laser may achieve some preservation of visual function and prevent blindness. Proliferative changes may be heralded by new retinal abnormalities characteristic of the pre-proliferative phase. In proliferative retinopathy (PR), abnormal new vessels grow into the vitreous originating from areas of local retinal ischaemia. Early treatment by laser may prevent its progression. If PR is not controlled, the new vessels will bleed into the vitreous; subsequent deposition of fibrous tissue will result in blindness. Vitreo-retinal surgery may improve visual acuity in those with such advanced diabetic proliferative complications.

Senile cataract occurs on average 10 years earlier than in non-diabetics.

Diabetic neuropathy

Diabetic neuropathy is thought to result from axonal damage secondary to microvascular ischemia in peripheral nerves. Abnormal nerve metabolism may also contribute. A classification of neuropathy in diabetes is given below.

1. A *chronic distal symmetric polyneuropathy* is most commonly found and is usually asymptomatic though evidence of impaired sensation of a glove and stocking distribution may be demonstrable. Lower limb deep tendon reflexes may be reduced or absent. There is no proven specific treatment.
2. *Acute painful neuropathy* is typically experienced in the lower limbs and may be very severe. Antidepressants can give symptomatic relief.
3. *Proximal motor neuropathy*, also called diabetic amyotrophy, leads to weakness and wasting of thigh muscles. It is often asymmetric and knee jerks are reduced or absent. The condition normally reverses within 2 years.
4. *Diabetic mononeuropathy* affects individual nerves. In some instances,

this relates to local pressure, e.g. carpal tunnel syndrome; in others, it results from a localised nerve infarction. More than one nerve may be affected (mononeuritis multiplex).

5. *Autonomic neuropathy* typically presents with diarrhoea, postural hypotension, impaired gastric emptying, bladder dysfunction and impotence.

Diabetic nephropathy (see p. 223)

1. Proteinuria develops in 40% of IDDM patients of whom two-thirds will develop renal failure.
2. Glomerular capillary basement membrane thickening can be detected within 2 years of diagnosis of IDDM and increases in time but does not cause clinical nephropathy per se. Its development in some patients is characterised by increasing proteinuria (sometimes with a frank nephrotic syndrome) decreasing GFR and hypertension and correlates with a progressive reduction of the filtration surface through expansion of the glomerular mesangium content. When plasma creatinine levels rise above normal, end-stage renal failure supervenes after an average of 5 years.
3. Microalbuminuria is a subclinical (Albustix negative) increase in urinary albumin excretion in the range 30–300 mg per 24 hours associated with a 20-fold increase in the risk of developing clinical nephropathy in IDDM.

Treatment

In patients with microalbuminuria, great attention should be paid to meticulous control of diabetes and hypertension if present. In those with frank proteinuria, perfect blood pressure control with diastolic levels below 85 mmHg may greatly delay the advent of uraemia. ACE inhibitors may have a particular role in treatment. Renal supportive therapy—transplantation, haemodialysis or continuous ambulatory peritoneal dialysis—may eventually be needed.

The diabetic foot

Neuropathy and ischaemia frequently act in combination, often with infection, to predispose to ulceration of the diabetic foot. The typical neuropathic foot is numb and warm with peripheral pulses. Complications include neuropathic skin ulceration and Charcot arthropathy. The ischaemic foot, in contrast, is cold and pulseless and prone to rest pain, ulceration and gangrene.

Management involves the correction of the relative contributions of neuropathy, ischaemia and infection in a collaborative teamwork exercise.

SURGERY

In diabetic patients undergoing surgery it is important to avoid extremes of hyper- or hypoglycaemia and to maintain normal hydration and electrolyte balance. In IDDM patients a glucose/insulin infusion with blood glucose monitoring is often used during the operation and for a variable time post-operatively until oral intake of food and water can be resumed.

PREGNANCY

Poorly controlled diabetes is associated with macrosomia, pre-eclampsia and hydramnios. The death of a fetus or neonate occurred in one-third of diabetic pregnancies 30 years ago. Current management with meticulous control of blood glucose levels has achieved results comparable to those with non-diabetic pregnancies.

Diabetes that develops during the course of pregnancy is termed gestational diabetes. Treatment is with diet in the first instance but some patients may require insulin during the pregnancy. NIDDM may develop later in life.

7

NEPHROLOGY
Charles R.V. Tomson

Renal disease may be either primary, which is relatively rare, or due to disturbances in renal function as a result of heart disease, liver disease, drug therapy, hypovolaemia or sepsis. Many multisystem diseases such as diabetes also affect the kidney. End-stage kidney failure is rare, but is important because of the availability of dialysis and transplantation, the cost of which raises ethical issues about resource allocation.

The effects of kidney disease reflect the various functions of the kidney:

1. excretion of waste products—failure of which causes 'uraemia'
2. control of systemic acid–base balance—failure of which may cause renal tubular acidosis
3. control of salt and water balance—failure of which may cause hypo-volaemia or hypervolaemia (resulting in hypertension and/or oedema)
4. 1-hydroxylation of vitamin D—failure of which causes calcium malabsorp-tion, osteomalacia and hyperparathyroidism.
5. erythropoietin production—failure of which causes anaemia
6. renin secretion—which may increase in many renal diseases, causing hypertension.

SYMPTOMS AND SIGNS OF KIDNEY DISEASE

Haematuria may be obvious (macroscopic) or only detected on dipstick testing or microscopy. The blood may come from anywhere between the glomeruli and the tip of the urethra. Important causes include bladder tumours, renal stones and glomerulonephritis.

Proteinuria is often detected on 'routine' urinalysis and may be due to increased glomerular permeability to protein or to decreased tubular reabsorption.

Pyuria, white cells in the urine, usually indicates infection.

Dysuria, pain on passing urine, is usually caused by infection of the lower urinary tract or prostatitis.

Polyuria (increased urine volume) and *nocturia* (passing urine at night) may reflect impaired urine concentrating ability, due either to renal disease, diabetes mellitus or diabetes insipidus. Urinary *frequency* may be due to polyuria, but may also indicate bladder instability caused by urological disease.

Oedema may be caused by increased capillary permeability, decreased plasma oncotic pressure or increased capillary pressure. It may occur in renal disease either as a result of sodium and water retention or heavy proteinuria causing hypoalbuminaemia (nephrotic syndrome).

Pruritis (itching) is a feature of chronic renal failure. Increased dryness of the skin and phosphate retention are responsible.

Anorexia, nausea and vomiting occur in chronic renal failure, although usually only in advanced disease.

Fatigue may be caused by anaemia.

Dyspnoea may be caused by pulmonary oedema (resulting from fluid retention and/or hypertension) or anaemia.

Investigations

Urinalysis and urine microscopy, for the presence of haematuria, proteinuria and tubular casts (cylindrical structures caused by agglomeration of whole or lysed cells in the tubules). Proteinuria is much more specific for the presence of renal disease; haematuria in the absence of proteinuria is as often due to urological disease (cancer, stones) as to glomerulonephritis.

Blood urea. Urea derives from protein catabolism and is excreted by the kidneys. Raised levels suggest increased protein catabolism (e.g. postoperative, gastrointestinal bleeding), or decreased renal excretion, which may be due to a decreased glomerular filtration rate (GFR) or decreased renal blood flow, e.g. in diuretic treatment for congestive cardiac failure.

Blood creatinine. Creatinine is produced at a constant rate from muscle, and filtered freely at the glomerulus, with little subsequent reabsorption or secretion by the tubule. In the absence of muscle disease or damage, therefore, blood levels vary inversely with GFR, high levels reflecting significant reduction in GFR. Plasma creatinine is a much more reliable marker of renal excretory function than plasma urea.

24-hour urine collection allows quantitation of total protein or albumin excretion and also allows estimation of GFR from creatinine clearance; this is calculated by dividing daily creatinine production rate by plasma creatinine. However, inaccurately timed or incompletely collected urine collections are common. Protein excretion may be more conveniently quantitated by measurement of the protein : creatinine ratio in a random urine specimen. If accurate estimation of GFR is required, the disappearance rate of injected ^{51}Cr ethylenediamine triacetic acid (EDTA) is measured.

Other blood tests. Tests for autoantibodies, monoclonal paraproteins and complement consumption may be indicated in suspected autoimmune disease, myeloma and amyloidosis. A full blood count and film are important in the diagnosis of haemolytic uraemic syndrome. Massive elevation of creatine kinase suggests skeletal muscle damage, which can cause renal failure. Raised lactate dehydrogenase measurements may occur in haemolysis and renal infarction.

Radiology. Renal ultrasound allows assessment of renal size, echogenicity and distension of the collecting systems (hydronephrosis—strongly suggestive of urinary tract obstruction). Plain radiography may also show calculi. Intravenous urography (IVU) gives more anatomical detail but is dependent on renal function. Sometimes it is necessary to proceed to pyelography, either by introducing a needle directly into the kidney ('antegrade') or by catheterising the ureter under anaesthetic ('retrograde'). CT scanning is useful in patients with renal masses or cysts and in suspected ureteric disease. Renal angiography is required for diagnosis of renal vascular disease. Isotope scanning is useful for assessment of renal blood flow, detection of focal scarring and exclusion of obstruction.

Renal biopsy is performed when knowledge of renal histology is likely to influence management, as in suspected acute glomerulonephritis, renal involvement in vasculitis, and progressive chronic renal disease. Samples are obtained by percutaneous siting of a biopsy needle in the lower pole under ultrasound guidance. Renal biopsy is seldom helpful if renal size is reduced, as this always reflects longstanding, and usually irreversible, renal disease. The procedure can cause life-threatening haemorrhage, and should only be performed if coagulation studies are normal.

HYPERTENSION AND THE KIDNEY

The kidney plays a crucial role in regulation of blood pressure via control of renin secretion and of salt and water balance. Hypertension is always associated with subtle alterations in renal function, and is commonly found in patients with overt renal disease. Less commonly, hypertension may cause kidney disease.

MALIGNANT (ACCELERATED) HYPERTENSION

Presenting features
This is a vicious cycle in which severe hypertension causes pressure-related arteriolar damage (fibrinoid necrosis) in the brain, retina and kidney. The latter results in renal ischaemia, with increased renin production and worsening hypertension. Severe renal damage may result, characterised on renal biopsy by damage to the intima and media of arterioles. Haematuria and proteinuria occur. Fibrinoid necrosis in the retinal vessels results in retinal haemorrhage and infarction ('soft exudates'), sometimes with papilloedema, resulting in visual impairment. The severe hypertension may cause acute left ventricular failure and pulmonary oedema.

Investigation
Renal function should be checked; serum creatinine above 300 μmol/l predicts progressive renal impairment and may reflect underlying renal disease, which may be shown by renal biopsy, e.g. glomerulonephritis or scleroderma; renal angiography may show renal artery stenosis.

Treatment and prognosis

Most patients can be managed with oral antihypertensive medication, such as beta-blockers or calcium-channel blockers. Patients with hypertensive encephalopathy or pulmonary oedema should be managed on ITU with short-acting parenteral agents, e.g. sodium nitroprusside. The long-term prognosis depends on the underlying cause and on the severity of target organ damage.

RENOVASCULAR HYPERTENSION

Narrowing (stenosis) of one or both renal arteries sufficient to cause renal ischaemia causes secondary hypertension by activating the renin-angiotensin–aldosterone system. In young adults, renal artery stenosis may occur as a result of fibromuscular dysplasia of the arterial wall. In older adults, it is usually due to atherosclerosis.

Symptoms and signs

Often, there are no symptoms but the presence of angina, claudication or cerebrovascular disease increase the likelihood of finding atherosclerotic renal disease. If both kidneys are affected, renal failure may develop, causing uraemic symptoms. Apart from hypertension, the only clinical sign is an abdominal bruit, which is found in a minority of cases only.

Investigations

Delayed excretion of contrast on IVU is suggestive but unreliable. Delayed transit on isotope renography, particularly after ACE inhibition, is more sensitive. Renal angiography is required to confirm anatomical narrowing, although magnetic resonance angiography may prove reliable in future.

Treatment

Medical treatment consists of antihypertensive drugs. Atherosclerotic renal artery disease is frequently associated with coronary, cerebral and peripheral vascular disease, warranting aspirin and lipid-lowering therapy. Preservation of renal blood flow in the presence of renal artery stenosis is dependent on intrarenal production of angiotensin II; ACE inhibitors prevent this, causing loss of renal function on the affected side, and should therefore be used with great care.

Revascularisation may be achieved either by transluminal angioplasty or stent insertion, or by surgical reconstruction or bypass grafting, depending on the anatomy and on local expertise. Revascularisation seldom cures hypertension in atherosclerotic renal disease, but may be curative in fibromuscular dysplasia.

HYPERTENSION IN CHRONIC RENAL FAILURE

Virtually all patients with renal impairment become hypertensive as renal function declines. The main causes are hypervolaemia from inadequate sodium and water excretion and excessive secretion of renin. It is established that hypertension itself hastens the progression of renal damage and dysfunction, and hence careful blood pressure control is essential.

Treatment

Loop diuretics control the hypervolaemia; high doses may be required. Thiazides are relatively ineffective as the GFR falls, and potassium-sparing diuretics (amiloride, triamterene, spironolactone) may cause dangerous hyperkalaemia.

Beta-blockers, calcium-channel blockers, vasodilators and converting enzyme inhibitors are used as needed to maintain a normal blood pressure.

GLOMERULAR DISEASES

A normal adult kidney has 1 million glomeruli. The extremely high rate of filtration of plasma constituents across the glomerular basement membranes makes them particularly susceptible to injury from circulating molecules such as immunoglobulins, which may be deposited in the basement membrane either as a result of filtration of preformed immune complexes, deposition of immunoglobulin on trapped antigen or, rarely, deposition of antibodies directed specifically at the collagen on the basement membrane. Once trapped, immune complexes may activate the complement pathway and promote invasion of inflammatory cells, leading to glomerular injury.

Other mechanisms of glomerular injury include endothelial damage causing thrombosis; small vessel vasculitis causing necrosis; and a maladaptive trophic response due to hyperglycaemia or loss of neighbouring nephrons, which leads eventually to deposition of fibrous tissue causing glomerulosclerosis.

Because the pathogenesis of most glomerular diseases is not well understood, they are classified according to the histological appearances on renal biopsy. However, because the same appearances may result from a wide range of diseases, there is only a limited correlation between the histological appearances and the clinical presentation. Fig. 7.1 shows the structure of the normal glomerulus and lists the abnormalities that are observed in common glomerular diseases. Glomerular abnormalities may be 'focal' (affecting some glomeruli but sparing others) or 'diffuse' (affecting all glomeruli), and may be 'segmental' (affecting some segments of the glomerulus but sparing the rest) or 'global'.

Correlation between clinical presentation and pathology

Proteinuria is caused by increased permeability of the basement membrane to protein. This may occur without any abnormality on light microscopy (as in 'minimal change' glomerulonephritis) or with evidence of damage, e.g. thickening as in diabetes, or immune complex deposition as in membranous glomerulonephritis and many other forms of chronic glomerulonephritis.

Haematuria is usually associated with glomerular inflammation, characterised by increased numbers of mesangial cells, as in proliferative glomerulonephritis and mesangial IgA disease (p. 222).

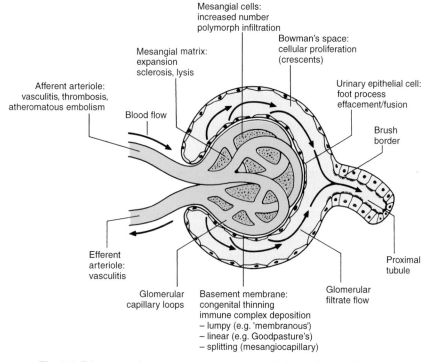

Mesangial cells:
increased number
polymorph infiltration

Bowman's space:
cellular proliferation
(crescents)

Mesangial matrix:
expansion
sclerosis, lysis

Urinary epithelial cell:
foot process
effacement/fusion

Afferent arteriole:
vasculitis, thrombosis,
atheromatous embolism

Blood flow

Brush
border

Efferent
arteriole:
vasculitis

Proximal
tubule

Glomerular
capillary loops

Basement membrane:
congenital thinning
immune complex deposition
– lumpy (e.g. 'membranous')
– linear (e.g. Goodpasture's)
– splitting (mesangiocapillary)

Glomerular
filtrate flow

Fig. 7.1 Diagrammatic representation of the normal glomerulus, and its repertoire of response to injury.

Chronic renal failure is associated with glomerulosclerosis and, more reliably, with interstitial scarring and tubular atrophy. It may complicate most forms of chronic glomerulonephritis.

The acute nephritic syndrome (acute renal impairment, fluid retention, hypertension, haematuria and proteinuria) is associated with acute glomerulonephritis, e.g. post-streptococcal diffuse proliferative glomerulonephritis or crescentic glomerulonephritis complicating systemic vasculitis.

The nephrotic syndrome (oedema, heavy proteinuria (> 3 g/24 hours) and hypoalbuminaemia) most often occurs in minimal-change glomerulonephritis, membranous glomerulonephritis and focal segmental glomerulosclerosis.

Table 7.1 lists some of the common categories of glomerulonephritis and their clinical presentation.

ACUTE GLOMERULONEPHRITIS

Diffuse proliferative glomerulonephritis

This occurs 10–14 days after streptococcal infection (e.g. pharyngitis) and results from immune complex-mediated glomerular damage. Its frequency is decreasing, possibly as a result of widespread antibiotic use for sore throats.

Table 7.1. Categories of glomerulonephritis (GN)

	Pathology	Immuno-fluoresence	Common clinical presentation
Proliferative GN	Endothelial and mesangial cell proliferation	C_3, IgG deposits	Acute nephritis, SLE
Minimal change GN	Normal	Absent	Nephrotic syndrome
Membranous GN	Thickening of GBM	IgG, C_3 deposits	SLE, nephrotic syndrome, chronic renal failure (33%)
Membrano-proliferative (mesangiocapillary) GN	Thickening of GBM, mesangial cell proliferation	C_3	Nephrotic syndrome, renal failure (50%)
Focal glomerulo-sclerosis	Segmental and focal sclerosis of glomeruli	? C_3, IgM	Nephrotic syndrome, renal failure (50%)
IgA nephropathy	Mesangial cell proliferation	Mesangial IgA	Recurrent haematuria, renal failure (20%)
Rapidly progressive GN	Crescents	Linear deposits IgG, C_3	Haematuria, proteinuria, renal failure (80–100%)

SLE = systemic lupus erythematosus; GBM = glomerular basement membrane.

It causes acute renal impairment, hypertension and oedema. Urinalysis shows proteinuria and haematuria. Investigation shows complement consumption, high titres of anti-streptolysin O and anti-DNAase B antibodies, and is confirmed, if necessary, by renal biopsy. Antihypertensive treatment, fluid restriction, diuretics and occasionally dialysis are required, but full recovery is the rule.

Henoch–Schönlein glomerulonephritis

This may complicate Henoch–Schönlein purpura, a skin vasculitis causing a purpuric rash on the extensor surfaces, arthralgia, and abdominal pain, which occurs most frequently in children. Renal involvement presents with haematuria, proteinuria and sometimes nephrotic syndrome. Mesangial IgA deposition is found on renal biopsy, together with focal segmental glomerulo-nephritis. Renal failure develops in a minority of cases. Henoch–Schönlein purpura is the name given to the rash, which frequently occurs without renal involvement. No treament is of proven benefit.

Rapidly progressive glomerulonephritis

This term is given to glomerulonephritis resulting in rapidly worsening renal function. It is most often caused by small vessel systemic vasculitis, causing glomerular capillary damage (p. 379), e.g. microscopic polyangiitis or Wegener's granulomatosis. Both diseases may affect other organs and cause a multisystem illness. Tests for serum antineutrophil cytoplasmic antibodies (ANCA) are usually positive. A similar clinical picture can be caused by anti-glomerular basement antibody disease (Goodpasture's disease), in which tests for antiglomerular basement antibodies are usually positive. Necrosis of glomerular capillaries ('necrotising glomerulonephritis') is associated with formation of epithelial crescents in Bowman's space. Untreated, these diseases progress to irreversible renal failure within days or weeks; however, aggressive immunosuppressive treatment with steroids and cyclophosphamide often results in recovery if started early enough.

CHRONIC GLOMERULAR DISEASES

The incidental finding of haematuria or proteinuria, or both, on medical examination of apparently healthy subjects is relatively common. Often these abnormalities are found to be due to chronic glomerulonephritis if investigated exhaustively. Chronic glomerulonephritis may also cause hypertension and chronic renal impairment.

IgA nephropathy

This is the most common cause of glomerular disease and is, by definition, associated with deposition of IgA in the mesangium. A variety of histological patterns of glomerular damage may occur; most common is an increase in mesangial matrix and cellularity. The cause is uncertain: the IgA deposited originates from the bone marrow and is abnormally glycosylated. The disease may be detected when haematuria with or without proteinuria is found on 'routine' urinalysis, but may also present with macroscopic haematuria, commonly following heavy exercise or within 1–2 days of an upper respiratory infection, with hypertension, or with nephrotic syndrome, and occasionally with acute renal failure. Progression to end-stage renal failuremay occur in up to 30% of patients in whom the diagnosis is confirmed by biopsy: progression is predicted by the presence of hypertension and proteinuria, and glomerulosclerosis and tubular damage on renal biopsy. There is no treatment of proven benefit, although recent evidence suggests that immunosuppressive treatment may be beneficial in carefully selected cases, and that fish oil may delay progression of established chronic renal impairment.

Membranous nephropathy

This is the most common cause of nephrotic syndrome in adults. It is defined by the presence of immune complexes in the glomerular basement membranes, which are irregularly thickened. It may be primary, or secondary to malignancy, autoimmune disease, drugs or chronic infection. Some patients with primary disease go into full remission; others follow a relapsing and remitting course, and others show progressive decline in renal function, which may be arrested by immunosuppressive therapy.

Mesangiocapillary glomerulonephritis (also called membranoproliferative)

This is a rare cause of nephrotic syndrome or renal failure characterised by proliferation of mesangial cells and disruption of the basement membrane, associated with immune complex deposition and persistent complement consumption. No treatment is of proven benefit.

Focal and segmental glomerulosclerosis (FSGS)

'Primary' FSGS is an important cause of nephrotic syndrome. Its cause is not understood, but there is evidence for an immune aetiology. Some patients respond to prolonged immunosuppressive treatment, but if remission from nephrotic syndrome is not obtained there is relentless progression to end-stage renal failure. A similar histological picture may occur as a late result of a wide range of renal diseases.

Diabetic nephropathy

This complicates the course of 30–40% of patients with diabetes mellitus, both IDDM and NIDDM (p. 213). It is caused by progressive deposition of extracellular matrix including collagen in the glomerular mesangium, causing a characteristic histological appearance ('nodular glomerulosclerosis'). Risk factors for the development of diabetic nephropathy include poor glycaemic control, smoking, and a family history of hypertension. It usually occurs in association with other microvascular and macrovascular complications. Affected patients develop increased urinary albumin excretion, hypertension and progressive renal failure. Blood pressure reduction, particularly with ACE inhibitors, reduces the rate of deterioration of renal function.

NEPHROTIC SYNDROME

The nephrotic syndrome is the combination of heavy proteinuria (> 3 g/day), hypoalbuminaemia and peripheral oedema. Several different glomerular diseases may cause the syndrome, including minimal change nephropathy, some forms of acute and chronic glomerulonephritis, diabetic nephropathy and amyloidosis. In all of these, there is loss of the normal sieving characteristics of the glomerulus leading to increased loss of plasma proteins into the glomerular filtrate, exceeding the capacity of the tubules to reabsorb protein. The proteinuria also causes intense renal sodium retention.

Symptoms and signs

Most patients complain of oedema, but some also have malaise or symptoms of chronic renal failure. On examination the oedema is pitting. Peripheral oedema worsens with upright posture; in the morning, facial oedema may be obvious. Ascites, pleural effusions and pulmonary oedema may also occur in severe cases.

Investigations

The diagnosis is confirmed by finding heavy proteinuria (> 3 g in a 24-hour urine collection, or > 300 mg/mmol creatinine on a random urine collection) and hypoalbuminaemia (< 30 g/l). Hypercholesterolaemia (due to increased hepatic synthesis in response to low plasma oncotic pressure) is nearly always present. Urinalysis, microscopy and tests for diabetes, autoantibodies, anti-streptococcal antibodies, complement consumption and monoclonal proteins may give clues to the underlying cause. However, renal biopsy is often necessary in adults, particularly in the presence of haematuria and/or renal impairment, as treatment depends on the histological findings.

Minimal-change nephropathy

This is the most common cause of nephrotic syndrome in children, but may occur at any age. By definition, there is minimal or no glomerular abnormality on light microscopy of a renal biopsy, although fusion of podocyte foot processes is seen on electron microscopy. The cause is unknown; there is an association with atopy and evidence for an abnormality of T-lymphocyte function. Untreated, there is a high morbidity and mortality from the complications of nephrotic syndrome (see below), but progression to renal failure does not occur. Remission can be induced with high-dose corticosteroid treatment, e.g. prednisolone 40–60 mg/day. In patients with frequent relapses, cyclosporin may be used to maintain remission. Alternatively, a 12-week course of cyclophosphamide reduces the risk of subsequent relapse.

Differential diagnosis

It is important to differentiate nephrotic syndrome from heart failure (which may cause moderate proteinuria) and liver disease. In heart failure the jugular venous pressure is high, whereas it is normal or low in nephrotic syndrome. Hypoalbuminaemia due to liver disease is usually associated with obvious signs of liver disease.

Complications

The nephrotic syndrome causes increased blood coagulability and is associated with an increased risk of deep venous thrombosis and renal vein thrombosis (which may cause acute renal failure). There is an increased risk of infection, particularly by pneumococci. Long-term nephrotic syndrome may increase the risk of atherosclerosis, but it is not yet known if cholesterol-lowering treatment alters this risk.

Treatment

General treatment of the nephrotic syndrome consists of diuretics (which may initially need to be given intravenously) and restriction of sodium and water intake. Prophylactic anticoagulation should be considered. Specific immunosuppressive treatment is available for some of the causes of nephrotic syndrome, particularly minimal-change nephropathy. If the underlying cause cannot be treated, protein excretion can be reduced by the use of ACE inhibitors in combination with dietary sodium restriction. Consideration should also be given to cholesterol-lowering therapy.

RENAL INVOLVEMENT IN SYSTEMIC DISEASE

In addition to systemic vasculitis and diabetes, other systemic diseases may also affect the kidney.

Systemic lupus erythematosus (SLE)

A variety of renal lesions may develop in patients with SLE; however, renal disease is seldom the first manifestation. Abnormal urinalysis or deteriorating renal function in a patient with active SLE should prompt renal biopsy, to help decide whether to advise intensive immunosuppressive treatment. This reduces the risk of progression to renal failure in active disease; in less active or burnt-out disease the risks (including infertility and opportunistic infection) outweigh the potential benefits.

Systemic sclerosis

Marked thickening of the arterial intima occurs and results in ischaemic glomerular damage and histological appearances indistinguishable from malignant hypertension. Adequate control of hypertension is very important in minimising renal damage.

Sickle cell anaemia

The kidney may be affected in several ways. Sickling of erythrocytes in the renal medulla, where oxygen tension is low, causes episodic macroscopic haematuria. Hypoxic tubular damage may cause nephrogenic diabetes insipidus. Glomerular damage may cause renal failure.

Haemolytic–uraemic syndrome (HUS) and thrombotic thrombocytopenic purpura (TTP)

These are related disorders in which there is intravascular haemolysis, sometimes triggered by infection, with fragmentation of red cells, fibrin deposition in small blood vessels and thrombocytopenia. In the kidney this process, called microangiopathic haemolytic anaemia, causes oliguria, haematuria and uraemia. Short-term support by dialysis may be required. Recovery from HUS is usual but the outlook is worse in adults, who often also develop neurological complications and failure of other organs.

Myeloma

Renal failure is common in this condition and has several possible causes, including hypercalcaemia, secondary hypovolaemia and tubular accumulation of myeloma paraprotein. Renal amyloidosis may complicate myeloma.

Amyloidosis

Tissue deposition of this insoluble protein may result from polymerisation of immunoglobulin light chains (AL amyloid) (with or without overt myeloma), or of serum amyloid A protein (AA amyloid), in chronic inflammatory conditions such as rheumatoid arthritis or osteomyelitis. In the kidney this produces refractory nephrotic syndrome and progressive renal failure.

Hepatorenal syndrome

This may complicate chronic ascites and liver failure. There is oliguria, hyponatraemia, intense sodium reabsorption and a reduction in GFR.

URINARY TRACT INFECTION

Urinary tract infection (UTI) is much more common in women than in men, probably because of the short length of the female urethra and proximity to the anal region, allowing ascending infection by bowel organisms. The most common infecting organism in UTI is *Escherichia coli*. Bladder infection (cystitis) is facilitated by poor bladder emptying, previous damage to the bladder epithelium and low urinary flow rates. Ascent of infection up the ureters is aided by vesico-ureteric reflux which occurs when normal valvular action at the uretero–vesical junction during bladder contraction is defective. Ascending infection results in renal parenchymal infection (pyelonephritis).

Symptoms

The symptoms of lower UTI are dysuria, cloudy and offensive-smelling urine and urgency of micturition. Suprapubic pain or tenderness, urinary frequency and nocturia are also present.

In pyelonephritis there may also be marked pyrexia and rigors, loin pain on the affected side, nausea and vomiting.

Investigation and treatment

The diagnosis is confirmed by urine microscopy, which shows pyuria, and by urine culture, usually obtained by collection of a midstream specimen. In symptomatic patients, 10^2–10^3 organisms/ml indicate infection; lower counts are usually due to contamination of urine from the vulva or foreskin during collection. Suprapubic aspiration or bladder catheterisation may be used to obtain uncontaminated bladder urine; in these specimens, any growth is significant.

Repeated infections in sexually active women do not usually warrant further investigation. Atrophic vaginitis is a treatable cause in older women. Persistent infection despite appropriate antibiotic treatment and genuine mixed growths warrants urography to look for an underlying abnormality. Infections in men are most often due to impaired bladder emptying or prostatitis.

Uncomplicated infections in women respond well to single dose or short courses of antibiotics. Acute pyelonephritis requires 10–14 days' treatment. Recurrent reinfection in women may be prevented by long-term low-dose prophylactic antibiotics.

Pyuria without bacterial growth on urine culture may be due to renal tuberculosis or papillary necrosis. Renal tuberculosis is confirmed by culture of early morning urine and treated with combination chemotherapy.

TUBULO-INTERSTITIAL NEPHRITIS

After chronic glomerulonephritis, chronic inflammation of the renal tubules and interstitium, with relative glomerular sparing, is the second most common finding in patients with chronic renal failure. It was once assumed that virtually all of these cases were caused by repeated urinary infection with reflux—'chronic pyelonephritis'. However, repeated infection with reflux in adult women does not cause renal impairment, although it may do so in infancy. In half of all adult patients who have histologically proven chronic tubulo-interstitial nephritis, no cause is established. Of the remaining 50%, a proportion are caused by infection and reflux in childhood.

Papillary necrosis accounts for another group of patients with tubulo-interstitial nephritis. In this condition there is ischaemic injury to the papillae, which may slough and pass into the ureter, causing obstruction. Diagnostic changes of calyceal clubbing are seen on IVU. The best-known cause of papillary necrosis is analgesic nephropathy—ingestion over years of large quantities of analgesics including salicylate, paracetamol and especially its metabolite phenacetin. Other causes of papillary necrosis are diabetes mellitus, sickle cell disease and toxin exposure, e.g. to lead or cadmium.

Acute increases in serum uric acid level (hyperuricaemia) occur when chemotherapy of lymphomas and other tumours leads to massive cell lysis and generation of urate. This may precipitate in the renal tubules, causing obstruction and uraemia. There is no strong evidence that chronic hyperuricaemia, the cause of gout, leads to renal failure. However, increased uric acid secretion may cause development of uric acid stones.

RENAL STONE DISEASE

Up to 5% of the population develop calculi at some stage. These may occur in the collecting system of the kidney (nephrolithiasis) or within the ureters and bladder (urolithiasis). Much more rarely, the renal parenchyma becomes calcified (nephrocalcinosis) as a result of hypercalcaemia, or as a consequence of medullary sponge kidney or renal tubular acidosis. Most calculi contain calcium and oxalate. Increased urinary concentration of calcium or oxalate, and decreased concentrations of inhibitors of stone formation such as citrate, are commonly found. Occasionally, increased urinary calcium excretion results from hypercalcaemia (hyperparathyroidism, sarcoidosis, vitamin D ingestion). Calcium oxalate stones are radio-opaque, in contrast to uric acid stones, which are radiolucent.

'Staghorn' calculi which enlarge slowly, outlining the renal pelvis, may develop in association with chronic UTI, especially with *Proteus mirabilis*. They also develop in cystinuria, an inborn tendency to excrete excessive urinary cystine.

Symptoms

Passage of a stone into the ureter causes renal colic with sharp severe flank pain radiating to the groin, and accompanying nausea, vomiting and sweating. There is no postural relief and it is worsened by increased urine flow rate.

Investigations

The diagnosis can be rapidly established by urine testing, microscopy and culture for haematuria, pyuria and coexistent UTI, renal ultrasound, abdominal X-ray and tomography for radio-opaque calculi, IVU to localise ureteric calculi. 24-hour urine is collected for excretion of calcium, oxalate and uric acid, and serum calcium is checked.

Differential diagnosis

This is wide and includes any cause of acute and severe abdominal pain, such as cholecystitis, pancreatitis or bowel pathology. In practice, the history of renal colic is usually typical and the diagnosis confirmed by abdominal X-ray demonstrating a stone, and coexistence of microscopic haematuria.

Treatment

Acute management of renal colic is conservative with adequate pain relief (opiates). Stones not passed spontaneously require urological removal. When possible this is endoscopic, involving percutaneous nephrolithotomy (kidney puncture), or ureteroscopic removal of lower ureteric stones.

Extracorporeal shock wave lithotripsy (ESWL) is increasingly performed; in this technique high-frequency shock waves are focused to shatter the calculus, enabling passage of fragments.

Prevention of recurrent stone formation involves ensuring a high daily fluid intake (3–4 litres per 24 hours) to reduce urinary mineral concentration. Dietary calcium restriction increases oxalate absorption, and is not useful. Thiazide diuretics reduce recurrence rates by reducing urinary calcium excretion.

URINARY TRACT OBSTRUCTION

Obstruction of urinary outflow may cause either acute or chronic renal

Table 7.2. Sites of urinary tract obstruction

Tubules	Precipitation, e.g. urate or sulphonamide crystals
Collecting system	Sloughed papilla
	Staghorn calculus
	Tumour
	Pelvic–ureteric junction obstruction
	Blood clot
Ureters	Stricture (previous calculus, tuberculosis)
	Calculus
	Blood clot
	Compression (retroperitoneal fibrosis, tumour)
Bladder	Tumour
	Blood clot
	Ureterovesical stricture
	Neuropathic bladder
Urethra	Prostatic hypertrophy (males)
	Stricture

failure. Acute obstruction may result in severe uraemia but full recovery is usually possible, provided the obstruction is rapidly relieved. In contrast, chronic obstruction, as in prostatic hypertrophy, may lead to unsuspected chronic renal failure with limited scope for recovery. Obstruction may occur at any point in the urinary tract, and potential sites are shown in Table 7.2. The blockage may be intraluminal (e.g. clot, calculus), or from abnormal urinary tract narrowing (stricture) or external compression (e.g. tumour). Obstruction above the level of the bladder must be bilateral to cause anuria or uraemia.

Acute obstruction causes dilatation above the blockage and back pressure which ultimately nullifies glomerular filtration pressure. If it persists, tubular and interstitial atrophy occur with eventual glomerular sclerosis. The tubular damage also interferes with urinary concentrating mechanisms, and many patients with prolonged obstruction have polyuria and nocturia.

Symptoms and signs
Loin pain and anuria occur in complete acute obstruction. Chronic partial obstruction causes polyuria, urinary retention and incomplete bladder emptying. Dysuria and frequency occur if there is accompanying infection.

The kidneys are palpable if they are enlarged by acute obstruction. Prostatic enlargement is present in prostatic hypertrophy. The bladder is enlarged and palpable in bladder outflow obstruction.

Investigations
In contrast to glomerulonephritis, urine microscopy shows no cellular casts. Renal ultrasonography will rapidly show whether a dilated collecting system is present, confirming obstruction. Cystoscopy with retrograde ureteric catheterisation will define precisely the site of a ureteric lesion. Alternatively, antegrade pyelography will visualise the upper ureter.

Abdominal CT scanning will demonstrate extrinsic compression from tumour or retroperitoneal fibrosis, a condition in which the ureters become encased in fibrous tissue, there is low back pain and the erythrocyte sedimentation rate (ESR) is raised.

Differential diagnosis
This is with the other causes of uraemia (p. 235).

Treatment
The principles are relief of the obstruction and decompression of the collecting system.

Prostatic obstruction is relieved by passage of a urinary catheter, until definitive prostate resection. Ureteric obstruction is bypassed with 'double J' stents at retrograde urography. If this is not possible, a percutaneous nephrostomy is inserted at antegrade pyelography, under local anaesthesia, with insertion of a drainage catheter into the renal pelvis. This will maintain urine flow and renal function pending a definitive procedure.

In retroperitoneal fibrosis the ureters are freed surgically (ureterolysis) or stented; steroid therapy may help prevent relapses.

Prognosis
There is complete recovery of renal function if acute obstruction is rapidly relieved. Unsuspected chronic obstruction may lead to irreversible renal failure, requiring long-term dialysis.

CYSTIC RENAL DISEASES

There are several forms of inherited or congenital cystic disease of the kidney. In all of them, cysts develop within the renal parenchyma but the outcomes differ greatly. Small renal cysts also arise with ageing, and in long-term dialysis patients.

ADULT POLYCYSTIC KIDNEY DISEASE (APKD)

APKD is an autosomal dominant condition and is by far the most common inherited cause of renal failure. Minute cysts, present from birth, progressively enlarge, causing loss of function. The cysts are apparent on ultrasound examination by late adolescence. Up to 60% of patients develop end-stage renal failure, usually after the age of 40.

Symptoms and signs
Bleeding or infection within the cysts causes fever, loin pain or tenderness. There is dull flank pain when the kidneys are large and ureteric colic from blood clots.

Grossly enlarged and irregular kidneys are usually easily palpable on abdominal examination. Hypertension is especially common in APKD. Associated hepatic cysts lead to liver enlargement.

Investigations

The diagnosis is readily made by ultrasound scanning, or alternatively by abdominal CT scan. Renal function is accurately assessed (serum creatinine or creatinine clearance). Urine culture is performed to exclude coexistent infection.

Treatment

The major principles of management in APKD are effective treatment of both urinary infection and hypertension, to maximise maintenance of renal function. Cyst infection may lead to severe septicaemia and requires parenteral antibiotics and cyst aspiration and drainage. Cyst debris or blood clots may cause acute ureteric obstruction.

A complication of APKD, in some families, is an association with berry aneurysms of the cerebral circulation, a potentially fatal cause of subarachnoid haemorrhage. Development of severe headache and focal neurological signs in a patient with APKD should always arouse suspicion of this complication. Mitral valve prolapse and sigmoid diverticular disease are also associated.

Prognosis

Patients with APKD and significant renal impairment will progress slowly but steadily to end-stage renal failure over a period of years.

Although antenatal diagnosis of APKD is now possible by genetic linkage analysis, the case for therapeutic abortion in this condition, in which the quality and duration of life may be near-normal, remains highly controversial.

MEDULLARY CYSTIC DISEASE

Inheritance may be recessive or dominant and end-stage renal failure develops in late adolescence. Development of small medullary cysts results in tubulo-interstitial scarring and secondary glomerular sclerosis.

In contrast, medullary sponge kidney is not inherited but is a sporadic and benign disorder in which medullary cysts develop and often calcify. Patients are prone to ureteric colic and urinary infection but renal function is preserved.

ACUTE RENAL FAILURE

Acute renal failure is characterised by rapid loss of renal function and the development of uraemia within hours or days. Usually, though not always, it is reversible. In contrast, chronic renal failure is the final outcome of many glomerular and tubulo-interstitial diseases and is slowly progressive, but irreversible loss of renal function occurs. The functional consequences of renal failure are similar whether acute or chronic and include uraemia, with loss of renal excretory function, loss of fluid and electrolyte balance, loss of acid–base balance, and abnormal endocrine function. However,

Table 7.3. Differentiation of acute and chronic renal failure

	Acute renal failure	Chronic renal failure
Duration of uraemic symptoms	Short (days)	Weeks or months Nocturia and cramps precede more severe symptoms
Signs		
Hypertension	Infrequent	Usual
Anaemia	Variable	Present (except polycystic disease)
Investigations		
Renal size	Normal	Small (except in amyloidosis, myeloma or polycystic kidney disease)
Secondary hyperparathyroidism	Absent	Present

the distinction between acute and chronic renal failure can usually be made using the guidelines summarised in Table 7.3.

In practice, the most useful pointers to longstanding chronic renal failure are demonstration of small echogenic kidneys on ultrasound scan and evidence of secondary hyperparathyroidism (phalangeal erosions, elevated serum parathyroid hormone) as neither occurs in acute renal failure. Tracing previous blood test results also helps.

Traditionally, the aetiology of acute renal failure is divided into pre-renal, renal and post-renal causes (Table 7.4). Although inexact, it is a useful categorisation, as it helps determine management. Pre- and post-renal failure (obstruction) in particular may respond rapidly to therapy if recognised and treated sufficiently early. The common factor in pre-renal failure is impaired renal perfusion, which causes a compensatory fall in the GFR and very avid sodium and water reabsorption. If renal perfusion remains impaired, acute tubular necrosis (ATN) supervenes. This is a progressive decline in both glomerular and tubular function, whose pathogenesis remains poorly understood. On renal biopsy there is patchy tubular necrosis and the glomeruli appear normal. Once ATN is established, there is an obligatory period of oliguria and renal failure, usually lasting 2–4 weeks, and followed by a diuretic phase as renal function recovers.

Symptoms and signs

These depend on the cause of acute renal failure, e.g. loin or back pain in urinary tract obstruction, haematuria and oedema in acute glomerulo-nephritis. Uraemic symptoms (anorexia, nausea, malaise, clouding of consciousness) may be marked in severe acute renal failure.

The signs also depend on the cause; hypotension and tachycardia are seen with haemorrhage or septicaemia, and hypertension and oedema in acute glomerulonephritis or rapidly progressive glomerulonephritis.

Table 7.4. Causes of acute renal failure

Pre-renal

Impaired renal perfusion	Hypotension, septic shock, volume depletion (haemorrhage, burns, gastrointestinal fluid loss)
Renal artery occlusion	Atherosclerotic thromboembolism, aortic dissection
Hepatorenal syndrome	

Renal

Glomerular disease	Acute proliferative GN (post-streptococcal), rapidly progressive GN, vasculitis, anti-GBM disease, haemolytic–uraemic syndrome
Acute interstitial nephritis	Penicillins, thiazides, non-steroidal anti-inflammatory drugs
Rhabdomyolysis + myoglobinuria	Trauma
Systemic infections	Viral infection, leptospirosis, legionella, HIV

Post-renal

Urinary tract obstruction	Intrarenal, renal pelvis, ureters, bladder, urethra

GN, glomerulonephritis; GBM, glomerular basement membrane.

Investigations

Assessment of volume status is crucial in patients with acute renal failure, to determine whether the intravascular volume is decreased (hypovolaemia) or increased (hypervolaemia). The guidelines for this are outlined in Table 7.5. The most sensitive parameter is the blood pressure (BP) and heart rate response to standing.

Urine microscopy shows urine virtually free of protein, cells or casts in pre-renal uraemia or obstructive uropathy. With ATN proteinuria, pyuria and tubular cell casts appear. Red cell casts indicate glomerulonephritis.

Urine of high osmolality and low sodium concentration (< 20 mmol/l) indicates intact tubular function and suggests hypovolaemia. Dilute urine

Table 7.5. Assessment of volume status

	Hypovolaemia	Hypervolaemia
Supine blood pressure	Normal or low	High
Postural BP fall	Present	Absent
Postural tachycardia	> 20/min	< 20/min
Tissue turgor	Reduced	Normal
Jugular venous pressure	Low	High
Pulmonary oedema	Absent	Present
Peripheral oedema	Absent	Present

with a higher sodium concentration occurs after diuretic treatment and in ATN.

Urgent ultrasound scanning is essential to determine kidney size and to exclude obstruction. An abdominal X-ray may show urinary tract calculi.

Renal biopsy is not indicated in obstruction and not necessary in ATN, unless the diagnosis is uncertain. It should be performed when rapidly progressive glomerulonephritis, accelerated hypertension or drug-induced acute interstitial nephritis is suspected.

Treatment

The need for urgency in evaluation of the cause of acute renal failure has already been stressed. This enables correct management.

Pre-renal uraemia

To minimise the likelihood of progression to ATN, hypovolaemia is corrected by volume expansion with saline, albumin or blood, as appropriate. Central venous pressure is monitored, and maintained in the range 5–10 cmH$_2$O. Frusemide and dopamine increase urine output but do not improve GFR or reduce the risk of established ATN.

Renal and post-renal acute renal failure

Outflow obstruction is relieved as soon as possible. If acute glomerulo-nephritis or vasculitis is diagnosed serologically or on renal biopsy, intensive immunosuppression is given.

Acute interstititial nephritis is a drug-induced hypersensitivity reaction, in which renal tubulo-interstitial inflammation may be accompanied by an erythematous skin rash, arthralgia and fever. The drug implicated is withdrawn and a short course of steroids is given. Complete recovery is usual.

Established acute renal failure

Meticulous management is essential, paying attention to several aspects.

Fluid and electrolyte balance. Stability is maintained by monitoring daily weight (1 litre of fluid lost/gained is 1 kg change in bodyweight), BP and pulse, central venous pressure and fluid balance. Plasma urea and electrolyte levels are measured daily. Salt and water intake are also adjusted daily to maintain normovolaemia. Potassium intake is restricted in the oliguric phase. In the polyuric phase, large volumes of i.v. crystalloids may be required to replace urinary losses.

Nutrition. Protein intake is reduced to minimise protein catabolism and urea load and 2000 kcal daily given as carbohydrate and fat.

Sepsis is avoided. Bladder catheterisation is unnecessary and should not be used.

Dialysis. If plasma urea and creatinine levels continue to increase despite the above measures, renal support is commenced. Other indications for dialysis are pulmonary oedema, pericarditis, hyperkalaemia (serum potassium > 6.5 mmol/l) and severe acidosis (pH < 7.2). Three main modes of renal support are used:

1. acute peritoneal dialysis
2. intermittent haemodialysis
3. continuous haemofiltration, which may be combined with dialysis (CAVHD, CVVHD). The patient's blood is circulated continually through a semipermeable membrane; up to 20 litres per 24 hours of plasma ultrafiltrate is removed and replaced by electrolyte solution.

Prognosis

With adequate dialysis support during the oliguric–uraemic phase, full recovery often occurs in acute renal failure. However, ATN often occurs as part of multiple organ dysfunction, and so the overall mortality of acute renal failure remains 50% or more.

CHRONIC RENAL FAILURE

Chronic renal failure is the end result of many of the different forms of renal injury already described. It refers to a progressive and usually irreversible loss of renal function. Once this is insufficient to sustain life (usually when GFR is 5% or less of normal), end-stage or terminal renal failure has occurred. The rate of decline depends on the underlying disease. It may be several weeks in rapidly progressive glomerulonephritis and many years in polycystic kidney disease and chronic pyelonephritis.

Although there are many possible causes of chronic renal failure, most fall into a few categories and the most common, in order, are chronic glomerulonephritis, chronic pyelonephritis/tubulo-interstitial nephritis, diabetic nephropathy, APKD and ischaemic nephropathy.

End-stage renal failure is rare, developing in 80–120 patients per million population per year. Resources for renal replacement therapy are limited. These limitations have led in the past to patients being denied treatment, often on the grounds of diabetes, age or coexistent morbidity, even though such patients can achieve satisfactory quality of life with dialysis or transplantation. The issue of how to prioritise spending on expensive treatments such as these continues to be the subject of intense ethical debate worldwide.

Prognosis

Chronic renal failure may remain stable, or may continue to progress to end-stage renal failure. Progression is usually characterised by a linear fall in GFR and, once a certain level of renal damage has occurred, appears to continue independent of the activity of the underlying disease, probably as a maladaptive response of remaining nephrons to renal injury. Such progression is usually characterised by hypertension, proteinuria, and progressive glomerulosclerosis and interstitial fibrosis. Because of the inverse relationship

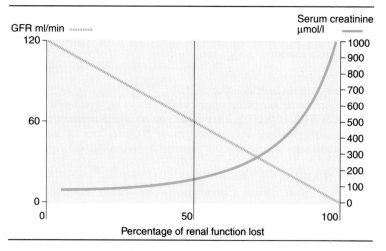

Fig. 7.2 Relationship between the linear decline in glomerular filtration rate (GFR) and exponential rise in serum creatinine levels as renal function is lost.

between GFR and serum creatinine, loss of renal function is best monitored by plotting serum creatinine or GFR against time (Fig. 7.2).

Symptoms

The onset of chronic renal failure is usually insidious and over half the renal function may be lost before any symptoms develop. Severe uraemia may cause symptoms referable to virtually every organ system (Table 7.6). The early symptoms of chronic renal failure (nocturia, polyuria, leg cramps) may give a guide to its duration. Nausea, fatigue and other characteristic uraemic symptoms arise relatively late.

Table 7.6. Clinical features of chronic renal failure

System	Symptoms
Cardiovascular	Hypertension, heart failure, pericarditis, oedema, ischaemic heart disease
Central nervous	Confusion, coma (severe uraemia), autonomic and/or peripheral neuropathy
Endocrine and metabolic	Hyperparathyroidism, amenorrhoea, infertility, glucose intolerance, hyperlipidaemia
Skin	Pruritus, pigmentation
Musculoskeletal	Muscle cramps, myopathy, bone pain (renal osteodystrophy), restless legs
Blood	Anaemia, platelet dysfunction

Signs

Signs may be few or absent in early chronic renal failure. In severe disease they are widespread and include oedema and hypertension from hypervolaemia, anaemia, peripheral neuropathy and uraemic fetor. In severe uraemia there may also be pericardial rub, confusion and metabolic flap.

Anaemia is largely caused by the failure of production of erythropoietin and accounts for much of the fatigue, lethargy and dyspnoea. It also worsens symptoms of ischaemic heart disease and causes left ventricular dilatation and hypertrophy.

Hypertension and hyperlipidaemia predispose renal failure patients to atherosclerosis; they also have a very high risk of stroke, myocardial infarction and heart failure.

Renal bone disease occurs for several reasons:

1. Decreased activation of vitamin D (cholecalciferol). Cholecalciferol normally undergoes 1-hydroxylation in the kidney and 25-hydroxylation in the liver. 1,25-dihydroxyvitamin D promotes bone mineralisation, increases calcium absorption, and directly suppresses production of parathyroid hormone (PTH); defective hydroxylation therefore results in defective bone mineralisation, calcium malabsorption and increased PTH secretion.
2. Phosphate retention is an early feature of chronic renal failure, and also causes increased PTH secretion.
3. Hypocalcaemia, resulting from calcium malabsorption, stimulates PTH secretion.
4. Increased PTH secretion results in increased mobilisation of calcium from bone, returning serum calcium towards normal.

The result is a combination of osteomalacia (due to defective bone mineralisation) and increased bone reabsorption with bone marrow fibrosis resulting from excessive PTH action. Both may cause bone pain and pathological fractures. Osteomalacia can only reliably be diagnosed by bone biopsy: hyperparathyroidism can be diagnosed by measurement of serum PTH (and alkaline phosphatase, which reflects bone turnover) and by radiology, which shows subperiosteal erosions in severe cases. Increased PTH secretion in chronic renal failure is termed secondary hyperparathyroidism, to distinguish it from primary hyperparathyroidism (p. 197). Prolonged secondary hyperparathyroidism may eventually result in resetting of the feedback control of PTH secretion by serum calcium, resulting in tertiary hyperparathyroidism, in which parathyroid overactivity results in hypercalcaemia.

Investigations

Ultrasound examination often shows decreased renal size (indicating irreversible loss of renal mass) and increased echogenicity. Focal scarring may also be seen, as in reflux nephropathy or renal embolism. The smaller the kidneys, the less likely that any disease found on renal biopsy will be reversible. For this reason, biopsies are seldom performed if the renal length on ultrasound is less than 9 cm. Renal asymmetry suggests reflux nephropathy, dysplasia or ischaemia.

Renal function is monitored initially by serial measurement of creatinine clearance or isotopic GFR and later by serum creatinine measurement.

The anaemia of renal failure is normochromic and normocytic, but haematinic deficiency, haemolysis and occult blood loss should be excluded if anaemia is unduly severe.

Regular measurements of serum calcium and phosphate are necessary: measurements of serum PTH are required for the diagnosis and monitoring of secondary hyperparathyroidism.

Treatment

Careful attention must be paid to avoidance of further renal damage, including avoidance of nephrotoxic drugs, relief of urinary tract obstruction and correction of hypovolaemia.

Effective control of hypertension is essential, because blood pressure reduction retards the progression of chronic renal disease. Correction of salt and water overload, which may require high doses of loop diuretics, is necessary for effective blood pressure control. In patients with proteinuria, ACE inhibitors offer better protection against progressive loss of renal function than other antihypertensive agents; however, these drugs are deleterious in ischaemic renal disease.

Dietary restriction of sodium and potassium intake is often necessary. Restriction of protein intake has theoretical benefits, and probably slows progression in proteinuric renal diseases. It also delays the onset of symptoms as renal failure approaches.

Correction of anaemia improves symptoms and prevents left ventricular hypertrophy. After exclusion of other causes, recombinant human erythropoietin, given by subcutaneous injection, is highly effective, although expensive. This treatment avoids the risks of blood transfusion, which include transmission of viral infections and sensitisation to HLA antigens, prejudicing later renal transplantation.

Phosphate retention is treated by dietary restriction and administration of calcium salts with meals, to retard phosphate absorption from the gut. Calcium supplementation also helps to correct hypocalcaemia. Early detection of secondary hyperparathyroidism and treatment with calcium and active vitamin D analogues (e.g. 1,25-dihydroxyvitamin D) may prevent later tertiary hyperparathyroidism.

END-STAGE RENAL FAILURE

When GFR is below 10 ml/min, patients develop increasingly severe symptoms of anorexia, malaise, fatigue and nausea. Renal replacement therapy should begin before this state is reached. This corresponds in general to a serum urea level of 30–40 mmol/l, a creatinine level of 800–1000 μmol/l, or severe hyperkalaemia or acidosis. The options for treatment are haemodialysis, CAPD and renal transplantation. Careful planning and an integrated approach are required for all of these.

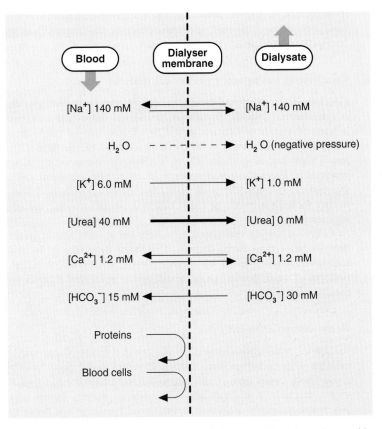

Fig. 7.3 The principle of haemodialysis. The dialysis membrane is semipermeable, allowing passage of water, ions and small molecules.

Haemodialysis

This involves circulation of the patient's blood and of dialysis fluid on opposite sides of a semipermeable dialysis membrane. The principle is shown in Fig. 7.3. The membrane allows the passage of water, electrolytes and small molecules, but not large molecules (> 20 kDa), proteins or cells. Urea, creatinine, other waste products and potassium diffuse down their concentration gradients. Water removal is achieved by applying negative pressure to the dialysis fluid circuit.

Access to the circulation is usually achieved by formation of an arteriovenous fistula between the radial artery and cephalic vein, which provides an accessible site for insertion of needles. Most patients undergo dialysis for 4–6 hours thrice weekly, usually in hospital, although sometimes home dialysis is possible. The dialysis machine controls blood flow and the composition and flow of dialysate. Many patients have now been maintained in relatively good health for 20–25 years by haemodialysis, although long-term complications have arisen such as aluminium overload and amyloidosis from deposition of β_2-microglobulin, which is not cleared from plasma by conventional dialysis.

Continuous ambulatory peritoneal dialysis

CAPD uses the peritoneal membrane as a natural semipermeable membrane. A soft silastic (Tenckhoff) catheter, implanted through the abdominal wall, is used to enable instillation of a 1.5–2.5 litre bag of sterile dialysis fluid into the peritoneal cavity. After dwelling for 4 hours, the fluid is drained out and a new bag drained in. These 'exchanges' are usually performed four times daily. Electrolytes and waste products equilibrate across the peritoneal membrane, between the fluid and adjacent blood vessels. Water removal occurs through osmosis, as CAPD fluid is available in varying strengths of hypertonicity.

CAPD is simple and effective, rapidly learnt, and allows greater patient independence than haemodialysis. The major drawback is the risk of peritonitis, which is treated by intraperitoneal antibiotics. Adequate overall removal of waste products can be difficult to achieve if there is no residual renal function.

Renal transplantation

Successful renal transplantation is the optimal mode of treatment for most patients with end-stage renal failure. It removes the need for dialysis and dietary restrictions and, if fully successful, returns renal function to normal with correction of anaemia and restoration of normal energy and fertility. When maintenance dialysis is commenced, patients are tissue-typed and placed on the transplantation waiting list. When a cadaver donor kidney is available, the most suitable recipient based on blood group compatibility and HLA tissue typing is chosen. Patients may also receive a kidney from a living donor and close relative, usually parent or sibling, of compatible tissue type.

The kidney is anastomosed to the recipient's iliac vessels, and the ureter is inserted into the recipient's bladder. Rejection is the major short-term risk, and occurs most frequently in the first few months. Cyclosporin, which interferes with recruitment of T-lymphocytes, is the basis of most immunosuppressive regimens, but is nephrotoxic and causes hypertension. Newer agents include Tacrolimus and Mycophenolate. Rejection is confirmed by biopsy and treated with high-dose methylprednisolone or, in resistant cases, antilymphocyte antibody preparations. One-year graft survival of 90% is achieved in most centres. In the long term, complications of transplantation include increased susceptibility to infections, including *Pneumocystis* and many viral infections, malignancy, particularly lymphomas and skin malignancy, and a high rate of cardiovascular mortality.

8

WATER, ELECTROLYTE AND ACID–BASE BALANCE

David Stansbie

Water accounts for over 60% of the body weight; the major part (70%) lies within the cells and constitutes the intracellular volume (ICV). The remainder, the extracellular volume (ECV), can be divided into an interstitial component (22%) and the plasma (8%). Water intake is mainly from food and drink but a small amount is produced by the oxidation of foodstuffs. Water is lost in urine, faeces, sweat and expired air. The distribution of body water in a 70 kg man is illustrated in Fig. 8.1.

The concentrations of the main intra- and extracellular ions are shown in Table 8.1. Sodium is the main extracellular cation and a 70 kg man contains 3000 mmol.

Potassium is the main intracellular cation; a 70 kg man has approximately 4500 mmol. Energy-dependent pumps maintain the gradient of sodium and potassium across the cell membrane.

WATER AND SODIUM BALANCE

Under normal circumstances the ECV is determined by the total body sodium and its distribution between the intra- and extracellular compartments. The maintenance of blood volume and the regulation of sodium and water homeostasis are controlled by aldosterone, antidiuretic hormone (ADH; also known as arginine vasopressin) and thirst.

Aldosterone and the renin–angiotensin system

A decreased ECV results in a decreased renal blood flow; this stimulates the release of renin from the juxtaglomerular apparatus of the kidney. Renin is an enzyme which acts on an alpha-2-globulin produced by the liver to produce the decapeptide angiotensin I.

Angiotensin-converting enzyme (ACE) cleaves angiotensin I to the octapeptide angiotensin II, which stimulates the release of aldosterone, a steroid produced by the adrenal cortex; this promotes the uptake of sodium in exchange for potassium or hydrogen ions in the distal tubule of the kidney.

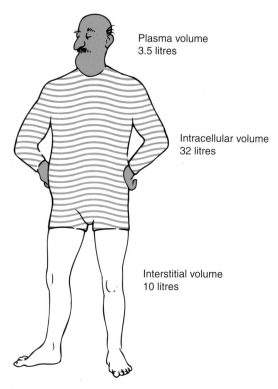

Fig. 8.1 Distribution of body water.

Table 8.1. Intracellular and extracellular ion concentrations

Intracellular concentration (mmol/l)		Extracellular concentration (mmol/l)	
Na⁺	10	Na⁺	145
K⁺	140	K⁺	5
H⁺	8×10^{-5}	H⁺	4×10^{-5}
Ca²⁺	1.5	Ca²⁺	2.5
HCO₃⁻	8	HCO₃⁻	25
Cl⁻	2	Cl⁻	100
SO₄²⁻	10	PO₄²⁻	1
Organic PO₄²⁻	50		

Antidiuretic hormone and thirst

ADH is normally secreted in response to changes in extracellular osmolality. An increase in plasma sodium concentration, the main determinant of plasma osmolality, results in the recognition by the osmoreceptors of an increase in the ratio of extracellular to intracellular osmolality and stimulates ADH secretion. The major effect of ADH is to increase the permeability to water of the distal tubules and collecting ducts of the kidney; in the presence of ADH, water is reabsorbed.

Thirst receptors, located near the osmoreceptors in the hypothalamus, stimulate drinking in response to an increased osmotic gradient across their cell membranes. Depletion of vascular volume may also stimulate thirst and ADH secretion independently of changes in osmolality.

Overall the net effect of a reduction in renal blood flow is to promote sodium retention which tends to increase ECV osmolality. This is turn stimulates ADH release which promotes water reabsorption and increases the circulating blood volume thus restoring renal blood flow.

DISORDERS OF WATER AND ELECTROLYTE BALANCE

Accurate measurement and recording of fluid intake and output is the key to understanding and resolving most fluid balance problems. Insensible loss of water in sweat and expired air is about 900 ml per 24 hours; 500 ml per 24 hours is produced by metabolic processes and, therefore, the net insensible loss is 400 ml per 24 hours. The daily requirement of water for an average adult is 2.5 litres, of which just over 2 litres is derived from food and drink.

Pyrexial patients or patients being ventilated have greater insensible losses.

Assessment of water and electrolyte balance requires the history, clinical and laboratory findings to be taken into account. Laboratory tests that are useful for assessing hydration are total plasma protein concentration and the haematocrit. The finding of elevated levels implies a loss of water. The estimation of sodium and potassium concentrations in plasma and urine is the basis for assessing electrolyte and water balance.

Hypernatraemia

The clinical effects of hypernatraemia are caused by the cerebral cellular dehydration that results when the brain is bathed in a hyperosmolal fluid, and depend more upon its rate of development than the absolute value of the plasma sodium concentration. Thirst, confusion, coma and ultimately death result.

Water deficit is the most common cause of hypernatraemia; a deficit of 2.5 litres in an adult will result in an increase in plasma sodium concentration of about 10 mmol/l. Some of the causes of hypernatraemia are given in Table 8.2.

Inadequate water intake
Failure of adequate water intake leads to the development of hypernatraemia, a hyperosmolal state and thirst. There is a shift in water from the cells to the extracellular space and consequently the plasma volume does not shrink unduly; blood pressure and renal blood flow are initially maintained. As the water deficit increases, renal blood flow falls and uraemia develops.

Table 8.2. Causes of hypernatraemia from water deficit

Inadequate water intake	Excess water loss
Lack of availability of water	Patients on a ventilator and/or with a fever and unable to replenish loss
Physical or mental illness which prevents drinking, e.g. stroke or coma	Diabetes insipidus
Neglect at the extremes of age	Vomiting or diarrhoea
Loss of appreciation of thirst	Osmotic renal loss

Excess water loss

In diabetes insipidus (DI) a lack of ADH results in excessive secretion of dilute urine and a failure to conserve water. It may be caused by a failure of secretion of ADH (cranial DI) or failure of the kidney to respond to ADH (nephrogenic DI). The kidneys lose the ability to produce concentrated urine.

The disorder is characterised by the production of dilute urine in the presence of hyperosmolal plasma due to hypernatraemia. Patients complain of thirst and polyuria; hypernatraemia usually only develops when the patient is deprived of water.

Loss of hypotonic fluids by vomiting, diarrhoea or through fistulae will lead to water loss and hypernatraemia. Loss of excess water in the urine because of a high solute load may also lead to hypernatraemia.

Sodium excess

This is usually iatrogenic from the administration of excessive amounts of sodium in the form of hypertonic intravenous infusions, or the use of oral sodium chloride solutions as emetics.

Investigation of hypernatraemia

The distinction between hypernatraemia from water depletion and that from sodium excess is most easily made from the clinical history. A raised haematocrit or total plasma protein concentration suggests water depletion. A failure to produce a concentrated urine (> 700 mosmol/l) in the presence of water deprivation (N.B. potentially dangerous), and the subsequent response to the synthetic ADH analogue desmopressin, will identify DI and allow a distinction to be made between its cranial and nephrogenic forms. Beware of artefactual causes of an elevated plasma sodium concentration as a result of blood being collected into a syringe containing sodium heparin or elevations caused by sampling from or near the cannula used to administer hypertonic sodium bicarbonate during resuscitation procedures.

Hyponatraemia

The clinical consequences are the result of the reduction in plasma osmolality that is normally a feature of hyponatraemia. This causes the osmotic uptake of water by cells, including those of the brain. Cerebral cellular oedema and a rise in intracranial pressure may occur if the hyponatraemia develops rapidly. As with hypernatraemia, the rate of development of hyponatraemia, rather than the absolute value of the plasma sodium concentration, is the main determinant of the clinical features. These may be present where the plasma sodium has fallen to 125 mmol/l over the course of a few hours, yet remain absent at 115 mmol/l if this level has been reached gradually over several days.

Clinical features of acute hyponatraemia are confusion and lethargy, nausea and vomiting, and seizures leading to coma and death.

Water excess (dilutional hyponatraemia)

Dilutional hyponatraemia occurs when the kidney is unable to dispose of a water load by producing a dilute urine. The increased ECV inhibits renin–aldosterone secretion and this condition is often known as the syndrome of inappropriate antidiuretic hormone secretion (SIADH) although serum ADH levels are not invariably increased.

Common causes of chronic dilutional hyponatraemia are ADH production by tumours, inflammatory lung disease, CNS disorders, trauma and surgery, and drugs, e.g. carbamazepine, chlorpropamide, cytotoxics, thiazides and tricyclic antidepressants.

The criteria for diagnosis are hypo-osmolal hyponatraemia with an inappropriately concentrated urine (urine osmolality > plasma osmolality) containing sodium at a concentration of > 20 mmol/l (implying no sodium deficit) in the presence of normal renal and adrenal function. The plasma urea and total protein concentrations and the haematocrit are usually low.

Acute dilutional hyponatraemia is often iatrogenic and most commonly occurs postoperatively following inappropriate fluid regimens. Compulsive water drinking is another cause and here the excessive fluid intake is associated with an impaired ability to excrete water.

Management of chronic hyponatraemia from water excess depends upon the clinical state. Water restriction to 500 ml per 24 hours is always effective if adhered to but changes take place slowly and sodium supplements may be required. Demeclocycline, which impairs the effects of ADH on the kidney, is useful in patients with inappropriate ADH secretion by tumours since this allows some relaxation in the water restriction schedule.

Patients who have the severe neurological manifestations of acute water intoxication often show a marked improvement in response to hypertonic saline but this treatment should be used with extreme caution since it may precipitate acute pontine myelinolysis and, in susceptible patients, heart failure.

Sodium depletion

Hyponatraemia is seen in Addison's disease partly as a result of a lack of aldosterone. In addition, these patients lack cortisol, which is necessary in order to excrete a water load. The hyponatraemia of Addison's disease is therefore due in part to relative water excess.

Hyponatraemia due to artefact

Pseudohyponatraemia may result from plasma with a high lipid or protein content, which leads to an underestimate of the sodium content in the plasma water. Spurious hyponatraemia commonly occurs when a blood sample is collected from an arm into which a dextrose drip is flowing.

Hyperkalaemia

Hyperkalaemia is a potentially life-threatening metabolic abnormality. Plasma levels > 6.5 mmol/l are associated with an increased risk of cardiac arrest; levels > 7.0 mmol/l must be reduced as a matter of urgency, by slow i.v. infusion of 5–10 ml of 10% calcium gluconate followed by 100 ml of 50% glucose with 20 units of short-acting insulin. Development of a cardiac arrhythmia may be the first clinical manifestation.

Pseudohyperkalaemia caused by release of potassium from cells in vitro is more common than true hyperkalaemia. Haemolysis of red cells, a high white cell or platelet count, storage of blood at 4°C or collection of blood from a 'drip arm' may all result in pseudohyperkalaemia.

Causes of true hyperkalaemia are excess potassium administration, renal failure, acidosis, drugs (e.g. spironolactone, amiloride, ACE inhibitors), hypoaldosteronism and tissue necrosis.

Several mechanisms lead to hyperkalaemia in vivo: cell destruction and release of intracellular potassium by trauma, burns or tumour chemotherapy; displacement of potassium from the intracellular compartment by acidosis; impaired excretion by the kidney because of acute or chronic renal failure; failure of exchange of sodium for potassium ions in the distal tubule caused by impairment of the aldosterone-mediated transport mechanism.

Hypokalaemia

Total body potassium depletion is the usual cause of hypokalaemia. The effects are muscle weakness, hypotonia, paralytic ileus and cardiac arrhythmias.

The potassium concentration in intestinal secretions may be 10 times that of plasma and loss by prolonged vomiting, watery or secretory diarrhoea or from fistulae leads to hypokalaemia. Villous adenomas of the rectum and laxative abuse are other causes of loss by this route. Diuretics increase renal losses of potassium by increasing the delivery of sodium to the distal tubule where potassium is lost secondarily to preferential sodium reabsorption. Hyperaldosteronism from Conn's syndrome and the mineralocorticoid effects of steroids administered or produced endogenously in Cushing's syndrome also result in hypokalaemia secondary to increased sodium reabsorption in exchange for potassium in the distal tubule.

Mild hypokalaemia is treated by oral potassium supplements and potassium-rich food (bananas). Severe hypokalaemia (≤ 2.5 mmol) may require intravenous KCl therapy. It should be given very cautiously at no more than 20 mmol per hour. In all cases, the cause of the potassium loss must be corrected. If diuretics are the cause, then potassium-sparing diuretics should be added to the existing potassium-losing drugs, e.g. amiloride to frusemide.

ACID–BASE BALANCE

The extracellular fluid (ECF) pH is maintained at about 7.4 (40 nmol/l of H^+) despite the daily adult production of up to 100 mmol of hydrogen ion (H^+). The H^+ is mainly derived from ureagenesis, anaerobic glycolysis and ketogenesis. Homeostasis is maintained by short-term mechanisms in the form of buffers; long-term compensation involves the kidney and depends on normal lung function. Buffering mechanisms in the blood include the bicarbonate and phosphate systems and haemoglobin. They are most effective at maintaining the free H^+ concentration when faced with an acid load. Acids dissociate to produce H^+; alkalis dissociate to form hydroxyl ions (OH^-). The action of the bicarbonate/carbonic acid system is illustrated below.

Bicarbonate/carbonic acid buffer system
$$H^+ + CO_3^- \rightarrow H_2CO_3 \rightarrow CO_2 + H_2O$$

An increase in H^+ concentration results in the combination of H^+ with HCO_3^- to form undissociated carbonic acid. The free H^+ concentration decreases as does the bicarbonate ion concentration. The carbonic acid dissociates in turn to produce carbon dioxide and water. Some cells, notably erythrocytes and renal tubular cells, contain an enzyme called carbonate dehydratase, which speeds this process.

The kidney is responsible for the elimination of H^+ produced during metabolism. It is able to secrete H^+ against a concentration gradient of about 800 : 1 and consequently the urine pH may fall to 4.5. The kidney's ability to secrete an alkaline urine is very limited and the maximum urine pH is 7.8. The H^+ in the urine is mainly buffered by the $HPO_4^{2-}/H_2PO_4^-$ buffer system.

Although the kidneys are responsible for H^+ elimination, whole body H^+ homeostasis also involves the lungs. The H^+ eliminated by the kidneys is derived from CO_2 which is hydrated to form carbonic acid which in turn dissociates to form H^+ and HCO_3^-. The secretion of H^+ is associated with the return to the circulation of HCO_3^-.

Investigation of acid–base balance

This is essentially an investigation of kidney and lung homeostatic mechanisms and depends upon the measurement of partial pressures of oxygen (PO_2) and carbon dioxide (PCO_2) as well as pH and HCO_3^- concentration in blood. Arterial blood is used for 'gas' measurements but PO_2 is not part of the acid–base assessment and will not be considered further.

The pH of blood determines absolutely whether the patient has an acidosis or an alkalosis. Compensatory mechanisms which act to restore blood pH towards normal always cease before normality is reached and over-compensation does not occur. The direction of the original pH perturbation may therefore be recognised.

The PCO_2 measures the respiratory component of an acid–base distur-bance. Part of a normal blood gas analysis is the standard bicarbonate. This is the HCO_3^- concentration which would be present in the blood sample at 37°C and normal barometric pressure if the PCO_2 was normal (40 mmHg or 5.3 kPa). It is a measure of non-respiratory or metabolic components of an acid–base disturbance. A change in PCO_2 or standard bicarbonate may be the primary event in an acid–base disturbance or a secondary compen-satory mechanism. It is not possible to determine which from an inspection of the PCO_2 or standard bicarbonate value alone.

In order to use these values to evaluate an acid–base disturbance the following simplified scheme may be helpful. The principal buffer in blood is the bicarbonate/carbonic acid system and PCO_2 is a reflection of the carbonic acid concentration. The lungs determine the PCO_2; the kidneys determine the HCO_3^- concentration. The relationship between them and pH may be expressed in the following way:

$$\text{pH} \propto \frac{[HCO_3^-]}{PCO_2}$$

This may be used to define the main acid–base disturbances found in practice.

Respiratory acidosis

Acute respiratory failure, e.g. from an impacted foreign body in the bronchial tree, will result in an increase in PCO_2 and decrease in pH.

$$\blacktriangledown \text{pH} \propto \frac{[HCO_3^-]}{\blacktriangle\, PCO_2}$$

Compensation leads to

$$\downarrow \text{pH} \propto \frac{\uparrow [HCO_3^-]}{\blacktriangle\, PCO_2}$$

If the cause of the respiratory failure is a long-term problem, e.g. chronic obstructive airways disease, the kidney compensates for the hypercapnia by excreting H^+ in the urine and, at the same time, secreting HCO_3^- into the blood, resulting in an increase in the standard bicarbonate.

Metabolic acidosis

Acute metabolic acidosis caused by lactic acid accumulation, for example, will lead to the production of H^+ which will be buffered by the bicarbonate/carbonic acid system and lead to a fall in HCO_3^- concentration. The H^+ will eventually be excreted by the kidney but in the short term the respiratory rate will increase (air hunger) and the PCO_2 level will fall; the blood pH will tend to return towards normal.

$$\blacktriangledown pH \propto \blacktriangledown \frac{[HCO_3^-]}{PCO_2}$$

Compensation leads to

$$\downarrow pH \propto \blacktriangledown \frac{[HCO_3^-]}{\downarrow PCO_2}$$

Respiratory and metabolic acidosis

A patient with respiratory failure and carbon dioxide retention who also develops a metabolic acidosis will have a raised PCO_2 associated with a decreased standard bicarbonate; blood pH will be depressed by both mechanisms.

$$\blacktriangledown pH \propto \blacktriangledown \frac{[HCO_3^-]}{\blacktriangle PCO_2}$$

The inter-relationship between blood pH, standard bicarbonate and PCO_2 is summarised in Table 8.3. It should be emphasised that while the student may find this approach useful it is didactic and simplistic and must only be used as an introduction to the understanding of acid–base disturbances in patients.

Table 8.3. Relationship between pH, standard bicarbonate (std HCO3⁻) and PCO_2

	pH	PCO_2	std HCO$_3^-$
Respiratory acidosis (compensated)	▼ ↓	▲ ▲	— ↑
Metabolic acidosis (compensated)	▼ ↓	— ↓	▼ ▼
Respiratory and metabolic acidosis	▼	▲	▼

9

GASTROENTEROLOGY
Ralph E. Barry

Gastroenterology includes the study of the gut and associated glands such as the liver and pancreas. Most of the gut, biliary and pancreatic ducts can be visualised or opacified using endoscopy, ultrasound and radiology. Absorption and breath tests can detect disorders of function within the gut and pancreas. Molecular virology is revolutionising our understanding of chronic liver disease.

DISORDERS OF THE OESOPHAGUS

OESOPHAGEAL REFLUX AND REFLUX OESOPHAGITIS
Reflux of gastric and duodenal contents into the oesophagus is common and may cause heartburn and pain. Oesophagitis, stricture formation and peptic ulceration can occur. It is encouraged by the following:

1. A defective lower oesophageal sphincter (LOS), as when a hiatus hernia destroys LOS function, or with relaxation of a normal LOS in the obese, in pregnancy, with smoking and stooping.
2. Impaired lower oesophageal 'clearing' which allows gastric juice retention in the oesophagus.
3. Impaired gastric emptying.

Pathology
There is oesophageal inflammation, ulceration and sometimes stricture formation. Gastric mucosal islands may be found in the lower oesophagus (Barrett's oesophagus) which may be premalignant. Ulcers may bleed, perforate and penetrate.

Symptoms and signs
1. Heartburn is a burning sensation from the epigastrium up to the neck and jaws. It is worse on lying, bending, straining, in pregnancy and after food, and is accompanied by acid regurgitation.

2. Dysphagia from oesophagitis, stricture or dysmotility.
3. Gastrointestinal (GI) bleeding may be from oesophagitis or an ulcer.
4. Severe pain may be caused by oesophageal spasm.
5. Aspiration into the lungs may cause wheezing and pneumonia. Usually there are no signs.

Investigations
Endoscopy reliably assesses the severity of oesophagitis, allows biopsy and detects complications such as stricture.

Radiology gives similar but less precise information; 24-hour oesophageal pH monitoring can be correlated with the patient's symptoms and is a valuable ambulatory method of establishing a diagnosis.

Treatment
This is initially medical (Table 9.1). Where symptoms are resistant or where complications occur, laparoscopic fundoplication restores the function of the LOS. Surgery for ulcers is seldom required since the advent of proton pump inhibitor drugs.

ACHALASIA OF THE CARDIA

This is caused by intramural autonomic nerve plexus degeneration and results in failure of LOS relaxation with dysphagia, oesophageal dilatation and retention oesophagitis. It occurs at all ages but is more common in young adults.

Symptoms and signs
There is a gradual onset of lower oesophageal dysphagia with regurgitation, initially relieved by drinking fluids with meals. Weight loss is moderate.

Severe attacks of central chest pain, often nocturnal and mimicking ischaemic heart disease, are caused by muscle hyperactivity in the denervated gullet. Cough, recurrent chest infections and wheezing from bronchial aspiration are seen. Rarely, clubbing of the fingers and chest signs are observed.

Table 9.1. Medical therapy of oesophagitis

Altered behaviour	Drugs
Stop smoking (it reduces LOS function) Lose weight	Simple antacids H_2-blocking agents, e.g. ranitidine 150 mg at night (to reduce gastric acid)
Avoid stooping Prop up head of bed at night	Cisapride 10 mg 8-hourly (releases acetylcholine and stimulates oesophageal clearing)
Avoid heavy meals (particularly at night) Avoid constipation (straining)	Omeprazole 20–40 mg per 24 hours (a proton pump inhibitor. Blocks gastric acid production almost completely)

Investigations

A chest X-ray may show a grossly dilated oesophagus, an absent gastric air bubble and possibly pneumonia or lung fibrosis. Barium studies confirm oesophageal dilatation and define the smoothly narrowed distal oesophagus (c.f. the irregularity seen with oesophageal cancer).

Endoscopy has little to offer except biopsy of the narrowed segment and may be dangerous (aspiration). Oesophageal manometry is diagnostic with raised LOS pressure and disorganised muscular activity.

Differential diagnosis includes lower oesophageal cancer and peptic oesophagitis. Ischaemic heart disease may be mimicked by the pain.

Treatment

Pneumatic dilatation of the LOS usually gives satisfactory relief and can be repeated.

Surgery for resistant or recurrent cases is by cardiomyotomy (Heller's operation) in which the muscular coat of the lower oesophagus is incised down to the mucosa.

Treatment relieves dysphagia, allows the oesophagus to return to normal size and prevents oesophageal cancer.

HIATUS HERNIA

Two major types of this common abnormality occur where part of the stomach is within the thoracic cavity. A sliding hernia (70%) is accompanied by an intrathoracic position of the LOS, and may cause major reflux while a rolling hernia in which the LOS is not displaced may or may not cause symptoms. It is more common in women in whom obesity, multiple pregnancies and ageing are important aetiological factors. Herniae contain gastric mucosa, and peptic ulceration may occur within them (Fig. 9.1).

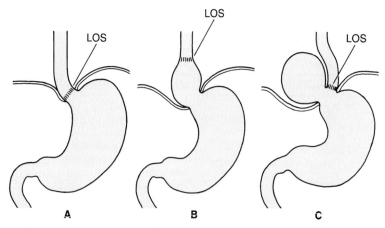

Fig. 9.1 (A) Normal structure; **(B)** sliding hiatus hernia; **(C)** rolling hiatus hernia.

Symptoms and signs

Large herniae are often asymptomatic but there may be attacks of severe chest pain, whilst complicating ulcers cause dyspepsia and vomiting. Bleeding, causing haematemesis or anaemia, also occurs. Small sliding herniae may cause severe heartburn and dysphagia from peptic oesophagitis.

Signs are usually absent.

Investigations

A barium meal demonstrates a pouch of stomach in the chest. With large herniae there may be a retrocardiac shadow on a plain chest film. Complications such as a stricture or ulcer within the gastric pouch are well demonstrated.

Endoscopy is valuable and allows a more precise identification of oesophagitis and its severity, and allows histology and cytology of ulcers.

Treatment

Control of symptoms is outlined in the section on reflux (Table 9.1). Rarely, surgery may be required. Hernia repair with laparoscopic fundoplication and highly selective vagotomy are the usual approaches; large rolling herniae may require surgery because of the risk of volvulus.

CARCINOMA OF THE OESOPHAGUS (see Table 9.6)

OTHER DISORDERS OF THE OESOPHAGUS (see Table 9.2)

DISORDERS OF THE STOMACH AND DUODENUM

The stomach acts as a hopper delivering premixed and predigested food to the small bowel. Lined with columnar epithelium forming pits or glands, it produces mucus, hydrochloric acid (HCl), pepsins and intrinsic factor (in the body of the stomach). The pyloric region produces gastrin from G cells.

HCl secretion is under humoral and vagal control. The final common stimulus to acid production is histamine while gastrin is an important intermediate. Released by vagal and food stimulation, it exists in several molecular forms. Gastrin release is inhibited by H^+ ions (HCl) and hormones like somatostatin. Vagal stimulation excites a gastrin response. The mucosa of the stomach is protected from acid damage by a thin layer of mucus through which bicarbonate is secreted.

PEPTIC ULCER

This includes both gastric and duodenal ulcers, acute or chronic. Peptic ulcer is common with still a significant mortality and 10% of adult males are sometime sufferers. The death rate is rising, particularly in elderly women, because of nonsteroidal analgesic consumption. The incidence of the disease varies from country to country. The 'cause' of peptic ulcer is unknown, but acid levels are generally high in duodenal ulcer and low or normal in gastric ulcer but with considerable overlap with normal subjects.

Table 9.2. Other diseases of the oesophagus

Lesion	Cause	Effect	Treatment
Candida oesophagitis	Candida infection of oesophagus in immunosuppressed, antibiotic treated or diabetic patients	Painful dysphagia Plaques of white material seen on endoscopy	Drug therapy nystatin, miconazole, fluconazole
Mallory-Weiss syndrome	Mucosal tear at the oesophagogastric junction, often following vomiting	Haematemesis Tear seen by endoscopy	Conservative
Barrett's oesophagus	Gastric mucosa lines part of the lower oesophagus	Caused by oesophageal reflux	Treatment of reflux Monitor for cancer
Systemic sclerosis	Involvement of oesophagus is common	Dysphagia Dilated aperistaltic oesophagus with secondary peptic oesophagitis	Conservative
Oesophageal web	Anteriorly placed shelf of epithelial tissue at level of cricoid cartilage Often associated with iron deficiency	Mild dysphagia May be a risk of subsequent carcinoma	Dilate endoscopically Treat iron deficiency
Diffuse oesophageal spasm	Uncertain—middle-aged and elderly patients show diffuse spasm of oesophagus on barium swallow (corkscrew oesophagus)	Chest pain mimicking angina Dysphagia	Nitrates or calcium channel blockers, e.g. nifedipine, occasionally dilatation

Cytoprotective mechanisms (mucus, prostaglandins, mucosal bicarbonate production) prevent acid/pepsin damage in normals but peptic ulcers may occur when these mechanisms are impaired by drugs (e.g. NSAIDs), *Helicobacter pylori* infection, alcohol or genetic factors.

H. pylori infection of the submucous layer of the gastric mucosa is almost universal in duodenal ulcer and common in gastric ulcer. Acute infection causes gastritis of variable severity, which becomes chronic and may impair mucosal cytoprotection and increase acid output by local alkalinisation of the submucous area through the action of bacterial urease.

Relapse of peptic ulcer after healing is extremely common, except where *H. pylori* infection is also eradicated.

Pathology

Chronic ulcers are commonly found on the gastric lesser curve and duodenal anterior wall and rarely occur in the second part of the duodenum. Chronic ulcers cause fibrosis and local deformity and can penetrate through the stomach or duodenal wall. The base of the ulcer often contains large blood vessels. Coexisting malignancy may be found in gastric ulcers, especially where atypically sited.

Symptoms and signs

Peptic ulcer may be asymptomatic. Often there is epigastric burning pain, usually well localised and periodic. Classically worse before or just after meals, and at night, it is relieved by food, alkalis and vomiting. Persistent and copious vomiting suggests pyloric outflow obstruction.

Heartburn, nausea and anorexia are further symptoms, and weight loss results.

Usually there are no signs except for epigastric tenderness. Physical signs result from complications.

Investigations

Peptic ulcers in the lower esophagus in a hiatus hernia or in the stomach or duodenum are readily demonstrated by a barium meal or endoscopy. Endoscopy also allows brush cytology and biopsy for all gastric ulcers to ensure they are benign. *H. pylori* infection is suggested by serum antibodies and confirmed by mucosal endoscopic biopsy or detection of urease activity by breath tests or mucosal incubation.

Anaemia and iron deficiency, and positive faecal occult bloods suggest ulcer bleeding.

Hypoalbuminaemia occurs in debilitated patients with large chronic gastric ulcers, and hypokalaemic alkalosis in those with vomiting.

The *differential diagnosis* is ulcerating gastric cancer which may be diagnosed by radiological appearance and proved by endoscopy and biopsy.

Complications

1. Penetration into the pancreas, posterior abdominal wall, etc. may cause back pain.
2. Perforation of an ulcer into the peritoneal cavity causes an abdominal emergency with severe pain, vomiting and shock.

3. Ulcers may penetrate large blood vessels with intestinal bleeding, either haematemesis, melaena or both, or chronic anaemia.
4. Local fibrosis and contraction of scar tissue results in hour-glass deformity from a lesser curve gastric ulcer, or more importantly pyloric obstruction with gastric outflow constriction. A history of ulcer dyspepsia then gives way to vomiting, which characteristically is copious, projectile and contains stale food eaten 48 hours or more before. Abdominal examination shows the outline of a distended stomach, visible peristalsis and a succussion splash.

Hypokalaemic alkalosis and mild uraemia is found in the blood. Gastric washouts, fluid replacement and surgical correction (gastroenterostomy and a highly selective vagotomy) are usually required.

Treatment
1. Patients should not smoke and should take regular small but tasty meals to ensure maximal food buffering.
2. Pain is helped by antacids, e.g. aluminium hydroxide 1–2 tablets chewed 3–4 times daily, and on retiring. Ulcerogenic drugs, e.g. aspirin and other non-steroidals, are avoided. In patients with gastric ulcer, malignancy must be excluded by biopsy or brush cytology and complete ulcer healing at endoscopic follow-up.
3. Ulcer healing requires a greater degree of acid suppression than is achieved with normal doses of antacids. Proton pump inhibitors (e.g. omeprazole, lansoprazole) or H_2 antagonists (e.g. cimetidine, ranitidine) are normally used either b.d. or as a combined night-time dose for 6–8 weeks.
4. Once healing has been achieved, relapse will occur in at least 80% unless maintenance treatment (e.g. H_2 blocker at night) is continued. However, eradication of *H. pylori* renders maintenance therapy unnecessary. *H. pylori* readily develops antibiotic resistance so triple therapy is normally used. Omeprazole 20 mg, amoxycillin 1 g and clarithromycin 250 mg twice daily by mouth for 1 week eradicates infection in more than 90% of patients. Omeprazole 20 mg b.d., bismuth subcitrate 120 mg q.d.s., oxytetracycline 500 mg q.d.s. and metronidazole 400 mg q.d.s. for 1 week has a similar eradication rate but compliance is poor due to intolerance.

Ulcers that fail to heal are treated with higher doses of ulcer-healing drugs, perhaps in combination, and by ensuring that smoking, alcohol intake, work stress, drug compliance and dietary indiscretions are controlled. The possibility of a Zollinger-Ellison syndrome (see Table 9.7) should also be considered. Relapse is most important in the elderly and in those with serious chronic diseases. Surgery is now rarely required.

GASTRITIS

Inflammation of the gastric mucosa may be acute or chronic.

Acute gastritis

Acute gastritis is caused by alcohol, aspirin and other non-steroidal drug ingestion, intracranial disease and subarachnoid haemorrhage. It is also common after major trauma, burns and shock. It can lead to serious bleeding from multiple acute gastric erosions and will require blood transfusion and treatment with proton pump inhibitor drugs.

Chronic gastritis

Two forms are recognised.

Atrophic gastritis in the antrum and body is an autoimmune lesion. Vitamin B_{12} malabsorption results from intrinsic factor deficiency causing pernicious anaemia. There is an associated increased incidence of gastric carcinoma and carcinoid tumours, and due to the achlorhydria, an increased incidence of bacterial infections of the gut.

Chronic superficial gastritis is virtually universal with ageing. It is common in the antrum after gastric surgery when it is due to reflux of bile into the stomach. It is not a primary autoimmune disorder, although patients may have parietal cell antibodies in the blood. The cause is usually infection with *H. pylori*, which causes an initial acute gastritis that progresses to a chronic phase with gastric atrophy. Non-infective causes include bile reflux, non-steroidal drugs and alcohol.

Symptoms vary from none to severe ulcer-type pain with nausea, vomiting and flatulence. Treatment is by eradication of *H. pylori* infection. Symptoms may respond to antacids or H_2-blocking drugs.

Ménétrièr's disease is a rare condition with rugal hyperplasia. The cause is unknown and there is a risk of malignant change.

THE SMALL BOWEL—MALABSORPTION

The small bowel digests and absorbs nutrients and is a major endocrine organ producing secretions that act locally or stimulate neural transmission.

Malabsorption can also affect haematinics such as iron, folic acid and vitamin B_{12} and electrolytes such as sodium, potassium and calcium.

Causes of malabsorption

1. liver or pancreatic disease, e.g. cirrhosis, obstructive jaundice, chronic pancreatitis
2. intestinal or gastric resection, short bowel syndrome, etc.
3. abnormalities of luminal environment, e.g. bacterial overgrowth, disaccharidase deficiency, abnormal small bowel pH (as in Zollinger-Ellison syndrome)
4. disease of the small bowel mucosa, e.g. coeliac disease, tropical sprue, Whipple's disease
5. disease of the small bowel wall, e.g. destruction of intramural nerve plexuses (aganglionosis), infiltration with lymphoma
6. systemic disease, e.g. amyloidosis, thyrotoxicosis, etc.

More than one cause may operate, as in extensive Crohn's disease where there may be mucosal disease and bacterial overgrowth from stricturing.

Symptoms and signs

Diarrhoea is the major symptom with pale, bulky, frothy, fatty, offensive stools (with excessive rectal wind), flushing with difficulty. Weight loss results from anorexia and malabsorption (though in some patients the appetite is preserved or even excessive, e.g. chronic pancreatitis).

Abdominal distension is due to excessive gas formation from fermentation of unabsorbed starches. There may be ankle oedema from hypoproteinaemia.

Anaemia, with dyspnoea and lassitude, is caused by deficiency of iron, folic acid and vitamin B_{12}. Iron and folate are absorbed in the upper small bowel, while vitamin B_{12} deficiency is a feature of ileal disease, resection, or small intestinal bacterial colonisation. Weakness and lassitude are also often related to electrolyte disorders such as hypokalaemia and hypomagnesaemia.

Tetany (painful cramps and paraesthesiae in the hands) is from hypocalcaemia and hypomagnesaemia. Metabolic bone disease, usually osteomalacia, is related to impaired absorption of vitamin D; sometimes there is osteoporosis. Adult coeliac disease commonly presents with mixed deficiency anaemia.

Other features are related to specific types of malabsorption, e.g. abdominal pain in Crohn's disease, lymphadenopathy in Whipple's disease, etc.

Investigations

1. Anaemia, either hypochromic (iron deficiency) or macrocytic (folate or vitamin B_{12} deficiency). Hypoalbuminaemia, a raised alkaline phosphatase and a low calcium level may signify the presence of osteomalacia, verified by bone biopsy.
2. Estimation of 24-hour faecal fat excretion on a high (100 g/day) intake of fat (fat balance). After an equilibration period, faeces are collected for 3–5 days (> 25 mmol fatty acid per day confirms malabsorption).
3. Radiology will show the non-specific changes of malabsorption, such as dilated small bowel. Specific features may suggest Crohn's disease, intestinal fistulae, a blind loop or coeliac disease.
4. Biopsy of the small bowel mucosa, either via a Crosby capsule or at upper gastrointestinal endoscopy, can diagnose coeliac disease, tropical sprue and Whipple's disease, etc.
5. Intestinal bacterial colonisation may be suggested by ^{14}C-labelled bile salt or hydrogen breath tests.
6. When items 3–5 above are normal, pancreatic failure is the likely cause and can be confirmed by oral pancreatic function tests, e.g. fluorescein dilaurate tests.

SPECIAL TYPES OF MALABSORPTION

Coeliac disease

This genetic disorder, in which small bowel mucosal damage (partial or sub-

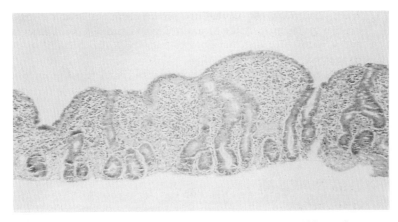

Fig. 9.2 The small bowel mucosa in coeliac disease. This jejunal biopsy shows blunting of villi, increased cellularity of the submucosa and crypt hyperplasia. Higher power changes include important epithelial disorganisation and lymphocytic infiltration. These changes are all corrected by a gluten-free diet.

total villous atrophy) results from exposure to dietary gluten, a protein found in wheat, rye, oats and barley, is found in about 1 in 2000 of the population in Western Europe. It is more common in women and sufferers are four times more likely than normals to have the histocompatibility antigens HLA B8/DW3. Mucosal damage is probably immunologically determined.

Biopsies of the small bowel show virtually diagnostic partial or total villous atrophy (Fig. 9.2). However, changes are found in cow's milk hypersensitivity, tropical sprue and some cases of intestinal lymphoma.

Seen classically in infancy with first exposure to dietary gluten, the disease may be delayed in onset until adult life. Weight loss, diarrhoea, anaemia, oedema and anorexia usually accompany a low red cell folate level. Anaemia, often chronic iron deficiency, worse with each pregnancy, is sometimes the only feature. Aphthous ulcers (small, painful, superficial ulcers) of the mouth and other autoimmune diseases can occur.

Complications

Dermatitis herpetiformis, a vesicular skin rash, causes severe itching. Lymphoma is the most serious complication and presents with abdominal pain, weight loss and perhaps intestinal perforation. Chronic ulceration of the small bowel may cause abdominal pain and intestinal obstruction due to stricturing.

Central nervous system disorders, including cerebellar and pyramidal tract damage, are of uncertain cause.

Atrophy of the spleen causes changes in the peripheral blood count, such as the presence of Howell-Jolly bodies (nuclear remnants).

Treatment

Coeliac disease is treated with a lifelong gluten-free diet. Wheat flour is present in bread, cakes, biscuits and many prepared foods such as sauces, soups, ice cream, etc. Gluten-free products are available and are marked for easy recognition. A few resistant patients may also need corticosteroids and a lactose-free diet, but poor compliance is the usual cause of failure to respond.

Biopsy appearances return to normal with complete gluten exclusion, and the risk of lymphoma is reduced.

Other causes of malabsorption

(See Table 9.3.)

GASTROINTESTINAL BLEEDING

Rapid bleeding from the GI tract may cause haematemesis (vomiting of blood) or melaena (passage of black, tarry stools) or both. Bleeding from the distal colon and anal region causes the passage of fresh blood, i.e. rectal bleeding. Insidious bleeding may cause anaemia, and although the stools appear normal they contain occult blood on stool testing. The causes of GI bleeding are given in Table 9.4.

UPPER GI BLEEDING

Symptoms and signs

The symptoms are haematemesis and melaena. If bleeding is severe, shock, faintness, nausea and sweating also occur. In elderly patients, loss of blood volume may cause stroke or myocardial pain.

The important signs are pallor, sweating, tachycardia and hypotension. If patients have underlying chronic liver disease, signs of liver cell failure (see p. 289) may appear.

Abdominal signs are usually absent unless there is liver disease (hepato-splenomegaly, etc.). Severe abdominal pain should suggest perforation as an accompaniment to bleeding. When taking the history, the following *must* be included:

1. Does the patient suffer from chronic dyspepsia? This may suggest peptic ulcer/hiatus hernia, etc.
2. Does the patient have a history to suggest chronic liver disease—previous jaundice, known alcoholism, etc.?
3. Does the patient take drugs such as aspirin, NSAIDs, anticoagulants, etc.?
4. Does the patient drink alcohol—was he or she drinking immediately prior to the bleed?
5. Has the patient bled before? If so:
   (a) When?
   (b) Was the patient in hospital and where?
   (c) Did the patient need a blood transfusion and how many units?
   (d) Was surgery performed?
   (e) What was the patient told concerning the cause?

Table 9.3. Other disorders causing malabsorption

Lesion	Cause	Symptoms and signs	Treatment
Tropical sprue	Acquired bacterial infection of small bowel causing villous atrophy Occurs after or during residence in tropical areas	Malabsorption with diarrhoea and anaemia Vitamin B_{12} deficient neuropathy	Antibiotics Vitamin B_{12} (curable)
Whipple's disease (Fig. 9.3)	Acquired bacterial infection of the gut and other tissues Causes villous atrophy with PAS+ve bacterial remnants in mucosa	Malabsorption Arthritis Lymphadenopathy Pigmentation	Antibiotics (curable but can relapse)
Intestinal lymphangiectasia	Genetic disorder with dilated lymphatics in gut and in other situations	Malabsorption Protein-losing Pitting oedema, e.g. of limbs Thickened yellow nails Pleural effusions	Low fat diet Medium chain triglyceride supplements (MCTs) Can be controlled
Radiation enteritis	Radiotherapy to gut, e.g. from irradiated cervix or abdominal lymph nodes Causes telangiectasia, bleeding, stricturing and obliterative vasculitis	Abdominal pain, diarrhoea, bleeding and malabsorption depending on situation	Resection if localised Otherwise symptomatic treatment
Stagnant loop syndrome	Bacterial colonisation of stagnant small bowel Follows surgery or complicates conditions like scleroderma or jejunal diverticulosis	Malabsorption Vitamin B_{12} deficiency	Antibiotics Vitamin B_{12} ? Corrective surgery

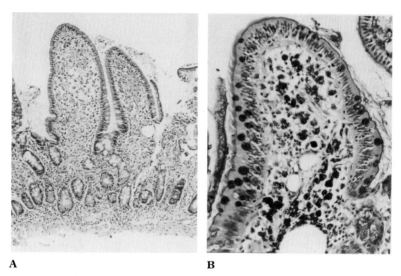

A   **B**

Fig. 9.3 Whipple's disease. **(A)** Ballooning of the villi which, in the PAS stained photograph **(B)**, show many bacteria.

Table 9.4. Causes of upper and lower gastrointestinal bleeding

Upper		
	Common	Acute erosive gastritis, e.g. NSAIDs, alcohol
		Severe oesophagitis
		Duodenal ulcer
		Gastric ulcer
		Mallory-Weiss syndrome (see Table 9.2)
	Rare	Gastric tumours
		Osler's disease (haemorrhagic telangiectasia) (hereditary—dominant inheritance with bleeding from GI tract and nose; facial, lip, tongue and hand telangiectasia)
		Pseudoxanthoma elasticum (hereditary—dominant inheritance; deficient elastic tissue in skin and in blood vessels; gastrointestinal bleeding, 'chicken breast' skin (pseudoxanthoma) and impaired vision (angioid streaks)
Lower		
	Common	Haemorrhoids
		Rectal and colonic polyps
		Rectal and colonic tumours
		Diverticular disease
	Rare	Angiodysplasia (dilated submucosal vessels—found in the elderly, sometimes associated with aortic stenosis, most common in the colon)
		Meckel's diverticulum—due to ulcer in contained gastric mucosa; treated surgically

6. Does the patient have any other serious disease, e.g. coronary artery disease?

Investigations

Providing the patient's condition is stable, an attempt should be made to determine the site of bleeding, but where bleeding has been severe (tachycardia > 100, blood pressure < 100 systolic) emergency supportive treatment is first required (see below).

The haemoglobin and packed cell volume (PCV) should be measured and blood sent for grouping and cross-matching. The patient's haemoglobin level may be misleadingly normal in the first 24 hours because of the lack of haemodilution. Estimation of the blood urea may help in the assessment of severity (pre-renal uraemia), but may also be high in proximal GI bleeding with subsequent small bowel metabolism and absorption of protein.

Liver function tests (LFTs) and coagulation studies are important in suspected liver disease.

The definitive tests to find out the source of bleeding are:

1. *Endoscopy*: upper GI endoscopy should be performed once the patient's condition is stable and certainly within 24 hours for maximal diagnostic yield. Where chronic ulcers occur, fresh clot or a prominent vessel in an ulcer suggests further bleeding is likely. Gastric ulcers should be brushed and biopsied if this is feasible.
2. *Barium studies*: these are valuable, particularly if endoscopy is not available. With double-contrast techniques the diagnostic yield is over 90%. Ulcers, both acute and chronic, erosions and small polyps are demonstrated.
3. *Angiography*: if after endoscopy and barium studies the source of bleeding is still uncertain, coeliac, superior mesenteric and inferior mesenteric angiography should be performed.
4. *Scintigraphy*: the patient's labelled red blood cells are given intravenously; this is indicated for chronic blood loss of uncertain cause.

Treatment

Resuscitation is vital. In severe cases, the foot of the bed is raised and i.v. plasma expanders such as Haemaccel are given before transfusion of cross-matched blood. In the elderly and those with serious bleeds a central venous line helps to monitor venous pressure and avoids overtransfusion. Transfusion aims to return the blood pressure, pulse rate and urine volume to normal. Sedation may be required but not in those with liver disease. Monitoring of the pulse rate, blood pressure and the patient's general condition is mandatory. About 80% of patients will respond to this treatment and not rebleed.

Bleeding is more likely to recur if the patient is elderly, suffering from chronic ulcers, particularly gastric, or bleeding from oesophageal varices.

Serious underlying disease, such as chronic bronchitis, heart failure, liver cell failure and the endoscopic features described above also increase the likelihood. Bleeding points may be endoscopically treated by laser photocoagulation or by adrenaline injection. Usually, early surgical consultation is required.

Acute erosive gastritis is treated with blood transfusion and H_2-blockers or omeprazole; gastric surgery may rarely be required.

If chronic ulcers fail to respond to conservative therapy, blood transfusion, a course of H_2-blockers (or omeprazole) and surgery are required. Local resection of the ulcer is performed or even ligation and oversewing, i.e. the simplest possible surgery that is likely to be effective.

Prognosis

The mortality remains at about 8% despite advances in investigation, post-operative care and endoscopic techniques because of the increasing number of elderly patients who have serious underlying disease and are unable to withstand bleeding or subsequent surgery.

DISORDERS OF THE GALLBLADDER AND BILE DUCTS

The gallbladder stores and concentrates hepatic bile via the biliary canaliculi and biliary duct system. Passage of bile down the biliary tree depends on osmotic forces from bile salts (bile salt dependent fraction) and partly on a sodium-dependent transport mechanism (bile salt independent fraction). Secretin, acting on bile ducts, contributes water and bicarbonate with a total flow of 500–600 ml per 24 hours. Gallbladder contraction is caused by food-released cholecystokinin.

GALLSTONES

These form in the gallbladder or the bile duct. They are composed of cholesterol alone (pure cholesterol stones), or are mixed with calcium salts (mixed cholesterol stones), or consist of bile pigments (pigment stones). The circumstances under which they are found are shown in Table 9.5. In the Western World, cholesterol stones and mixed cholesterol stones are the most important. Cholesterol stones develop because bile becomes supersaturated

Table 9.5. Gallstones—risk factors

Cholesterol-containing stones
  Obesity ⎫
  Diabetes ⎭ Increased hepatic cholesterol synthesis
  Female sex/multiple pregnancies
  Drugs—oral contraceptives (c.f. pregnancy), clofibrate
  Ileal disease—reduction of bile salt level
Pigment stones
  Haemolysis—increased pigment load
  Liver disease—increased pigment load (minor haemolysis)

with cholesterol, the bile salts being insufficient to keep it in solution. They are more common in females and increase with age, so at the age of 60 years 15–20% of normal women will have them. Pigment stones occur where there is excessive haemolysis and in cirrhosis. Important differences are seen in stone composition and site of formation in the Far East, where mixed duct stones result from duct infection and infestation.

Symptoms and signs
Patients may be asymptomatic, or pain may occur when stones occlude the cystic duct, migrate into the common bile duct or cause pancreatitis. Pain is then severe, constant, in the right upper abdomen and epigastrium, radiating to the back and angle of the right scapula, with vomiting.

Obstructive jaundice may occur with migration into the common bile duct. Flatulence and dyspepsia are common.

Important signs are right upper abdominal tenderness and guarding. A positive Murphy's sign, when the patient experiences inspiratory right upper abdominal pain on palpation, may be found. Rarely, a mucocele or empyema makes the gallbladder palpable. Fever, rigors, jaundice and collapse with hypotension may occur from complicating cholangitis and septicaemia.

Investigations
Plain films of the abdomen may show mixed but not pure cholesterol or pigment stones. Ultrasound is the best way of demonstrating gallbladder stones.

Routine LFTs are often normal, though mild elevations of alkaline phosphatase and gamma glutamyl transferase may occur. With cholangitis, more florid changes occur, e.g. raised bilirubin, alkaline phosphatase, etc. The blood count may show a polymorph leukocytosis. A serum amylase is required to rule out accompanying pancreatitis.

Complications
See Fig. 9.4.

Treatment
Symptomless gallstones, despite possible complications, are generally not treated. Gallstone cholecystitis is treated conservatively with analgesics, including non-steroidals, and sometimes with antibiotics. Once the attack has settled, a decision is made on procedure. Cholecystectomy is a safe operation which relieves acute symptoms with a low mortality, even in the elderly. It is commonly carried out at laparoscopy, thus often reducing hospital stay.

Non-surgical treatment of gallbladder stones
1. Bile salts (chenodeoxycholic) or (chenodeoxyocholic plus ursodeoxycholic acid) continuously by mouth will dissolve cholesterol gallstones 15 mm or less in diameter after 18 months. Relapse is common.
2. Methylene terbutyl ether (MTB) is repeatedly infused directly into the gallbladder under ultrasound control. After the contents have been

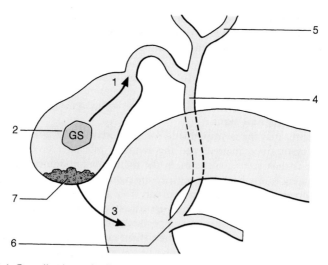

Fig. 9.4 Complications of gallstones. (1) Acute cholecystitis (migration to the cystic duct); (2) empyema or mucocele; (3) rupture into the duodenum—gallstone ileus, or peritoneal cavity—biliary peritonitis; (4) common bile duct migration (obstructive jaundice); (5) ascending sepsis (hepatic abscess, cholangitis, septicaemia); (6) pancreatitis; (7) carcinoma of the gallbladder.

aspirated, infusion is repeated. Again, cholesterol stones only can be treated. Further, follow-up therapy with oral bile salts may be required.
3. Stones may be fragmented by shock waves produced by an external lithotripter, or under laparoscopic control the gallbladder may be punctured, the entry point dilated and endoscopic examination of the gallbladder carried out. Stones may be removed, broken up with forceps or by a lithotripter introduced into the gallbladder.

Gallstones in the common bile duct or common hepatic ducts may cause biliary obstruction with jaundice and pain. Complications include hepatic abscess formation, cholangitis and septicaemia. Detection of common duct stones may not be conclusive with ultrasound and visualisation of the duct system by endoscopic retrograde choledochopancreatography (ERCP) or fine-needle cholangiography may be required. Surgical removal and T-tube drainage with choledochoduodenostomy or sphincterotomy under endoscopic control are ways of removing or facilitating the removal of duct stones.

CHOLANGITIS

This is an infection of the biliary tree with pyogenic organisms. It occurs where there is a nidus of infection in the obstructed biliary tract, most usually with common duct stones. Patients are usually ill with a high swinging fever and obstructive jaundice. There is tender hepatomegaly. Investigations show a polymorph leukocytosis and LFTs, an obstructive pattern. Hypotension, tachycardia and septic shock indicate septicaemia. Treatment is with i.v. antibiotics such as gentamicin and/or a cephalosporin such as cephradine, fluid replacement and, where required, relief of biliary obstruction either surgically or by endoscopic stenting.

ACUTE CHOLECYSTITIS

This is an acute inflammation of the stone-containing gallbladder, often with a stone impacted in the cystic duct. Rarely, pus may form to produce an empyema, or a stone may ulcerate through the gallbladder into the duodenum later to obstruct the ileum (gallstone ileus). Patients are likely to have the risk factors for gallstones (see Table 9.5), but no group is immune.

Symptoms include abdominal pain, sometimes radiating to the shoulder or angle of the right scapula, with vomiting. Signs are of right upper abdominal tenderness with a positive Murphy's sign. Ultrasound detects gallbladder thickening and the presence of stones. Treatment consists of analgesia, non-steroidals for their anti-inflammatory action, and antibiotics. Generally, patients who are not too ill are treated conservatively and subsequent treatment of gallstones is usually by cholecystectomy. When patients are very ill, urgent surgery may be required and is essential when complications such as perforation of the gallbladder or empyema are suspected.

OTHER DISORDERS OF THE GALLBLADDER

Sclerosing cholangitis is an immunological disorder with thickening, stenosis and dilatation of the biliary tract, causing obstructive jaundice with or without cholangitis. Diagnosis is by ERCP. It is associated with inflammatory bowel disease and AIDS.

Choledochal cyst is a congenital dilatation of the common bile duct, causing obstructive jaundice, fever and abdominal mass. Cancer risk is increased. Treatment is surgical.

Carcinoma of bile ducts. Slowly growing adenocarcinoma is associated with ulcerative colitis, choledochal cyst and, in the Far East, with liver fluke infestation. It causes progressive obstructive jaundice. Surgical removal (rare), stenting and internal radiotherapy are possible treatments.

Carcinoma of the gallbladder is usually a complication of chronic cholecystitis with gallstones. It causes progressive obstructive jaundice and is usually inoperable but partial hepatectomy is a possibility.

THE PANCREAS

The presence of food in the upper small bowel which leads to the release of secretin and pancreozymin (cholecystokinin, CCK). Secretin is released in response to acid in the duodenum with the production of pancreatic fluid rich in bicarbonate. CCK is particularly stimulated by fat in the small bowel lumen and results in the production of fluid rich in pancreatic enzymes.

ACUTE PANCREATITIS

This is an acute inflammation of the pancreas with a high mortality. The inflammation and necrosis are caused by activation of destructive pancreatic enzymes. In the UK, there are two common causes of acute pancreatitis: alcoholism and the presence of gallstones. Rarer causes are trauma (particularly postoperative trauma), drugs (e.g. corticosteroids, oral contraceptives, thiazide diuretics), hyperparathyroidism, hyperlipidaemia (types IV, V or I) and infections such as mumps.

Symptoms and signs
Severe abdominal pain, usually epigastric, radiating to the back, shoulders or generally throughout the abdomen, is persistent and sometimes relieved by sitting forward. Vomiting is almost universal and there may be haematemesis.

Signs are of abdominal tenderness and rigidity. Abdominal swelling may occur, usually caused by small bowel distension (paralytic ileus), or more rarely by the presence of fluid in the lesser sac or abdominal cavity (pancreatic ascites). Jaundice may be present, particularly in alcoholics or from gallstones. The pulse may be rapid and the patient hypotensive.

Rare physical signs include a pleural effusion on the left side. Grey-Turner's sign (a violaceous discoloration in the flanks) and Cullen's sign (a similar appearance around the umbilicus), both due to the extravasation of inflammatory pancreatic fluid, can occur.

Patients may be short of breath because of pulmonary adult respiratory distress syndrome (ARDS) with low arterial PO_2 levels. Cardiac dysrhythmias, hypotension and ECG changes may also occur.

Investigations
1. The serum amylase is elevated, usually > 1000 Somogyi units/l. Levels twice this are pathognomonic of the disease but other intestinal disorders cause moderately elevated levels.
2. LFTs may be abnormal, particularly in alcoholics.
3. Abdominal or pleural fluid may show very high amylase levels.
4. The serum calcium level may be low from loss into the inflammatory exudate and the glucose level may be raised due to transient insulin deficiency.
5. Blood urea and electrolyte levels may be abnormal because of fluid losses and hypotension.
6. Serial estimations of arterial gases detect and monitor complicating ARDS.
7. Ultrasound shows the enlarged pancreas, the extravasation of fluid and associated abnormalities, e.g. cirrhosis, gallbladder stones.

Complications
The complications of acute pancreatitis are shown in Fig. 9.5.

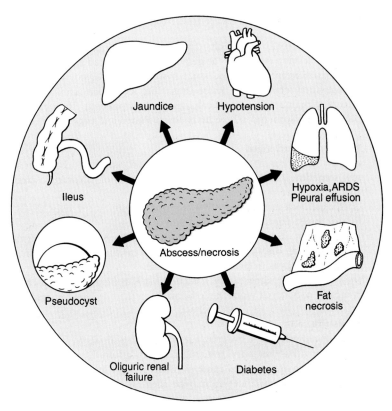

Fig. 9.5 The complications of acute pancreatitis.

Treatment

Treatment is supportive and includes intestinal rest. Pain is treated with pethidine, and shock is vigorously treated by fluid replacement with blood if there has been intra-abdominal bleeding. Monitoring of the pulse, blood pressure and urine volume (catheter) is important, and a central venous line helps. Abnormal levels of blood calcium and glucose need treatment. Nasogastric suction allows gastrointestinal rest and helps to control ileus. Oxygen is administered and ventilatory support (PEEP) may be required.

Where the course is prolonged, intravenous feeding will be required. Surgery and manipulative endoscopy may be needed when there are common duct stones or pancreatic necrosis.

Prognosis

The disease has a 20% mortality. Adverse signs include hypocalcaemia, hypotension, a raised blood urea level and tissue hypoxia. Recurrent attacks are a possibility unless a cause is found and eradicated.

CHRONIC PANCREATITIS

This is not usually the result of recurrent attacks of acute pancreatitis and seems to develop de novo. The gland becomes fibrosed and possibly calcified. The parenchyma, islets and duct system are involved, and pseudocystic changes may occur. The major causes are alcoholism and, worldwide, the effects of malnutrition when calcification is prominent. Rare causes include pancreas divisum and a hereditary form. Pancreatic cancer may develop.

Symptoms and signs

Attacks of abdominal pain, usually epigastric and episodic, with vomiting are sometimes exacerbated by food and alcohol. Diarrhoea and severe steatorrhoea are often seen.

Weight loss is occasionally a marked feature but it may be caused by food-induced pain, malabsorption and diabetes.

Attacks of obstructive jaundice may occur from constriction of the lower end of the bile duct in the thickened pancreas, or in alcoholics from intra-hepatic cholestasis or parenchymal disease.

There are few signs; rarely, a pseudocyst may be palpable, otherwise there is merely abdominal tenderness. Sometimes there is hepatomegaly.

Investigations

1. Reduced pancreatic exocrine function can be shown by tubeless screening tests, e.g. Pancreolauryl test, backed up by a Lundh or pancreozymin test. Glycosuria and a raised random blood glucose level indicate diabetes.
2. Characteristic calcification may be seen on a plain abdominal X-ray and fibrosis and pseudocyst formation on CT scanning.
3. A definitive diagnosis can also be made at ERCP when stricturing, dilatation and ectasia of the pancreatic ducts are seen.

Treatment

Control of this disease is difficult. Alcohol is forbidden and pain treated without rendering the patient addicted to strong analgesics. Antidepressants may be helpful. Steatorrhoea is treated with a low-fat diet and enteric coated replacement therapy such as Nutrizym GR, Creon or Pancrease taken with meals. Adequate vitamins, including A, D and K, are given. Diabetes is treated by carbohydrate restriction, oral hypoglycaemic agents and sometimes insulin. If pain is severe, a coeliac axis block may be tried and repeated if successful.

If symptoms are intractable, surgery should be considered. The gland can be resected (pancreatectomy), when long-term insulin is required, or where there is pancreatic duct obstruction, drainage proximal to a strictured area can follow partial resection and pancreatico-jejunostomy.

MALIGNANT TUMOURS OF THE GASTROINTESTINAL TRACT, LIVER AND PANCREAS

See Table 9.6.

NEUROENDOCRINE TUMOURS

These tumours secrete one or more hormones (Table 9.7). It has been suggested that, because of their neuroendocrine properties, they are derived from embryonic neural crest cells. They are also referred to as APUD tumours (amine precursor uptake decarboxylation) because of their content and staining properties, although others argue a local (gut) origin. They all have malignant potential.

HEPATOMA

See page 292.

INFLAMMATORY BOWEL DISEASE (IBD)

This section includes Crohn's disease (CD) and ulcerative colitis (non-specific proctocolitis, NSP). Although there are differences (see Table 9.8), sometimes a definite diagnosis may be impossible.

Major epidemiological similarities exist. Both are more common in Whites, in urban as opposed to rural dwellers and in Jews. Both show a familial tendency in up to 30% of cases. Both are more common in young adults but occur, and may be serious, in the elderly. Both demonstrate humoral and cellular immunological abnormalities, of uncertain role in disease initiation and progression. Changes include the presence of anti-colon antibodies and of circulating lymphocytes cytotoxic to cultured colon epithelial cells. IBD has defied a search for an infective cause. In CD, atypical acid-fast bacilli are noted in some cases.

The incidence of the two diseases is different and variable: in North Europe CD has an incidence of $2–5/10^5$ population and a prevalence of about 30; NSP figures are about three times higher. In Third World countries IBD is rare. There are differences in eating and smoking habits. Refined carbohydrate consumption is higher and fibre intake lower in CD, whilst patients with NSP are less likely than normals to smoke. Smoking may actually be more common in Crohn's patients.

Pathology (see Table 9.8)

CROHN'S DISEASE

The symptoms of CD are usually colicky-abdominal pain, most often in the right iliac fossa, diarrhoea, sometimes with features of malabsorption (blood is noted by 25% of patients, particularly in colonic disease), and abdominal distension, weight loss, fever and general ill health.

Signs include anaemia, weight loss, sometimes finger clubbing, fever and a tender right iliac fossa mass. Ankle oedema may occur with hypoproteinaemia. Retarded growth is seen in children.

Table 9.6. Malignant tumours of the GI tract

	Type	Aetiological factors
Oesophagus	Squamous cell carcinoma, also secondary invasion of lower third by gastric adenocarcinoma	Iron deficiency, smoking, alcohol, coeliac disease ?Barrett's oesophagus. Common in China and Transkei in South Africa
Stomach	Adenocarcinoma Ulcerating, polypoid or superficial (confined to mucosa). Rarely linitis plastica (Fig. 9.6) (leather bottle stomach) or infiltrating	High nitrate content of food (smoked) and water, chronic gastritis, pernicious anaemia. Commonest in Japan
Colon and rectum	Adenocarcinoma From pre-existing adenomatous polyp (60% in rectum and sigmoid)	Familial polyposis coli Relatives with large bowel cancer. Large adenomatous polyps Chronic IBD ?Cholecystectomy
Pancreas	Adenocarcinoma of pancreas, also from ampulla of Vater or duct	Chronic pancreatitis ?Smoking, diabetes, coffee

ERCP = endoscopic retrograde cholangiopancreatography; IBD = inflammatory bowel disease FOBs = faecal occult blood tests.

The following should always be examined:

1. the mouth for ulceration or hypertrophic gingivitis
2. the perineum for ulceration, fistulae and skin tags
3. the joints and spine for arthritis and spondylitis
4. the skin and eyes for pyoderma or erythema nodosum and iritis
5. the rectum for palpable thickening of the anal and rectal mucosa.

CD can also present as a pyrexia of unknown origin or symptomless weight loss, or with fistulae into the perineum, bladder or another part of the gut. Patients with colonic disease have a higher incidence of rectal bleeding, more perianal disease and more diffuse abdominal pain.

Investigations
A blood count shows mild anaemia, a leukocytosis and elevated platelets.

Symptoms and signs	Diagnosis	Treatment	Prognosis
Progressive dysphagia, profound weight loss, signs of mediastinal and hepatic secondaries	Endoscopy Cytology Biopsy	Radiotherapy for upper third Resection and colonic transplantation	Poor
Ulcer type dyspepsia, GI bleeding, wasting, anaemia, epigastric mass, possibly pelvic masses	Endoscopy Cytology Biopsy	Surgical resection	Poor, except superficial cancer
Abdominal pain, anaemia, bowel upset, rectal bleeding or bloody discharge, abdominal or rectal mass	Sigmoidoscopy, colonoscopy, biopsy, barium enema, FOBs, surgical resection	Surgical resection	Quite good in early stage diagnosis
Head Obstructive jaundice, weight loss, intestinal bleeding *Body and tail* Weight loss, abdominal and back pain, thrombophlebitis migrans	Ultrasound with guided biopsy ERCP	If resectable, Whipple's operation. If not, ?endoscopic stending or cholecystenterostomy	?Very poor

The plasma protein levels may be low and with oedema, the serum albumin may be 30 g/1 or less.

Barium studies may show thickening and narrowing of the ileum with caecal and ascending colonic deformity. There may be deep ulceration and a cobblestone mucosa. A barium enema detects colonic involvement (Fig. 9.7). Changes similar to those in the small bowel are seen and small multiple ulcers of the mucosa are readily demonstrated.

Sigmoidoscopy or colonoscopy, will demonstrate inflammation, aphthoid ulceration, and thickening and inflammation of the bowel. In CD, comparatively normal areas (skip areas) may be interspersed between areas of Crohn's inflammation. Endoscopy allows biopsies to be taken, crucial in the diagnosis of CD; granuloma formation and deep inflammation are helpful findings.

Activity of the disease is assessed by measuring the erythrocyte sedimentation rate (ESR), plasma viscosity or acute-phase proteins such as C-reactive

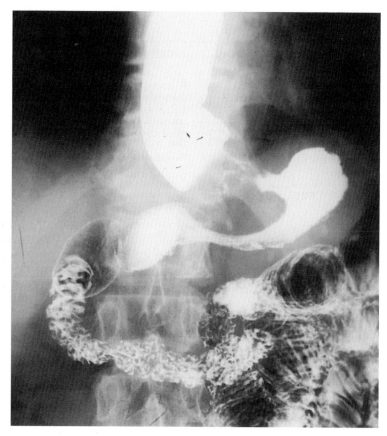

Fig. 9.6 A barium meal radiograph showing an invasive carcinoma of the stomach (linitis plastica). The lumen of the stomach is narrowed due to the thickened rigid infiltrated gastric wall. The oesophagus is dilated because of oesophagogastric involvement.

protein. A further technique is the injection of the patient's indium-labelled white cells which 'home' to areas of active inflammation where they can be detected by scanning.

Differential diagnosis
1. infective dysentery (i.e. *Shigella, Salmonella,* enteroinvasive *Escherichia coli,* amoebiasis), *Campylobacter enteritis,* pseudomembranous enteritis, gonococcal enteritis
2. vascular—ischaemic colitis
3. post-radiotherapy radiation colitis
4. Others: diverticular disease, carcinoma.

Treatment
Treatment is either medical or surgical by a joint team.

Table 9.7. Neuroendocrine tumours of the gut

Tumour	Site	Secretion	Effects	Treatment
Carcinoid	Gut, lung May metastasise to liver causing 'carcinoid syndrome'	5-hydroxytryptophan Histamine and others	Flushing Diarrhoea Right-sided heart lesions Bronchospasm (carcinoid syndrome)	Serotonin antagonists for diarrhoea, e.g. methysergide—consider somatostatin Hepatic artery embolisation
Insulinoma	Pancreas	Insulin	Fits/attacks of stupor due to hypoglycaemia	Resection or streptozotocin and somatostatin
Zollinger-Ellison syndrome	Pancreas	Gastrin	Duodenal and jejunal ulceration Diarrhoea/steatorrhoea	Omeprazole (to inhibit gastric acid production)
Vipoma	Pancreas	Vasoactive intestinal polypeptide	Profuse watery diarrhoea Hypokalaemia Acidosis	Resection or streptozotocin and somatostatin
Somatostatinoma	Pancreas	Somatostatin	Steatorrhoea Diabetes Gallbladder stones	Resection and/or streptozotocin
Glucagonoma	Pancreas	Glucagon	Steatorrhoea Weight loss ++ Diarrhoea Diabetes Characteristic skin rash of perineum, thighs, etc.	Resection

Table 9.8. The pathology of Crohn's disease (CD) and ulcerative colitis

	Crohn's disease	Ulcerative colitis
Site of disease	Ileocaecal most common Small bowel and upper GI tract sometimes	Total or left-sided, proctocolitis may extend proximally Rectum invariably involved
Inflammatory process	Transmural (all layers of gut) Walls thickened, deep ulcers, lumen narrowed, normal 'skip' areas between involved segments	Confined to mucosa with continuous shallow ulceration
Histology	Transmural inflammation, deep fissures, granulomata, crypt abscesses	Superficial mucosal inflammation Crypt abscesses Mucus (goblet cell) depletion
Pathological consequences	Intestinal obstruction, abscess formation, fistulae, carcinoma	Carcinoma Pseudo (inflammatory) polyps

1. Immunosuppressant drugs. Corticosteroids, usually given as oral prednisolone, suppress but do not cure this disease. Abdominal pain, fever and diarrhoea may all respond to short courses of corticosteroids, providing abscess formation can be excluded. It may be difficult to withdraw therapy because symptoms return. The side-effects of corticosteroids in this largely young group of patients are serious and the dose can be reduced by using azathioprine as a corticosteroid sparing agent.

2. Other drugs. Azathioprine may be effective in severe cases, particularly for fistulae. Sulphasalazine and other 5-amino-salicyclic acid derivatives are helpful, particularly in Crohn's colitis. Metronidazole sometimes produces healing of troublesome perineal ulceration.

3. Surgery. Resection is only used where there is a failure to control symptoms by medical treatment or where complications such as abscess, fistulae or carcinoma have occurred. The standard operation for CD is a right hemicolectomy and ile-ectomy with ileo-transverse colostomy. Stricturoplasty is helpful in subjects who have had previous resections.

4. Nutrition is preserved by encouraging the appetite and adding high calorie, high protein liquid feeds; in addition enteral, elemental diet will induce remission in active CD.

5. Symptomatic treatments with anti-diarrhoeals and antispasmodics are used, and anaemia is treated appropriately.

Prognosis

Despite many complications, the long-term prognosis is surprisingly good.

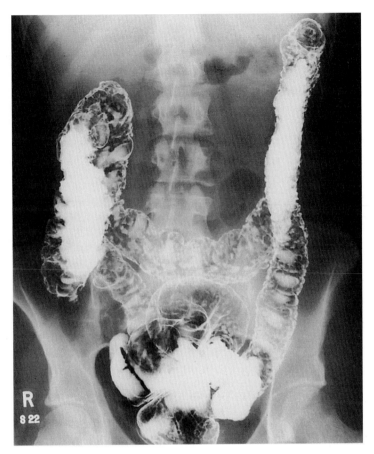

Fig. 9.7 Barium enema showing gross mucosal ulceration throughout the colon and ileum caused by Crohn's disease.

Once surgery is required, however, the chances of further symptoms and surgery are about 50%. Many patients have a long and chronic course before their disease eventually burns itself out.

ULCERATIVE COLITIS

Symptoms vary with the amount of colon involved (Fig. 9.8) but usually include diarrhoea with blood mixed in the stools many times per day, cramping abdominal pain relieved by bowel actions, anorexia, lethargy and weight loss.

Signs include weight loss, anaemia, fever and occasionally finger clubbing. There is often abdominal tenderness. On inspection of the anus there may be soreness, piles and abscess formation. Sigmoidoscopy shows mucosal reddening, loss of the normal vascular pattern, granularity with touch bleeding and purulent discharge.

Crohn's disease

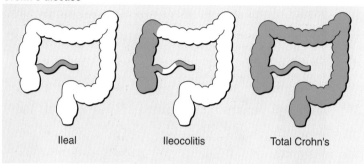

Ileal   Ileocolitis   Total Crohn's

Ulcerative colitis

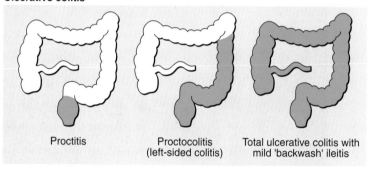

Proctitis   Proctocolitis   Total ulcerative colitis with
                   (left-sided colitis)   mild 'backwash' ileitis

Fig. 9.8 Crohn's disease and ulcerative colitis: the site and pattern of gut involvement.

In less severe cases, although diarrhoea with blood is still the major symptom, there is less constitutional upset, whilst in the least extensive cases (proctitis) bleeding may be accompanied by constipation.

Investigations

A blood count may show anaemia, usually from iron deficiency, leukocytosis and increased platelets. C-reactive protein, the ESR and plasma viscosity are raised because of inflammatory activity. LFTs are often abnormal as a variety of liver disorders may accompany ulcerative colitis (Table 9.9).

The diagnosis rests essentially on the endoscopic appearances of the colonic mucosa supplemented by biopsy and histology. The classical histology is of superficial mucosal inflammation, crypt abscesses and goblet cell (mucus) depletion.

A double-contrast barium enema shows fine mucosal granularity of variable extent. In total chronic cases the bowel may be shortened and featureless due to lack of haustra, with stricturing or the presence of pseudopolyps (Fig. 9.9).

Table 9.9. Complications of ulcerative colitis and Crohn's disease

Local	Abscess, fistula, haemorrhage, perforation, toxic megacolon, carcinoma, stricture

General
(1) Related to disease activity

Skin	Erythema nodosum, pyoderma gangrenosum
Eyes	Scleritis, iritis
Joints	Arthralgia, arthritis of large joints, spondylitis (HLA B27 +ve)
Blood	Hypercoagulability of blood, risk of pulmonary emboli

(2) Not related to disease activity

Kidney	Renal stones, right hydronephrosis from ileocaecal mass
Liver	Hepatitis, cholestasis, cirrhosis, sclerosing cholangitis, bile duct cancer
Others	Amyloidosis

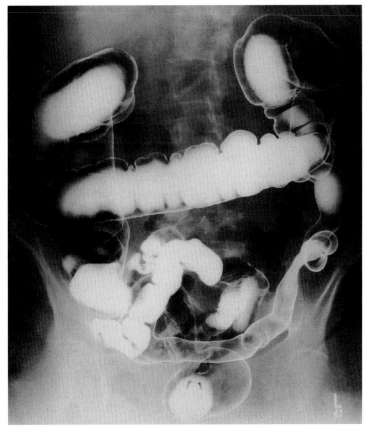

Fig. 9.9 Ulcerative colitis in the rectosigmoid region. The colon here is narrowed and featureless, contrasting with the rest of the normal-looking bowel.

Treatment

Patients with proctitis may respond to treatment of underlying constipation with a high-fibre diet. More diffuse disease is treated with anti-inflammatory drugs: long-term sulphasalazine or mesalazine are useful. Sulphasalazine has many side-effects, including headache, anorexia, skin rashes and in males temporary azoospermia, all due to the sulphapyridine portion. The modern approach is to use drugs lacking this portion, such as mesalazine. These drugs suppress colonic inflammation and although relatively ineffective in treating acute disease, they prevent relapses. Corticosteroids can be given locally by enema foam or suppository, and are useful for treating proctitis and left-sided disease. Corticosteroids given systemically are required in patients who are ill. Short courses are preferred, but there are problems, as in CD, in weaning patients off corticosteroids. Symptomatic treatment of pain, diarrhoea and anaemia is also important.

Surgery must be considered when disease is not controlled by medical therapy, and also for the treatment of some complications (see Table 9.9). Total proctocolectomy with ileostomy is used (as patients with severe symptoms invariably have total colonic involvement) but is now being replaced by a so-called 'pouch' operation. This procedure forms a reservoir from the distal ileum which allows continence and preserves the normal route of evacuation, thus avoiding the need for a permanent ileostomy. Recurrence and sepsis prevent its use in Crohn's colitis.

Ileostomy is well tolerated; adhesive bags are used and emptied regularly several times a day and most patients lead a totally normal life. A patients' self-help society, the Ileostomy Association, and stoma nurses are of great help.

Complications of NSP and CD

These are listed in Table 9.9. However, one or two need further explanation:

1. Toxic megacolon is a serious disorder, usually seen in patients with extensive ulcerative colitis. It is sometimes precipitated by instrumentation of the bowel and the use of antispasmodic and anti-diarrhoeal drugs. Abdominal distension, pain accompanied by vomiting and clinical deterioration occur, although diarrhoea may lessen. The pathology is a spreading inflammation into the muscle walls of the colon and destruction of the autonomic plexuses. Regular abdominal radiographs assess colonic and subsequent small bowel dilatation.

Treatment is as a medical emergency: high-dose steroids, intravenous nutrition and fluids, nasogastric suction, and antibiotic cover may reverse the situation. Otherwise, total colectomy and ileostomy is required as a surgical emergency.

2. Carcinoma. This is a complication of longstanding, extensive colitis. It is also seen in the colon and small bowel with longstanding CD. An estimate of the likelihood of cancer can be made by colonoscopic monitoring of patients looking for warning histological dysplastic change in the mucosa. Cancer is highly invasive and multicentric; the symptoms are no different from those of colitis and therefore clinically it is often missed.

3. Sclerosing cholangitis is described on page 267. An increased incidence of bile duct cancer in patients with NSP and CD occurs even in patients who have had total removal of their diseased bowel.

OTHER DISORDERS OF THE GASTROINTESTINAL TRACT

THE IRRITABLE BOWEL SYNDROME

This is extremely common. One survey showed that 14% of apparently normal subjects have symptoms but do not seek medical advice. Symptoms are thought to be caused by abnormal intestinal motility and pressure generation. There is no pathological change in the bowel. Some patients have purely colonic symptoms, but in others there is evidence of small bowel, gastric or oesophageal dysfunction.

Patients are more likely than controls to be anxious, depressed or neurotic, and in some there is an increased sensitivity to intestinal pain. Diverticular disease of the colon may represent an end stage of the disease. Irritable bowel syndrome may also follow an acute attack of gastroenteritis and symptoms may be grafted on to those of another disease such as IBD.

Symptoms and signs

There is abdominal pain and disturbance of bowel function—either diarrhoea, constipation or both. The diagnosis in many patients is one of exclusion, but the following positive features are often present.

1. Pain is usually lower abdominal, colicky and relieved or rarely worsened by a bowel action. The pain may be upper abdominal and related to the taking of food and be mistaken for dyspepsia.
2. The stools may be small and pellety, or there may be diarrhoea. Often these alternate.
3. The patient may pass mucus from the rectum.
4. There may be abdominal distension and a sensation of incomplete bowel evacuation.
5. Proctalgia fugax (attacks of severe rectal pain) can occur.

Signs, apart from abdominal tenderness, are absent. There may be evidence of neurotic or depressive illness and identical pain may occur with air insufflation on sigmoidoscopy.

Investigations

1. If the patient is young and a normal clinical, rectal and sigmoidoscopic examination is accompanied by a negative faecal occult blood test, no further investigation is necessary.
2. In middle-aged or elderly patients, if symptoms are of short duration and if weight loss is a feature, then additionally radiological examination of the large bowel (barium enema), and possibly of the stomach and small bowel, are required. Small bowel radiology is important for the detection

of CD, and barium enema for the detection of colonic polyps, carcinoma and IBD.

3. A full blood count, plasma viscosity or ESR, together with LFTs, are helpful in excluding organic disease.

Treatment

A positive attitude must be taken by the clinician and an explanation of how symptoms arise and the fact they are not due to organic disease, including cancer, must be conveyed to the patient. Reassurance and explanation are essential and may have to be repeated. Factors that seem to aggravate symptoms are identified and corrected. These include fear of cancer, anxiety, depression, the stresses of work and family life, and food allergy. The latter has led to the use of exclusion diets with subsequent identification and exclusion of offending foods. Some patients may become malnourished and totally neurotic. They often seek many medical opinions and repeated unnecessary investigation must be resisted.

Symptomatic treatment. Diarrhoea is treated with Ioperamide and codeine phosphate, and constipation with a high-fibre diet and a stool-bulking agent such as ispaghula (Fybogel, Isogel, etc.). Abdominal pain may be relieved by antispasmodics such as mebeverine and propontheline. Hypnosis may be helpful.

Prognosis

Symptoms tend to be recurrent and troublesome but about 25% will respond completely to simple explanation, dietary and medicinal therapy.

DIVERTICULAR DISEASE

This common condition found particularly in the middle-aged and elderly causes outpouching of the colonic mucosa through the colonic muscle to occur along the length of the colon, maximally in the sigmoid colon.

Symptoms and signs

Symptoms may be absent or identical to those of the irritable bowel syndrome with attacks of lower abdominal pain accompanied by diarrhoea, constipation, or both. Complications can produce dramatic symptoms:

1. Bleeding from dilated peridiverticular arteries causes anaemia with positive faecal occult bloods, or severe rectal bleeding with shock and collapse. This is treated conservatively, although emergency resection of the diseased bowel may be required.
2. Perforation causes acute abdominal pain and evidence of local or generalised peritonitis. Emergency surgery is required.
3. Abscess formation is by local extension of peridiverticular inflammation with abdominal pain and a tender mass. Drainage and resection of the affected area of colon are required.
4. Portal pyaemia from infection spreading from a diverticular abscess and

causing septic embolisation of the portal circulation may result in hepatic abscesses or septic portal vein thrombosis and portal hypertension.

JAUNDICE

Jaundice, the retention of bilirubin in the tissues, can be caused by:

1. haemolysis, when breakdown of red blood cells overwhelms hepatic conjugating capacity
2. obstruction, where the exit of conjugated bilirubin from the biliary tree is prevented
3. liver cell or hepatocellular dysfunction, where there is defective cellular metabolism of bilirubin by the liver cells.

HAEMOLYTIC JAUNDICE

Haemolytic jaundice is mild, with bilirubin levels < 85 mmol/l. The bilirubin is unconjugated and does not appear in the urine, but excessive urobilinogen does. LFTs, apart from the raised serum bilirubin, are normal but pigment stones may cause a secondary obstructive picture. Causes are those of haemolytic anaemia (see Chapter 11).

OBSTRUCTIVE JAUNDICE

Obstructive jaundice may be mild, moderate or severe. The urine is dark because of the presence of conjugated bilirubin, and the stools are pale from steatorrhoea (bile salt deficiency) and diminished stercobilinogen. Usually there is pruritus. Signs include hepatomegaly, an enlarged palpable gall-bladder when obstruction is below the cystic duct, and occasionally splenomegaly. LFTs show raised serum bilirubin and alkaline phosphatase levels and moderately elevated serum transaminases. The obstruction may be:

1. Extrahepatic, i.e. of the common bile duct or common hepatic duct
   (a) duct stones
   (b) malignant tumours of bile ducts, gallbladder, head of pancreas, or ampulla of Vater
   (c) sclerosing cholangitis
   (d) biliary strictures (usually following surgical injury).
2. Intrahepatic, i.e. at the level of the biliary canaliculi, and also has several causes. Acutely it may be caused by viral hepatitis or by certain drugs; it is sometimes seen in the third trimester of pregnancy, or it may be recurrent and of uncertain cause (recurrent idiopathic cholestasis). Chronic causes of intrahepatic cholestasis include primary biliary cirrhosis (see p. 294) and some persistent cholestatic drug reactions (e.g. chlorpromazine).

The site of biliary obstruction cannot be reliably detected clinically although pancreatic tumours can cause intestinal bleeding, and lesions obstructing below the cystic duct may cause gallbladder enlargement. Patients with gallstones may have attacks of biliary pain and fever, and with tumours there is often striking weight loss and back pain.

Investigations
Hepatic ultrasound shows dilatation of the intrahepatic bile ducts in extrahepatic obstruction. Occasionally patients with extrahepatic obstruction from gallstones may not show this change. Ultrasound may also show a cause for obstruction, such as a pancreatic mass or gallstones.

CT scans also show bile duct dilatation in extrahepatic obstruction and demonstrate causes such as hepatic or pancreatic tumours, pancreatitis, etc.

ERCP identifies the site of obstruction, e.g. from bile duct stones, or can place the lesion in the head of the pancreas by identifying pancreatic duct obstruction. Endoscopic ultrasound through the duodenum may allow more detailed visualisation.

Fine-needle cholangiography will also demonstrate the biliary tree above an obstructive lesion and thus help to define its extent and site.

In patients with intrahepatic obstruction, liver biopsy offers the only possible way of identifying the cause—apart, that is, from the history and viral studies. Even then, distinction between drugs and hepatitis may not be clearcut. An ERCP in such cases would confirm a patent but non-dilated biliary tree.

Surgery and biliary obstruction
Patients with extrahepatic obstruction may require surgery. Although ampullary tumours may be resectable, other cancers often are not and a cholecystenterostomy is performed to relieve jaundice. In the elderly and weakened patient, a stent may be placed endoscopically through a stenosing tumour. Adequate hydration and vitamin K therapy are important before surgery so that renal failure and bleeding are prevented. Cholangitis and septicaemia are other possible complications.

Intrahepatic biliary obstruction is not amenable to surgery.

Chronic biliary obstruction
The important cause of this is primary biliary cirrhosis. Patients with chronic biliary obstruction develop:

1. Severe itching, treated by bile salt chelation, e.g. with cholestyramine.
2. Secondary melanin pigmentation of the skin.
3. Metabolic bone disease, both osteomalacia from vitamin D deficiency (malabsorption and the effects of skin pigmentation) and osteoporosis. Prophylactic supplements of vitamin D and calcium are given.
4. Bleeding, spontaneous and postoperative from prothrombin deficiency and vitamin K malabsorption, treated with prophylactic i.m. vitamin K.
5. Hypercholesterolaemia with xanthoma formation and occasional peripheral neuropathy, and bone cholesterol deposits. Treatment is difficult and may require plasmapheresis.
6. Night blindness and dry skin from malabsorption of vitamin A, treated with vitamin A prophylaxis.

7. Postoperative renal failure.
8. Neuropathy and brain disease from vitamin E deficiency, particularly likely in children.

HEPATOCELLULAR JAUNDICE

Two types of disorder are seen:

1. jaundice without light microscopic liver cell damage, i.e. the congenital hyperbilirubinaemias
2. that due to generalised liver cell disease, e.g. viral hepatitis or cirrhosis.

The congenital hyperbilirubinaemias are caused by defective metabolism of bilirubin. The retained pigment may be unconjugated bilirubin (as in Gilbert's syndrome and Crigler-Najjar syndrome), in which case no pigment is seen in the urine, or conjugated bilirubin (as in Dubin-Johnson syndrome and Rotor syndrome), where pigment is present in the urine. In both types, the serum bilirubin levels are raised.

1. Gilbert's syndrome is a common (5% of population) autosomal dominant condition. LFTs are normal. Bilirubin uptake and conjugation may be defective. Bilirubin rises with fever, trauma and starvation.

2. Crigler-Najjar syndrome is a rare inherited disorder. Severe cases are fatal because of kernicterus; less severe cases are compatible with life.

3. Dubin-Johnson syndrome is a rare inherited disease. The liver contains black (melanin) pigment. Serum alkaline phosphatase levels are raised.

4. Rotor syndrome is a variant of Dubin-Johnson syndrome but the liver does not contain melanin pigment.

Hepatocellular jaundice from liver cell disease

The jaundice is mild, moderate or severe. Stools are pale and the urine dark. Itching, if present, is usually transient. The liver may be enlarged, of normal size or smaller than usual. Splenic enlargement is common and in chronic cases the cutaneous signs of hepatocellular disease occur (see Table 9.13).

LFTs show raised serum bilirubin, greatly raised transaminase and normal or somewhat raised alkaline phosphatase levels. The prothrombin time is prolonged. The diagnosis of the cause of liver cell jaundice (Table 9.10) rests on a full history, clinical examination, immunological tests for causative viruses, an autoimmune profile and, if no clotting problems, a liver biopsy.

VIRAL HEPATITIS

Several viruses cause hepatitis, and viruses A, B, C, D and E are the most important. Viral hepatitis is a worldwide condition and, in the case of B and C infection, probably accounts for much of the chronic non-alcoholic liver

Table 9.10. Some common causes of hepatocellular jaundice

Acute	Hepatitis (viral, drugs and alcohol)
	Fatty infiltration (drugs and alcohol)
	Hepatic necrosis (viruses, drugs)
Chronic	
Chronic hepatitis	Autoimmune, viral, drug induced
Cirrhosis	Alcoholic, post-viral, metabolic

Table 9.11. The main causes of viral hepatitis

Virus	Type	Incubation period	Detecting infection
A	Picornavirus (RNA)	2–3 weeks	Virus A IgM antibody
B	DNA	4–26 weeks	HBsAg HBeAg anti-HBc
D	RNA (incomplete virus)	?	anti-Delta + anti-HBc
C	RNA	6–9 weeks	anti-virus C antibody Reverse transcriptase PCR
E	?RNA	—	Nil
EBV	DNA (herpes)	—	Antibody to viral capsid antigen (VCA) EB virus specific IgM
CMV	DNA (herpes)	2–6 weeks	Complement fixation IgG CMV IgM (fluorescent antibody test)

EBV = Epstein–Barr virus; CMV = Cytomegalovirus; PCR = polymerase chain reaction.

disease and primary hepatic cancer. Despite the number of viruses involved, the clinical picture and some of the complications are common to all. The incubation period is, however, variable (Table 9.11).

Types of viral hepatitis (see also Table 9.11)

Virus A causes infective hepatitis. This is common in childhood within the family unit. Epidemics are common where hygiene is poor. It is spread by oral–faecal contamination. It does not cause chronic liver disease, although fatal acute hepatic necrosis occasionally occurs.

Virus B (HBV) (Table 9.12) is spread by contaminated blood and blood products. Subjects at special risk include homosexuals, those given infected

Table 9.12. The immunology of virus B infection

Blood test	Significance
HBs antigen +ve	Indicates infection or carrier state
HBs antibody +ve	Indicates past infection and immunity
HBe antigen +ve	Indicates infectivity and, if persistent, chronicity
HBe antibody +ve	Indicates low infectivity and recovery
HB core antigen +ve	Not detected in serum
HB core antibody +ve	Indicates recent infection (IgM) even if other tests are −ve. If persistent (IgM), chronic liver disease
HBV DNA +ve	The most sensitive test of viral replication and chronicity

blood or blood products, intravenous drug users, the newborn of infected mothers, patients and staff of mental deficiency and renal dialysis units, and the immunocompromised. The disease is widespread in the Third World and approximately 300 million chronic carriers may exist. Virus B is an important cause of chronic liver disease and hepatic cancer. About 0.1% of subjects in the UK carry the virus, but in Africa and the Far East the rate reaches 15%. The important immunological tests used in the monitoring of virus B infection are shown in Table 9.12. Mutants of hepatitis B have been described and are of importance in HBV vaccination.

Virus C (HCV). Transmission is parenteral by infected blood, tissue and blood products. Sexual and vertical transmission seem rare. Most (> 90%) post-transfusion (non-A, non-B) hepatitis is now known to be caused by HCV. Transfused blood is now screened for HCV as for HBV. Subjects at risk include parenteral drug abusers, haemophiliacs, patients transfused with blood prior to screening and health care workers. Unidentified routes of transmission exist (sporadic).

Infection is usually asymptomatic but a few develop typical, but relatively mild, hepatitis. Eighty per cent of infected patients fail to clear the virus and develop chronic hepatitis. The insidious development of cirrhosis occurs in about 30% of chronic HCV infections over 20–30 years. Hepatoma may be an important sequel.

Antibody tests for several epitopes of the putative viral protein are used for diagnosis. Definitive confirmation is by reverse transcriptase PCR.

Prevalence is high at 0.1–1.0% of Europeans.

Virus D (delta) only exists in association with virus B. It therefore occurs as a combined infection or as a secondary delta infection in a virus B carrier. It is particularly related to intravenous drug abuse, causes acute hepatitis and renders the virus B carrier more likely to develop hepatic cirrhosis.

Virus E is found in India and the Far East and behaves like virus A. It does not cause chronic liver disease but can cause fulminant hepatitis in pregnancy.

Symptoms and signs

These are of fairly sudden onset. In the pre-icteric phase the symptoms are malaise, fever, upper right abdominal and epigastric pain, and discomfort with nausea and vomiting. After a few days, these symptoms remit and the patient becomes jaundiced. However, jaundice may be absent (anicteric hepatitis). Hepatitis C is commonly anicteric and asymptomatic.

Apart from jaundice, the signs are tender, moderate hepatomegaly, splenomegaly, and sometimes enlarged lymph nodes in the neck. The urine contains bile, even before there is jaundice.

Jaundice lasts 7–10 days, improvement is then rapid, appetite returns and LFTs normalise. Many patients, however, suffer from continuing debility, lethargy, abdominal discomfort and fat intolerance: 'post-hepatitis syndrome'.

Investigations

The blood count shows a normal haemoglobin level with leukopenia and a relative lymphocytosis. The ESR and plasma viscosity are raised.

LFTs are abnormal, the serum bilirubin is raised, and serum transaminases elevated, sometimes markedly so (1000–2000 iu/l). The serum albumin level is normal in uncomplicated cases, but total globulin level is raised, with hypergammaglobulinaemia.

A liver biopsy, performed only if coagulation is normal, shows hepatic damage to be maximal in the centrilobular areas with a scattered lobular and portal lymphocytic infiltration.

Complications

Resolution without chronic changes in the liver is usual and invariable in virus A or E infection. Chronicity is a feature of virus C (80%), B (12%) and D.

1. Acute fulminant hepatitis. An acute and severe necrosis of the liver can complicate hepatitis caused by any virus with deepening jaundice, hepatic coma, bleeding and renal failure. The liver becomes smaller and there is an 80% mortality without hepatic transplantation.
2. In virus B infection, immune complex disease may occur either in the preicteric phase, with arthralgia and skin rashes, or later as an acute polyarteritis nodosa or glomerulonephritis. Virus C may cause cryoglobulinaemia. Bone marrow involvement with severe aplastic anaemia is also a rare complication of any viral hepatitis. Patients with viral hepatitis can also develop an obstructive picture—cholestatic hepatitis—which may cause diagnostic difficulty.
3. Chronic active hepatitis. Here symptoms continue, there is hepatosplenomegaly and the cutaneous signs of liver disease (see Table 9.13). LFTs do not normalise, liver biopsy shows piecemeal necrosis, bridging necrosis between portal tracts and the centrilobular areas, fibrosis and cellular infiltration.

Treatment

Bedrest and a sensible nutritious diet usually lead to uneventful resolution of the disease. The treatment of acute liver failure is discussed below. Patients with chronic hepatitis following viral infection with virus B, C or D may require antiviral therapy. This is currently carried out by injections of alpha-interferon three times weekly over a 3–6 month period.

Prophylaxis

Vaccines are available for virus A and, more importantly, for virus B. A recombinant yeast-derived virus B vaccine is used. Large-scale vaccination of children in the Third World is an important but expensive way of reducing hepatic cirrhosis and cancer. At present vaccination is with three injections, given at 0, 1 and 5 months, to those at risk, e.g. family and contacts of sufferers, uninfected homosexuals, medical and dental personnel, etc. There is no vaccine for HCV.

Liver cell failure

Impaired hepatocyte function leads to hepatocellular jaundice, fluid retention, bleeding and hepatic encephalopathy. Other important associations include abnormal drug sensitivity, certain endocrine changes and the development of cutaneous signs of liver disease.

Hepatocellular jaundice. This is variable, depending on the severity of liver cell damage. There is no specific treatment.

Fluid retention. This causes ankle oedema, ascites, particularly if portal hypertension exists, and is sometimes generalised. Although hypoalbuminaemia is a factor, the major cause is excessive renal sodium retention.

Treatment is by bedrest, sodium restriction and the use of potassium-sparing diuretics (potassium deficiency is common in liver cell disease). Despite this precaution, electrolyte disturbances are common. Hyponatraemia and a rising blood creatinine level herald the onset of renal failure. Ascites drainage by repeated paracentesis with salt-poor albumin infusions are beneficial in resistant cases. A LeVeen shunt, which drains ascitic fluid into the major veins in the neck, is occasionally useful in refractory cases.

Acute cases clear easily with improvement in liver function but diuretics may be required.

Bleeding. Spontaneous bleeding may occur into the skin or from mucous membranes. Important causes include failure of hepatic synthesis of coagulant factors, particularly vitamin K-related ones, thrombocytopenia and increased thrombolytic activity.

Clotting defects are treated with fresh frozen plasma plus platelet infusions if required.

Hepatic encephalopathy. Confusion, somnolence leading to coma, a flapping tremor of the outstretched hands and a sweetish smell of the breath (fetor hepaticus) are the main features. It is caused by the intoxication by protein-derived breakdown products of the reticular formation and basal ganglia of the brain. The syndrome can occur with rapid onset of coma from acute hepatic necrosis, but in more chronic conditions consciousness is retained, whilst dysarthria, tremor, confusion and constructional apraxia are more obvious.

Alimentary bleeding, infection (anywhere), surgical trauma, paracentesis, a high protein meal, and drugs (analgesics, sedatives and diuretics) may precipitate hepatic encephalopathy.

Protein restriction to < 40 g per day, and the use of non-absorbable antibiotics reduce bacterial protein breakdown in the gut. Drugs known to aggravate hepatic encephalopathy, such as diuretics and all sedative drugs, are stopped. Lactulose, a non-absorbable liquid carbohydrate, soften the stools, lower faecal pH and inhibit ammonia-producing organisms (NH_3 is one of the known toxic nitrogenous breakdown products).

Abnormal drug metabolism. Patients with liver cell disease are sensitive to drugs, particularly to sedatives. The reasons for this include slower hepatic metabolism, altered binding to serum albumin, altered distribution volume and diminished first-pass metabolism. The sensitivity to sedative drugs is also related to latent hepatic encephalopathy. Drug therapy needs to be carefully monitored in subjects with liver disease and reduced dosing is advised.

Endocrine changes. Both feminisation and impotence occur in males with chronic liver cell failure; changes in females are less obvious. The initial event in males appears to be testicular atrophy with low serum testosterone values. FSH and LH are not appropriately elevated after clomiphine. Hyperoestrogenaemia also occurs, but oestrogen turnover is normal. An increase in numbers of cell oestrogen receptors is a likely explanation for gynaecomastia and some vascular abnormalities. Diabetes with insulin resistance is also common in cirrhosis, and in alcoholics pseudo-Cushing's syndrome occurs. Here physical features of Cushing's syndrome with high non-suppressable levels of corticosteroids are reversed when drinking stops.

Cutaneous signs of liver disease. See Table 9.13

Hepatic transplantation is the only successful treatment for end-stage liver failure.

Table 9.13. Cutaneous signs of liver disease

Nails	Clubbing
	White (opaque) nails
	White bands (hypoalbuminaemia)
Skin	Paper money skin (facial telangiectasia)
	Vascular spiders
	Palmar erythema
	Jaundice
Others	(Males)
	Gynaecomastia
	Testicular atrophy
	Loss of secondary sexual hair

CIRRHOSIS OF THE LIVER

Cirrhosis is a chronic generalised liver disease resulting from necrosis and regeneration of liver cells. It is characterised by:

1. a variable element of liver cell (hepatocyte) dysfunction
2. increased hepatic fibrosis
3. nodule formation (nodular regeneration).

The latter is most important as nodules are functionally less effective than normal liver tissue, they have an abnormal blood supply and they constrict hepatic venous outflow to produce portal hypertension. Further, malignant, change (hepatoma) may occur within them.

Causes

1. Alcohol excess
2. Viral hepatitis (viruses B, D and C)
3. Non-viral (autoimmune) chronic active hepatitis
4. Primary biliary cirrhosis
5. Haemochromatosis (primary genetic iron overload)
6. Cystic fibrosis
7. Alpha-1-antitrypsin deficiency
8. Wilson's disease (excessive copper retention).

Symptoms and signs

Patients can be asymptomatic and present with abnormalities found on clinical examination, e.g. hepatomegaly, or with abnormal investigations. Presenting symptoms may include:

1. intestinal bleeding, often severe from oesophageal varices caused by portal hypertension
2. jaundice from liver cell failure
3. fluid retention, either as ascites with abdominal distension and dyspnoea, or with ankle oedema
4. hepatic encephalopathy with confusion, tremor and coma
5. excessive bleeding, purpura, bruising and nose bleeds
6. fever, confusion and abdominal pain from *E. coli* infection of ascitic fluid with resultant septicaemia
7. weight loss, abdominal pain, ascites and bleeding from a complicating hepatoma.

The signs are variable; any or none of the following can be present:

1. The skin is pigmented and/or jaundiced.
2. There may be purpura and bruising due to a bleeding tendency.
3. The patient's palms may be warm and reddened (palmar erythema).
4. There may be finger clubbing and white (opaque) nails.
5. There may be spider naevi, i.e. dilated arterioles usually on the face, arms, shoulders and trunk, or facial telangiectasia (paper money skin).

6. The liver may be enlarged, firm and nodular, or may be smaller than normal, by percussion.
7. There may be splenomegaly.
8. There may be ascites, often with an umbilical hernia and, due to portal hypertension, enlarged abdominal veins around the umbilicus.
9. There may be peripheral oedema.
10. Signs of hepatic encephalopathy may be found.
11. Male patients may show feminisation.

Investigations

Mild anaemia, leukopenia and thrombocytopenia are caused by hypersplenism. The prothrombin time may be prolonged.

An ultrasound scan of the liver confirms that it is enlarged or small, diffusely abnormal and nodular.

Tests of previous and continuing virus B, D and C infection may be positive. LFTs are usually abnormal, but in compensated cases abnormalities are minimal. A raised serum bilirubin level, moderately raised transaminases and alkaline phosphatase, reduced serum albumin and increased serum globulins, particularly the gammaglobulins, all occur.

Liver biopsy, which should be routinely stained for iron, alpha-1-anti-trypsin and copper, shows fibrosis, nodule formation, liver cell damage and fragmentation. There is invariably a periportal cellular infiltrate.

Table 9.14 gives the major features of the various types of cirrhosis.

PRIMARY LIVER CANCER

Cancer derived from hepatocytes is a hepatoma. In 70–80% of cases it complicates cirrhosis and is most commonly seen in Africa, the Middle East and the Far East, where cirrhosis is widespread. The type of cirrhosis is variable, but preceding virus B and C infection are particularly important and incorporation of virus B into hepatocyte DNA seems a common consequence of virus B infection. Whether this mechanism or the cellular hyperactivity of the cirrhotic process is responsible for hepatoma is uncertain. Males who have well-compensated cirrhosis, e.g. haemochromatosis, may have a risk as high as 15%. Aflatoxin, a carcinogenic product of the mould *Aspergillus flavus* which contaminates stored cereals in some countries, is a further risk factor.

Hepatoma in a cirrhotic liver is commonly multiple, but in non-cirrhotic patients a single neoplasm is usual.

Symptoms and signs

These include vague ill health, weight loss and hepatic pain in a patient with previously diagnosed cirrhosis, bleeding from oesophageal varices (hepatomas tend to invade portal venous radicles), ascites, often bloodstained, and/or of high protein content, and rupture of the tumour into the peritoneal cavity with shock and pain.

The liver may be nodular, tender and perhaps increasing in size. LFTs show no specific change, but a rising alkaline phosphatase may be suggestive.

In 60% of patients the serum alpha-fetoprotein level is raised; this is negative, however, in non-cirrhotic (fibrolamellar) growths and in cholangiocarcinoma.

Tissue diagnosis is by ultrasound-guided needle biopsy. Arteriography shows the tumour circulation, size and number of tumours.

Hepatomas can produce erythropoietin (polycythaemia), lipids (hyper-lipidaemia), insulin (hypoglycaemia) or parathormone-like protein (hyper-calcaemia), thus widening the clinical features. Secondary spread to neighbouring structures, bone and lymph nodes and occurs early.

Differential diagnosis is from decompensated cirrhosis and secondary hepatic cancer.

Treatment

Resection by hepatic lobectomy may be possible with a single tumour in one lobe in a non-cirrhotic liver. Otherwise chemotherapy, e.g. adriamycin, or embolisation of the tumour via its arterial blood supply lessen pain. Hepatic transplantation is a further possibility but secondary tumour recurrence is common.

Cholangiocarcinoma

This is another form of primary hepatic cancer with growth from bile duct cells. Obstructive jaundice results. There is an association with ulcerative colitis.

PORTAL HYPERTENSION

Raised pressure within the portal circulation (Fig. 9.10) of > 10 mmHg

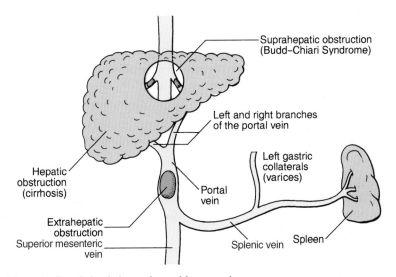

Fig. 9.10 Portal circulation and portal hypertension.

Table 9.14. Cirrhosis of the liver

Type	Cause	Diagnosis
Cryptogenic F>M (macronodular)	Unknown ?virus C	Elimination of other causes
Primary biliary cirrhosis F>M++9:1 (micronodular)	Autoimmune destruction of septal bile ducts	M antibodies in blood Granulomata around bile ducts on biopsy ERCP shows patent non-dilated biliary tree
Chronic active hepatitis (macronodular) F>M (usually young)	Autoimmune liver disease 60% HLA-B8+ve	Usually grossly deranged LFTs Hypergammaglobulinaemia Biopsy shows piecemeal necrosis, plasma cell infiltration +ve DNA antibodies +ve Smooth muscle antibodies
Wilson's disease (macronodular/ variable) F>M (usually young)	Genetic Autosomal recessive Disorder of copper metabolism Tissue copper overload	Kaiser-Fleischer rings in eyes Serum caeruloplasmin usually low Urinary copper increased Increased copper content in liver biopsy
Haemochromatosis M>F (micronodular)	Genetic Autosomal recessive Link with HLA-A3	Raised serum iron Raised hepatic tissue iron
Alcoholic M>F (micronodular but variable)	? due to toxicity of acetaldehyde	History Liver biopsy may show fat, central hyaline sclerosis or acute alcoholic hepatitis with polymorph infiltrate and Mallory's alcoholic hyaline, etc.
Post-viral	Virus C or B	+ve tests for virus C or B Often from high-risk group – drug abuse (B or C) – previous transfusion (C) – homosexual, promiscuous (B) – immunosuppressed (B or C)
Alpha-1-antitrypsin (AT) deficiency	Genetic Autosomal recessive AT is a protease inhibitor	Suspect in young and adults with liver disease ± emphysema PAS +ve granules in periportal hepatocytes Confirmation by immuno- precipitation and phenotyping

Effects	Treatment
Bleeding varices Liver cell failure Mild obstructive jaundice Bone disease Other autoimmune disorders, e.g. renal tubular acidosis CREST syndrome (scleroderma)	Fat-soluble vitamin supplements, ursodeoxycholate Transplantation
Liver cell dysfunction Part of multisystem disease, e.g. ulcerative colitis, skin rashes, arthralgia (c.f. SLE)	Corticosteroids and azathioprine
Liver failure Haemolysis Bone disease CNS involuntary movements Personality deterioration	Oral *D*-penicillamine to remove copper
Hepatomegaly Skin pigmentation Diabetes Cardiomyopathy Gonadal failure Arthralgia Hepatoma risk ++	Venesection to remove iron
May be deeply jaundiced Fever Hepatomegaly Liver cell failure Delirium tremens Peripheral neuropathy Dupuytren's contractures	Forbid alcohol; treat liver cell failure
Mild liver cell failure or portal hypertension May be silent	May be suitable for antiviral treatment (alpha-interferon)
Neonatal hepatitis with cholestasis Childhood and adult cirrhosis Panacinar emphysema	AT can be given therapeutically for lung disease

results in changes that include splenomegaly, formation of oesophageal and gastric varices and opening up of venous connections between the portal and systemic circulation. The three major types of portal hypertension are:

1. suprahepatic, resulting from obstruction of sinusoidal outflow, e.g. thrombosis of hepatic veins or a vena caval web
2. hepatic, resulting from sinusoidal distortion due to hepatic disease, e.g. cirrhosis
3. prehepatic, resulting from portal vein obstruction, usually thrombosis.

Portal hypertension causes:

1. splenomegaly, sometimes with pancytopenia, i.e. hypersplenism
2. bleeding from oesophageal and gastric varices, either as haematemesis and/or melaena, or chronic anaemia
3. the shunting of protein blood products through the portosystemic collaterals around rather than through the liver resulting in hepatic encephalopathy
4. shunting of gut bacteria through similar collaterals, causing *E. coli* septicaemia and endotoxemia.

Hypersplenism
Usually, there are no symptoms, and splenomegaly may be the only sign. A blood count shows pancytopenia, although not severe enough to be associated with spontaneous infection or bleeding. Splenectomy is not recommended.

Bleeding from oesophageal varices
This is an important condition because bleeding can be massive and repeated. Bleeding in those whose portal hypertension is caused by liver disease may precipitate liver cell failure with jaundice, ascites and hepatic encephalopathy.

The mortality is high; about 50% of those bleeding from oesophageal varices complicating liver disease die as a result of their first bleed.

Differences between suprahepatic and extrahepatic portal hypertension (Fig. 9.10)

Suprahepatic portal hypertension (the Budd–Chiari syndrome) causes blockage of hepatic venous outflow, variceal bleeding, tender hepatomegaly and the rapid onset of ascites and liver cell failure. Unless obstruction of hepatic veins is partial, the mortality is > 80%. It has many causes, e.g. polycythaemia, membranous obstruction of the inferior vena cava, contraceptive pill use.

In extrahepatic portal hypertension the prognosis from bleeding varices is better because there is no liver cell disease or liver cell failure. The cause is usually a septic portal endophlebitis, arising in childhood from an infected appendix, or in adults from septicaemia or septic diverticulitis. Occasionally a clotting disease like polycythaemia or antithrombin-3 deficiency is the cause.

Symptoms and signs

Symptoms include haematemesis, melaena and those of acute or chronic anaemia.

There may be tachycardia and hypotension; if there is liver disease the cutaneous signs such as spider naevi may be present but are difficult to detect in hypovolaemic subjects. Fluid retention, particularly ascites and signs of hepatic encephalopathy, i.e. fetor, stupor, confusion, etc., develop quickly. There may be splenomegaly.

Investigations

A blood count confirms the effects of bleeding and may show a pancytopenia. LFTs are abnormal where there is hepatic disease. Prothrombin time and other coagulation tests are prolonged where there is hepatic disease.

Endoscopy is vital to diagnose the presence of varices and to commence sclerotherapy. Hepatic ultrasound may be helpful, if feasible, to diagnose chronic liver disease.

Treatment

1. Blood volume must be restored by adequate transfusion.
2. Sedative drugs must be avoided.
3. Impending hepatic encephalopathy is treated by stopping oral protein and giving oral neomycin to prevent intestinal bacterial protein breakdown. This can be supplemented with oral lactulose.
4. Injection sclerotherapy is performed through the endoscope. A sclerosant such as phenylethanolamine is injected directly into the varices. Injections are repeated every 3–4 weeks until all varices have been thrombosed. In those with active bleeding, cessation can usually be achieved with a Sengstaken–Blakemore tube (Fig. 9.11) and intravenous vasopressin or glypressin which constricts arterial flow into the portal circulation. Somatostatin is an effective but expensive alternative drug. Beta-blockers prevent recurrent variceal bleeding in the long term.
5. Surgery for those fit enough may be required if bleeding continues. The usual operation is a transection of the oesophagus and re-stapling using a staple gun, although some surgeons favour an emergency portocaval shunt. In patients with extrahepatic portal hypertension, variceal sclerotherapy is preferable as surgery does not produce lasting benefit.

DISEASES OF THE LIVER IN CHILDHOOD ALSO OCCURRING IN ADULTS

Neonatal hepatitis

Neonatal hepatitis causes neonatal jaundice and may be due to viruses or protozoa or be 'idiopathic' (75%) or familial. The long-term prognosis is fairly good although cirrhosis may develop.

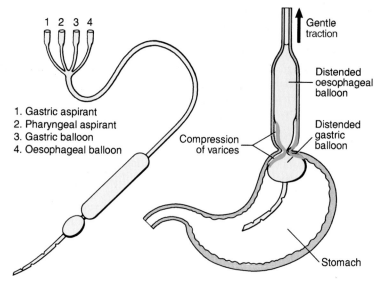

Fig. 9.11 The Sengstaken–Blakemore tube.

Biliary atresia

This results from failure of development or damage to the biliary tree in utero. It may be variable in completeness and causes progressive obstructive jaundice. The prognosis is poor but a Kasai operation (hepatic porto-enterostomy) performed early can prevent disease progression. For others, transplantation may be possible. Prophylactic fat-soluble vitamins A, D, E and K are given.

Reye's syndrome

A fine fatty infiltration of the liver of childhood occurs following a viral infection. Cerebral oedema develops with vomiting and coma in severe cases. It can also follow aspirin administration in children.

Indian childhood cirrhosis

This is seen in middle-class Indian children. There is often a family history. The prognosis is poor. Copper overload may be a factor in the aetiology.

Fibrocystic disease (see Table 9.16)

Wilson's disease (see Table 9.14)

Cystic fibrosis (see p. 77)

DISEASES OF THE LIVER SPECIFIC TO PREGNANCY

Idiopathic cholestasis

Obstructive jaundice develops in the third trimester with pruritus and disappears with delivery. It reappears with subsequent pregnancy and with oral contraceptives. It is probable that cholestasis is induced by oestrogens.

Acute fatty liver

Microvesicular fatty infiltration of the liver of uncertain cause is seen in the last trimester. It causes vomiting and liver cell failure. The white cell count and normoblasts in peripheral blood are raised. There is severe bleeding. Treatment is of liver failure and/or renal failure. Caesarean section may be necessary.

DRUG-INDUCED LIVER DISEASE

Drugs may cause any type of hepatic disease, including benign and malignant tumours. In some patients there is a known (allergic) hypersensitivity, whilst others probably depend on the production of reactive metabolites. The most important drug-induced lesions produce cholestasis, hepatocellular damage or a mixed picture (cholestatic hepatitis) (Table 9.15).

Table 9.15. Some examples of drug-induced liver disease

Cholestatic	Oral contraceptives
	17-alpha alkyl substituted testosterones and nortestosterones
	Chlorpropamide
Hepatocellular	Paracetamol
	Ketoconazole
	Carbon tetrachloride
	Amiodarone
	Methotrexate
Cholestatic hepatitis	Chlorpromazine
	Erythromycin
Fatty infiltration	Sodium valproate
	Tetracycline
Chronic active hepatitis	Alpha methyldopa
	Nitrofurantoin
Hepatic tumours	
Adenoma	Oral contraceptives
Carcinoma	Oral contraceptives
	Androgens
	Vinyl chloride
Peliosis (dilatation of sinusoids)	Oral contraceptives
	Androgens

OTHER IMPORTANT DISEASES OF THE LIVER

Table 9.16. Other diseases of the liver

Cause	Effect	Investigation/treatment
Non-viral infections		
Schistosomiasis		
Migration of ova from S. mansoni and S. japonicum (adult worms) in mesenteric veins	Portal hypertension due to portal fibrosis around ova No true cirrhosis	Diagnosis: ova in rectal snip or stools Praziquantel 40–60 mg/kg or oxamniquine but needs control of water supply (snails) Sclerosis of varices
Hydatid disease		
Cystic stage of dog tapeworm (*Echinococcus granulosa*) —intermediate host sheep	One or several hepatic cysts May be visible and palpable Usually right lobe Cysts also possible in lung, kidney, etc.	Ultrasound confirms cystic nature Eosinophilia and +ve antibody tests Surgery required for complete cyst removal following cyst sterilisation Mebendazole and derivatives may help
Metabolic disease		
Fatty infiltration		
(a) Macrovesicular (large fat droplets) due to alcohol, diabetes (b) Microvesicular (fine fat droplets) due to drugs like tetracycline and in pregnancy and in Reye's syndrome	Smooth non-tender	LFTs mildly abnormal Generalised—sometimes localised—change Biopsy diagnostic Treatment is of the cause
Amyloidosis		
Fibrillar glycoprotein material either AA—due to chronic suppuration (rare) or rheumatoid arthritis (common) or familial Mediterranean fever AL—associated with myeloma or no underlying disease	Firm hepatomegaly Often proteinuria/renal failure and evidence of splenomegaly	Biopsy of liver diagnostic Biopsy of rectal mucosa helpful and of kidneys for renal involvement Treatment nil or of the cause

Table 9.16 *continued.* **Other diseases of the liver**

Cause	Effect	Investigation/treatment
Polycystic liver disease A genetic disorder with either multiple hepatic cysts, extensive fibrosis or dilatation of biliary tree	Multiple cysts—nodular liver Extensive (congenital hepatic) fibrosis—portal hypertension Dilatation of biliary tree—recurrent cholangitis and possible carcinoma	Ultrasound shows all three Biopsy helpful for fibrosis and ERCP for congenital bile duct dilatation LFTs normal except in presence of multiple cysts. Portal hypertension requires sclerotherapy Resection for bile duct dilatation

10

NUTRITION AND OBESITY
Kenneth W. Heaton

DIET AND HEALTH

Rising public concern and awareness of diet–health interactions demands that tomorrow's doctors know more about nutrition than most of their teachers. Regrettably, doctors must be able to counter disinformation from vested interests, excitable reporters and cranks of all sorts.

Features of a health-preserving diet

Many official bodies have issued guidelines to healthy eating and there is a worldwide consensus, summarised in Table 10.1.

Table 10.1. Characteristics of a health-preserving diet

Desirable feature	Main problem(s) in UK
Enough energy for normal physiological processes but no more	Most people fail to limit their intake Overnutrition fosters many diseases
Enough micronutrients (vitamins, minerals, trace elements) and essential fatty acids	Possibility of subclinical deficiencies fostering chronic disease
Saturated fat not more than 10% of calories	Excess is common, raises serum LDL cholesterol
Enough fibre (cell-wall material) to allow easy defecation and stool weight > 150 g per 24 hours	Deficiency is common, may lead to symptomatic constipation, bowel cancer
Not too much rapidly digested carbohydrate, esp. extracellular sugars ('refined carbohydrates')	Dental disease, obesity
Salt limited to 5 g per 24 hours, preferably less	UK average of 10 g per 24 hours fosters hypertension in susceptible people

Practical implications

1. Minimise intake of intermeal snacks, puddings, especially sugar–fat mixtures, and sugary drinks.
2. Fill up on unprocessed or lightly processed starch foods, especially bread (preferably wholemeal), rice, pasta, legume seeds or pulses (peas, beans, lentils), root vegetables and potatoes.
3. Minimise fried food, pastry, cold prepared meats; use vegetable oils, especially olive oil.
4. Use lean cuts of meat, poultry and fish freely. Milk, cheese and yoghurt should be consumed in moderation.
5. Eat several helpings of fruit and vegetables a day.
6. Eat breakfast.
7. Use salt sparingly in the kitchen and at the table.

MALNUTRITION IN DEVELOPED COUNTRIES

Diet-related diseases are caused by incorrect food choices or eating practices (or infected food). Overnutrition is much more common than undernutrition in terms of energy balance but suboptimal intake of protective factors in fruit, seeds and vegetables is common, especially fibre (cell-wall material) and, perhaps, anti-oxidant vitamins A, C and E and essential fatty acids.

OVERNUTRITION

Besides obvious obesity, lesser degrees of excess body fat are almost universal. With age, muscle mass and bone mass tend to decrease so people whose weight stays the same may be laying down fat. Excess fat has many metabolic consequences, especially if it is intra-abdominal. In fact, 85% of people in Britain gain weight during adult life; serious consequences of this include 'essential' hypertension, hyperlipidaemia, insulin resistance resulting in hyperinsulinaemia or hyperglycaemia, and gallstones. Furthermore, several common cancers are linked with overnutrition, especially carcinomas of the colon, breast, uterus (endometrium) and ovary. It is for these reasons that the World Health Organization and many other bodies begin their guidelines to healthy eating with 'maintain desirable body weight'. Unfortunately such advice is too vague to be helpful: more practical and effective would be 'keep your waist measurement unchanged from early adulthood'.

Avoiding overnutrition is difficult in a society where food is abundant and relatively cheap and many manufactured foods and drinks are laced with extra calories in the form of sugars or fats. Such foods and drinks are inherently attractive, heavily promoted and associated with positive emotions like affection and gratitude. Much eating and drinking occurs for social reasons and some for emotional rather than physiological reasons.

Success in the battle of the bulge always requires self-discipline and is aided by peer pressure and vigorous exercise.

UNDERNUTRITION

In a welfare state, chronic undernutrition (a low total food intake) has psychological causes or is secondary to organic disease. Aversion to food occurs in some teenagers (anorexia nervosa, see p. 508) and in some depressed people, especially the lonely and old. The latter may maintain an adequate energy intake but, because they live mainly on white bread, biscuits and sweetened tea, they develop deficiencies of ascorbic acid, folic acid and iron. Substance abuse is often associated with neglect of food. Alcoholics are especially prone to folic acid and thiamine deficiency. Smokers tend to be slim.

Acute undernutrition

Acute undernutrition, especially of protein, is liable to occur with any major illness or trauma, including burns and surgical operations. Not only is food intake reduced but catabolism of protein is increased. Recovery from major illness or trauma is aided by adequate diet. This may require enteral or parenteral nutrition using nutritionally complete liquid feeds. The expertise of a dietitian or, better, a nutrition team is very desirable here.

FOOD INTOLERANCE

Adverse reactions to food are uncommon (other than infected food and psychological food aversion) but can be serious. There are three main types:

1. reactions to pharmacologically active substances in foods, such as caffeine, causing tachycardia and tremor, and tyramine in certain cheeses, causing vascular headaches
2. idiosyncratic reactions due to lack of enzymes, e.g. deficiency of lactase in small bowel mucosa resulting in osmotic diarrhoea when milk is ingested
3. true allergy with immunological hypersensitivity, usually acute and IgE-mediated, but occasionally delayed as in coeliac disease (gluten enteropathy). Important causes are eggs, fish, cow's milk and peanuts.

Table 10.2 shows the main recognised syndromes of food allergy.

Table 10.2. Syndromes of true food allergy

Systemic	Anaphylaxis
Gastrointestinal	Lip swelling, vomiting, diarrhoea, malabsorption (coeliac disease)
Skin	Urticaria, eczema
Respiratory	Rhinitis, asthma

UNDERNUTRITION IN POOR COUNTRIES

Starvation

When food intake stops, the body lives on its energy reserves. These are mostly triglycerides (fat) in the adipose tissue but protein is also used. In a normal, non-obese man it take 40 days on average for the available energy stores to be exhausted and death to occur. Women tend to last longer because their fat stores are twice as large (26% of bodyweight in a healthy young woman). The very young and very old are most vulnerable. During starvation all tissues and organs shrink except the brain. The heart can shrink to a third of its normal weight before it fails. The small intestine becomes paper-thin and inefficient at absorption. Unfortunately, this counteracts the benefits of re-feeding and can prejudice recovery. Re-feeding must be cautious and gradual.

With partial starvation, as in famines, symptoms include feeling cold, nocturia, amenorrhoea and impotence. People become irritable, apathetic or vicious. The pulse is slow and blood pressure low, the ECG low voltage. Oedema is common and not just because of hypoalbuminaemia. The abdomen distends. Terminally there is diarrhoea, and intercurrent infections are common. Treatment is simply provision of food; this should be done gradually, restricting salt. Severely underweight people (weight for height < 70% of standard; weight in kg/[height in m]^2 < 15.7) need hospital-type treatment. Most starvation is political and social rather than medical in origin.

MALNUTRITION IN CHILDREN

Because growing children have higher protein requirements per calorie and are more at risk of being given a low-protein diet than adults, they are more liable to protein deficiency. This is common in poor countries. The World Health Organization has estimated that about 100 million children are suffering from it at any one time (up to a quarter of Third World children). The most common and most regrettable form, which is called marasmus, is simply starvation of babies. It is usually caused by ignorant, very poor mothers weaning their babies on to too-dilute formula feeds. Poor hygiene leads to gastroenteritis and a vicious circle starts as the ill baby loses its appetite. Losing more weight, its small intestine atrophies and malabsorption exacerbates the diarrhoea.

KWASHIORKOR

Kwashiorkor ('first-second' in the Ga language of Ghana) is the sickness of a child which is displaced from its mother's breast by the arrival of a new baby and is weaned on to a gruel which is relatively adequate in energy but too low in protein. Such gruels or porridges are based on cassava, plantain, maize, rice or banana which are the staple foods of villagers in Africa, West Indies, Indonesia, etc.

The biochemistry is complex but seems to involve preservation of insulin

Table 10.3. The physical signs of Kwashiorkor

Failure to grow	Muscle wasting
Misery, apathy	Skin peeling
Sparse, thin hair	Depigmentation or patchy pigmentation
Anaemia	Enlarged liver
Smooth tongue	Watery diarrhoea
Angular stomatitis	Oedema of legs

secretion (unlike marasmus) and, perhaps, zinc deficiency. Because hypoalbuminaemia and oedema are prominent features the child may not look thin or be underweight, but reduced circumference of the upper arm is always present (e.g. under 12 cm at 1–5 years). Mild to moderate cases are 7–10 times more common than the severe, classical ones (Table 10.3); their most obvious manifestations are failure to grow and frequent infections, learning problems and slow motor development. Subclinical cases lead to nutritional dwarfism. Treatment of severe cases is difficult, involving rehydration, repletion of electrolytes, correction of acidosis, hypothermia and hypoglycaemia, and treatment of acute and chronic infections and infestations. Gradual re-feeding is essential, as is nutritional education of the mother to prevent recurrence.

VITAMIN DEFICIENCIES AND EXCESSES

All vitamins are co-factors for metabolic enzymes. The variety of names and daily requirements are given in Table 10.4. Vitamins have caught the popular imagination and are now big business. In the West, deficiencies are rare and unwise self-medication can lead to overdosage.

Table 10.5 summarises the effects of deficiency and overdosage and the metabolic roles of vitamins. A sensible mixed diet should provide enough vitamins; however, most processed foods, especially those rich in sugars and fats, are deficient in vitamins.

Diets high in the antioxidant vitamins A, C and E are associated with decreased rates of cancer and atherosclerosis. Vitamin E supplementation slows progression of atherosclerosis. However, antioxidant supplementation has not been shown to prevent cancer; indeed, beta-carotene supplements increased cancer mortality in two recent studies.

NUTRITIONAL SUPPORT

In seriously malnourished patients, perhaps $\geq$ 10–15% below ideal weight, supplementary feeding may be required. These subjects have other hallmarks of malnutrition, including anthropometric abnormalities such as reduced skinfold thickness measured at standard sites and reduced concentrations of

Table 10.4. The vitamins: average requirements for healthy non-pregnant adults

Recommended name	Alternative name	Usual pharmaceutical preparation	Daily requirement
Water-soluble			
Thiamine	Vitamin B$_1$	Thiamine hydrochloride	1 mg
Riboflavin	Vitamin B$_2$	Riboflavin	1.3 mg
Niacin	Nicotinic acid Nicotinamide	Nicotinamide	15–20 mg
Vitamin B$_6$	Pyridoxine	Pyridoxine hydrochloride	1.4 mg
Folate	Folacin	Folic acid	200 μg
Vitamin B$_{12}$	Cobalamin	Hydroxo-cobalamin	1.5 μg
Vitamin C	Ascorbic acid	Ascorbic acid	40 mg
Fat-soluble			
Vitamin A	Retinol	Vitamin A	700 μg
Vitamin D	Vitamin D2, Vitamin D3	Calciferol, alfacalcidol, calcitriol	10 μg*
Vitamin E	Tocopherols	Alpha tocopheryl acetate	10 mg
Vitamin K	—	Menadiol sodium phosphate, phytomenadione	100 μg

*Up to age 50 years, no dietary requirement when adequate exposure to sunlight.

serum proteins such as albumin, transferrin and retinol binding protein (RBP).

The choice of method for giving increased nutrition will depend on:

1. whether the small bowel is accessible (e.g. not obstructed) and has a normal absorptive mucosa
2. whether the intention is to 'rest' the bowel as for an intestinal fistula or Crohn's disease
3. how long extra nutrition will be required, e.g. over the span of a corrective operation or of recovery from burns, or permanently because of small bowel resection.

METHODS

Oral carbohydrate and protein and whole-food liquid formulae can be used to supplement a nutritious diet. Preparations include Isocal or Ensure (complete feeds), Caloreen or Fortical (carbohydrate preparations) or Casilan (whole protein).

Table 10.5. Effects of deficiency and excess of the major vitamins

Vitamin	Chief metabolic role	Effects of deficiency	Effects of excess
Thiamine	Metabolism of carbohydrate (esp. pyruvate)	Beri-beri (heart failure) Wernicke-Korsakoff syndrome Peripheral neuropathy	—
Riboflavin	Cellular oxidation (FAD)	Angular stomatitis, cheilosis Facial erythema Oro-genital syndrome	—
Niacin	Cellular oxidation (NAD, NADP)	Pellagra (maize eaters) Scaly dermatitis Glossitis, stomatitis, dementia	Flushing Lowers plasma cholesterol
Vit B_6	Transamination, decarboxylation	Hyperhomocystinaemia Prevents isoniazid neuropathy	Peripheral neuropathy
Folate	Haemopoiesis	Megaloblastic anaemia Hyperhomocystinaemia	
Vit B_{12}	Haemopoiesis	Megaloblastic anaemia Hyperhomocystinaemia Subacute combined degeneration of the cord	—
Vit C	Collagen synthesis, antioxidant	Impaired healing Scurvy and bleeding into tissues and joints Perifollicular haemorrhages Swollen bleeding gums, loose teeth	Increased urinary oxalate
Vit A	Night vision, epithelial function, antioxidant	Night blindness, xerophthalmia (major cause of blindness in SE Asia) Perifollicular hyperkeratosis	Raised intracranial pressure, liver damage, skin changes
Vit D	Calcium metabolism	Rickets and osteomalacia (associated with sunlight deprivation, malabsorption)	Hypercalcaemia
Vit E	Red cell function, antioxidant	Mild haemolytic anaemia Neuropathy in children	—
Vit K	Synthesis of clotting factors (II, VII, IX, X)	Bleeding diathesis	—

Oral elemental/peptide diets

These low-residue preparations contain amino acids, peptides or whole proteins, triglycerides and glucose or glucose polymers. They may be of value when it is required to 'rest' the small bowel, e.g. in active Crohn's disease. Many formulations and flavours are available.

Enteral feeding

A fine-bore nasal tube (2 mm diameter) is passed into the stomach or even positioned endoscopically and is used together with a pump to allow continuous feeding. Complications include tube displacement, gastro-oesophageal reflux, abdominal discomfort and diarrhoea.

Percutaneous endoscopic gastrostomy (PEG)

This method is used when normal swallowing is impossible. The endoscopist distends the stomach with air and transilluminates it so that an assistant can push a trocar into it through the abdominal wall. A string is passed down the trocar, which the endoscopist grasps with forceps, pulls out through the mouth and ties to a flanged tube. The assistant then pulls the string until the tube emerges and its flange is flush with the stomach wall. Formula feeds or liquidised food can be given conveniently and safely for long periods.

Parenteral nutrition

This major procedure is used only when the GI tract is either unavailable or inadequate. A silicone catheter is passed into the superior vena cava using strict aseptic technique. A 3-litre container of amino acids, glucose and other sugars, and lipid is given each 24 hours, supplemented with vitamins and minerals.

The major complications are sepsis (septicaemia), hyperglycaemia and cholestasis, the latter possibly caused by gallbladder immobility and bile sludging. Trained patients can manage this technique at home, long term, for example, for the short bowel syndrome.

OBESITY

Obesity is best measured by the body mass index (BMI), also known as the Quetelet index. This measures weight for height and is calculated as the weight in kilograms divided by the square of the height in metres. A normal BMI is that associated with maximum life expectancy and is 20–24.9. Overweight is 25–29.9, obesity 30–34.9 and morbid obesity ≥ 35. The prevalence of obesity in British adults is high and rising: 13% in men and 16% in women. It is a major public health problem. It is more common in lower social classes and has a familial tendency, which may be genetic or cultural.

Aetiology is both obvious and controversial. Weight can be gained only when energy intake exceeds energy expenditure but this imbalance can result from low output or physical inactivity as well as from excessive intake. Factors probably include an inactive lifestyle and the extreme availability and palatability of high-calorie foods and snacks. Overweight people under-report their food intake, especially of sugary and fatty foods. Psychological problems mount with increasing obesity and can be both cause and effect.

Rare causes include endocrine diseases (hypothyroidism, Cushing's syndrome, hypogonadism) and hypothalamic disease or trauma. Leptin is a newly discovered hormone which signals the mass of adipose tissue to the brain. Obese patients have high serum leptin levels, prompting speculation that obesity is associated with down-regulation of CNS leptin receptors.

Symptoms and signs

The most common physical symptoms of severe obesity are joint pains (ligamentous strain rather than arthritis) and exertional dyspnoea. Other symptoms arise from the many diseases caused by obesity, some of which shorten life (Table 10.6). Depression, poor self-esteem, marital or sexual dissatisfaction, unemployment, social isolation and poverty may be caused by obesity or by the attitudes of society and doctors to fat people.

Metabolic effects

These are greatest when fat is distributed in and around the abdomen (central obesity), as shown by a high waist–hip ratio. There is insensitivity to the action of insulin with glucose intolerance, raised blood pressure, raised plasma triglycerides and uric acid, and low plasma HDL cholesterol (syndrome X). Bile is overloaded with cholesterol, favouring gallstone formation.

Treatment

The younger the patient and the more severe the obesity, the greater the urgency of treatment. Mild to moderate static obesity of middle age is rarely cured. Unfortunately, failure of treatment or—more often—recurrence after initial success reinforces the patient's depression and poor self-esteem. Motivation is all-important. Cure demands lifelong self-discipline and sensitive support from family, friends and GP. Doctor and patient should agree a series of written contracts, each specifying a target weight and a realistic date for achieving it.

Table 10.6. Disorders associated with obesity

Stroke	Cancer of breast, ovary, endometrium, colon
Respiratory failure	Arthritis
Coronary heart disease	Varicose veins and
Hypertension	thrombo-embolism
Gallstones	Clumsiness hence accidents
Diabetes	Increased risk of suicide

Conservative treatment options

Reducing diet. Energy intake is kept at 800–1500 kcal/day and energy expenditure is increased by regular exercise. The major problem is compliance but this can be maximised by regular visits to a dietitian or a slimming group, and a close-fitting waist-band.

Diet plus anorectic drugs. Anorectic drugs produce additional weight loss which is rarely of clinical significance. These drugs are rarely justified. Almost all are modified amphetamines with greater or lesser undesirable CNS effects, including habituation.

Behaviour modification. An individualised programme supervised by a clinical psychologist helps the patient to recognise and avoid 'triggers' that precipitate eating. However, prolonged 1 : 1 therapy is expensive.

Very low calorie diets are suitable for short-term use only. There is an increased incidence of sudden cardiac death.

Radical treatment options

These are suitable only for highly selected young grossly obese patients.

Vertical banded gastroplasty. Weight loss can be large and permanent but there may be problems with vomiting, tolerance and patient selection.

Jejunoileal bypass. Weight loss can be large and permanent but there is a high incidence of both long- and short-term metabolic complications. Diarrhoea may also be present. These patients require high quality long-term postoperative follow-up.

Jaw wiring. Weight loss can be large but it is only a short-term measure. It can be highly dangerous (e.g. with vomiting) and the long-term results are poor.

All successful regimens lose adipose and lean body mass in the short term. The main danger is prolonged cardiac repolarisation.

11

HAEMATOLOGY

Geoffrey L. Scott

Diseases of the blood fall into three main groups: red cell disorders, mainly anaemia, which is one of the most common diseases in the world; white cell disorders, principally the leukaemias; and disorders of clotting.

ANAEMIA

Anaemia (low haemoglobin concentration) occurs in many disease. It causes symptoms of fatigue, dyspnoea on exercise, and palpitations. Signs include pallor and those of cardiac failure. Haemopoiesis occurs in the bone marrow. Exceptionally, the liver and spleen may be involved (extramedullary haemopoiesis). Haemopoiesis depends on the presence of stem cells, which generate functional cells (Fig. 11.1), and is governed by growth factors that control

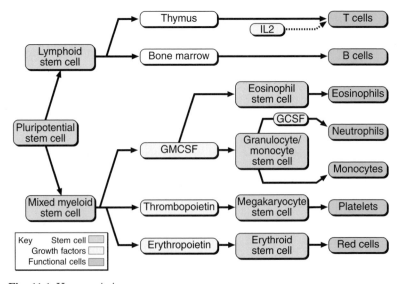

Fig. 11.1 Haemopoiesis.

Table 11.1. Normal red cell values

	Haemoglobin (g/dl)	Red cell count ($\times 10^{12}/1$)	PCV ratio	MCV (fl)	MCH (pg)
Adult male	13–18	4.5–6.5	0.40–0.54	80–96	27–32
Adult female	11.5–16.5	3.8–5.8	0.37–0.47	80–96	26–31
Children (10–12 years)	11.5–14.5	4.0–5.2	0.38–0.45	79–93	24–30

Reticulocytes 0.2–2.0% assuming normal red cell count.
Absolute numbers 0.025–$0.085 \times 10^{12}/1$.

production of the major cell lines. Manipulation of growth factors has exciting therapeutic potential in the treatment of haematological malignancies.

Normal red cell values are shown in Table 11.1. The use of modern, automated cell counters has simplified the diagnosis of anaemia. Mild abnormalities may be detected before they are visible on a blood film. Morphologically, anaemia can be divided into three types:

1. *Normochromic, normocytic* (normal mean cell volume (MCV), normal mean cell haemoglobin (MCH), e.g. anaemia of chronic disease, malignancy, renal failure, aplastic anaemia.
2. *Hypochromic, microcytic* (low MCH, low MCV), e.g. iron deficiency, thalassaemia, sideroblastic anaemia, anaemia of chronic disease (severe).
3. *Macrocytic* (raised MCV), megaloblastic anaemia but also reticulocytosis (haemolysis or haemorrhage), liver disease, alcoholism, sideroblastic anaemia, cytotoxic therapy, aplastic anaemia, hypothyroidism.

The main causes of anaemia are shown in Table 11.2.

IRON DEFICIENCY ANAEMIA

Iron deficiency anaemia is the most common cause of anaemia in the world. It usually results from a combination of inadequate intake and excessive blood loss either from the uterus or gastrointestinal tract; iron malabsorption is another cause. Premenopausal women and children are particularly susceptible and in some underdeveloped countries, it is almost universal from a combination of poor diet and chronic blood loss from parasitic infestation.

The normal iron requirements are approximately 1 mg per day for men and 2 mg per day for premenopausal women. Pregnancy and lactation cause an average net loss of 500 mg. The average Western diet contains 15–20 mg of iron per day but only about 10% of this can be absorbed. The principal site of iron absorption is the duodenum and factors that promote absorption include acidity, iron deficiency and active erythropoiesis. Absorption is impaired following partial gastrectomy, by the presence of dietary phosphates and phytates, and by H_2 antagonists.

Table 11.2. Causes of anaemia

Decreased red cell production (low reticulocyte count)
Failure of haemoglobin synthesis (hypochromic, microcytic)
Iron deficiency
Thalassaemia
Sideroblastic anaemia
Anaemia of chronic disease (severe)
Failure of DNA synthesis (macrocytic)
Megaloblastic anaemia from vitamin B_{12} folate deficiency
Cytotoxic drug therapy
Other rare causes (congenital enzyme deficiency)
Bone marrow failure or replacement (usually normocytic but may be macrocytic)
Aplastic anaemia
Infiltration caused by leukaemia, myeloma, lymphoma, carcinoma or
myelofibrosis (usually leukoerythroblastic)
Miscellaneous (usually normocytic)
Hypothyroidism (sometimes macrocytic)
Erythropoietin lack (chronic renal failure)

Decreased red cell survival (increased reticulocyte count)
Haemolysis
Chronic blood loss (usually leads to iron deficiency) e.g. ulcers, menorrhagia,
haemorrhoids

Symptoms and signs

In addition to anaemia, severe iron deficiency causes atrophy of the oral and gastric mucosa (angular stomatitis, glossitis), the formation of an oesophageal web, and brittle spoon-shaped nails ('koilonychia'). Symptoms are usually those of anaemia.

Investigations

Hypochromic anaemia is usually due to iron deficiency. If proof is required, serum ferritin is a reliable indicator of iron stores and is reduced in iron deficiency. It is essential to establish the cause: in men and post-menopausal women this usually requires investigation of the gastrointestinal tract.

Differential diagnosis

Iron deficiency anaemia which is not responsive to treatment with iron must be distinguished from other causes of hypochromic anaemia.

The anaemia of chronic disease. This is the most important and occurs in chronic infection, chronic inflammatory disease, e.g. rheumatoid arthritis, and malignancy. The serum ferritin level is invariably low in iron deficiency and normal or raised in chronic disease. An acute-phase response (raised erythrocyte sedimentation rate (ESR), plasma viscosity or C-reactive protein) is often found.

Thalassaemia minor. See Thalassaemia, p. 325.

Sideroblastic anaemia. This may also be hypochromic. It is usually associated with dimorphic red cells. The serum ferritin level is high and the diagnosis is confirmed by the presence of ring sideroblasts in the bone marrow. It is predominantly a disease of the elderly.

Treatment

Most cases of iron deficiency will respond to oral iron therapy. Ferrous sulphate 200 mg 8-hourly after meals is the cheapest and most effective. Ferrous gluconate may be used as an alternative. Failure of oral iron therapy to induce a rise in haemoglobin level of 1 g per week suggests poor compliance, which may be due to intolerance of gastrointestinal side-effects. In this situation, intramuscular iron can be used.

MEGALOBLASTIC ANAEMIA

Megaloblastic anaemia is the result of defective DNA synthesis and is caused by deficiency of vitamin B_{12} or folate or both. B_{12} and folate are both co-factors in the synthesis of thymidine. B_{12} is one of the cobalamins, the physiological form being methylcobalamin. It is contained in most animal produce. The average daily intake is 30 µg and the average daily need is 2 µg. Body stores in the liver are around 3 mg. For absorption, B_{12} must combine with intrinsic factor secreted by the gastric parietal cells. Absorption occurs via specific receptors in the terminal ileum.

Folic acid is present in most green vegetables, yeast and liver in the form of polyglutamates, which are split to monoglutamates for absorbtion throughout the small intestine. The active form is methyl tetrahydrofolate (THF). The average daily requirement is about 100 µg. Folate needs are increased where there is rapid cell proliferation, e.g. haemolysis, malignancy and pregnancy. The body stores, mainly in the liver, are about 10–15 mg. The main causes of B_{12} and folate deficiency are shown in Tables 11.3 and 11.4.

Table 11.3. Causes of vitamin B_{12} deficiency

Inadequate intake (normal Schilling test)*	Strict vegetarianism—vegans, extreme malnutrition, food faddism
Gastric lesions (abnormal part 1 Schilling test)	Pernicious anaemia, partial or total gastrectomy, congenital intrinsic factor deficiency (very rare)
Intestinal lesions (abnormal parts 1 and 2 Schilling test)	Blind loop syndrome, tropical sprue (indicate bacterial overgrowth), Crohn's disease, coeliac disease, ileal resection (absence of specific receptors), fish tapeworm (rare except in Scandinavia), congenital B_{12} malabsorption (very rare)

*Vitamin B_{12} absorption test measures absorption of a small dose of radioactive B_{12} without (part 1) and with (part 2) exogenous intrinsic factor.

Table 11.4. Causes of folate deficiency

Inadequate intake	Malnutrition, old age ('tea and toast' diet), poverty, psychiatric disturbance, alcoholism (other factors, cirrhosis, haemolysis)
Malabsorption	Coeliac disease (may be only manifestation), tropical sprue, dermatitis herpetiformis enteropathy
Excess demands	Pregnancy, lactation, prematurity, chronic haemolysis, malignancy (widespread carcinoma, leukaemia and lymphoma, myeloproliferative disorders, e.g. myelofibrosis, polycythaemia), exfoliative skin disorders, inflammatory diseases, e.g. rheumatoid arthritis
Drugs	Anticonvulsants (often combined with inadequate intake), alcohol (several actions), oral contraceptives (rare, mainly high oestrogen), folate antagonists (methotrexate, pyrimethamine, cotrimoxazole)

Pathology

B_{12} and folate deficiency affect all rapidly proliferating cells. The nuclei show a characteristic open chromatin pattern.

The main cause of B_{12} deficiency is pernicious anaemia, which is an autoimmune disease leading to gastric atrophy and reduced intrinsic factor production.

Symptoms and signs

Early megaloblastic anaemia is asymptomatic and may be discovered accidentally by finding a raised MCV.

Symptoms of more advanced disease include those of anaemia, jaundice from ineffective erythropoiesis and painful glossitis.

B_{12} deficiency can also cause neurological complications, peripheral neuritis, spastic paraplegia, posterior column signs, confusion, dementia and optic atrophy.

In pernicious anaemia, associated autoimmune diseases are common and include hypothyroidism, vitiligo and Addison's disease.

Investigations

Megaloblastic anaemia must be distinguished from other causes of macrocytosis. Serum B_{12} and red cell folate levels must be measured before treatment.

In severe cases, other haematological findings include oval macrocytes, hypersegmented polymorphs and reduced white cell and platelet counts. Characteristic changes are found in the bone marrow but this is rarely needed as a routine procedure.

The presence of gastric parietal cell antibodies is of little diagnostic value. Intrinsic factor antibodies are present in 60% of cases of pernicious anaemia.

Most cases of megaloblastic anaemia in older patients are caused by pernicious anaemia and a B_{12} absorption test (Schilling test) is rarely required; however, it is useful in problem cases or in younger patients.

Further investigations of the GI tract are often needed in younger patients; unexplained folate deficiency should prompt tests for antigliadin antibodies and/or small intestinal biopsy to exclude coeliac disease.

Differential diagnosis
Other causes of macrocytosis (see p. 313).

Treatment
Treatment is of the cause if possible; otherwise, replacement therapy is needed. B_{12} deficiency is treated with hydroxycobalamin. In acute cases, particularly with neurological complications, six intramuscular injections of 1 mg are given over a 2-week period, followed by 1 mg in alternate months. Patients with pernicious anaemia should be kept under surveillance because of the risk of the development of hypothyroidism or gastric carcinoma.

Folic acid deficiency is treated by oral folic acid 5 mg daily. Folic acid can correct anaemia caused by B_{12} deficiency but does not prevent the neurological complications (p. 138) although there is no evidence to support the long-held belief that these may be precipitated or accelerated by folate supplementation.

ANAEMIA FROM BONE MARROW FAILURE

This form of anaemia is caused by either the failure of haemopoietic stem cells or their replacement by other tissue, usually malignant. It results in a reduction of all haemopoietic cell lines, i.e. pancytopenia (Table 11.5).

Table 11.5. Causes of pancytopenia

Cellular bone marrow

Normal maturation with excess destruction
    Hypersplenism
    Felty's syndrome (rheumatoid arthritis)
    Systemic lupus erythematosus (SLE) (antibody formation)

Abnormal maturation
    Megaloblastic anaemia
    Myelodysplasia

Infiltration
    Carcinoma (usually leukoerythroblastic picture)
    Myelofibrosis (splenomegaly, tear drop poikilocytes)
    Acute leukaemia
    Myeloma

Hypocellular bone marrow

Aplastic anaemia
Paroxysmal nocturnal haemoglobinuria

Note: bone marrow examination (usually a trephine) is essential in all cases.

Aplastic anaemia

This is caused by a reduction in the number of haemopoietic stem cells in the presence of all the essential factors required for normal haemopoiesis. Usually, all cell lines are involved but selective reduction may occur.

Many cases of aplastic anaemia are the result of damage to marrow from drugs, chemicals or viruses although some cases are idiopathic. Individual susceptibility is important. The known causes of aplastic anaemia can be classified as follows:

1. Marrow-suppressant drugs, e.g. cytotoxic drugs, especially alkylating agents. Their effect is dose related.
2. Other drugs, reaction to which is unpredictable. Only a small percentage of patients receiving them will react adversely. Usually several courses are needed although the total dose received may be small. At present, there is no known way in which the susceptible subject may be identified by laboratory tests. Many drugs have been suspected of causing aplastic anaemia although there is difficulty in establishing a causal relationship. Known high-risk drugs include chloramphenicol, phenylbutazone and derivatives, gold, penicillamine, anticonvulsants and oral hypoglycaemic agents.
3. Chemicals: benzene, toluene, DDT, etc.
   All chemicals, particularly solvents, insecticides and weed killers, are capable of producing aplastic anaemia and should be handled with extreme caution.
4. Viruses: aplasia following viral hepatitis is well recognised. The hepatitis is often mild and aplastic anaemia develops several months after recovery. The fatality rate is high. Parvovirus B19 is known to be a cause of aplasia in patients with haemolytic anaemia.
5. Excessive radiation.
6. Miscellaneous, including:
   (a) *Congenital aplastic anaemia.* Several rare varieties exist, e.g. Diamond Blackfan syndrome (red cell aplasia).
   (b) *Pure red cell aplasia.* Red cell series alone is affected. It may have an immunological basis as it is often associated with autoimmune disease and a thymoma.

Symptoms and signs

The symptoms and signs are those of anaemia: neutropenia, causing infection, especially of the throat and tonsils; and thrombocytopenia, causing bruising, purpura, and bleeding from mucous membranes.

Investigations

Anaemia is invariable and may be severe. It is usually normocytic although macrocytosis may occur. Reticulocytes are low or absent. Granulocytes and platelets are variable although usually low.

Bad prognostic features are platelets $<20 \times 10^9/1$, neutrophils $<0.5 \times 10^9/1$ and reticulocytes $<0.010 \times 10^{12}/1$.

It is usually impossible to aspirate bone marrow and a *trephine is mandatory* in all cases. This shows hypoplasia with the marrow replaced by fat spaces.

Paroxysmal nocturnal haemoglobinuria should be excluded.

Treatment

1. For younger patients with severe aplastic anaemia, bone marrow transplantation is the treatment of choice, if they have a compatible sibling. Exposure to blood products should be limited as far as possible to avoid sensitisation.
2. An exhaustive search should be made for a toxic cause and any drugs suspected should be withdrawn immediately. Chelating agents are of use in gold or heavy metal poisoning.
3. The basis of treatment is supportive therapy to prevent death from anaemia, haemorrhage or infection until spontaneous recovery occurs, usually, if at all, within 6 weeks.
4. Patients in whom anaemia is a major problem may be maintained for many years by regular blood transfusions, although difficulty may arise from lack of veins, antibody production and haemosiderosis.
5. Haemorrhage may be prevented by platelet transfusions but antibody formation may lead to resistance. Infections should be treated vigorously with broad-spectrum antibiotics.
6. Androgenic steroids may have a beneficial effect on anaemia. Oxymetholone is the most widely used because of its low androgenic effect. It must be used in a high dose (2–5 mg per kg per 24 hours) and treatment may be needed for several months before any effect is seen. Regular liver function tests (LFTs) are needed to detect impending liver damage.
7. Some patients, particularly when an immunological mechanism is involved, may respond to antilymphocyte globulin (expensive).

Prognosis

Aplastic anaemia is a serious disease. For those with bad prognostic features, the mortality rate at 5 years is 90% in the absence of bone marrow transplantation.

Anaemia from bone marrow infiltration

Carcinoma and other malignancies may infiltrate the bone marrow and cause anaemia. The blood picture is usually leukoerythroblastic, i.e. both immature white cells and normoblasts are seen. Although lymphomatous infiltration may respond to cytotoxic therapy, the prognosis in carcinoma is usually very poor.

ANAEMIA FROM MISCELLANEOUS CAUSES

In uraemia, bone marrow function is depressed partly because of a direct toxic effect but mostly from a lack of erythropoietin.

The anaemia of liver disease is complicated and includes marrow depression as well as haemolysis, hypersplenism and iron and folate deficiency.

In hypothyroidism, a normocytic anaemia is commonly seen although it may be macrocytic. The main factor is diminished tissue needs for oxygen.

HAEMOLYTIC ANAEMIA

Haemolytic anaemia occurs when the red cell lifespan (normally 100–120 days) is shortened by premature destruction and the capacity of the bone marrow to compensate is exceeded. Premature destruction of red cells may be caused by intrinsic abnormalities of the red cells or by extracorpuscular factors, e.g. antibodies (Table 11.6).

Pathology

Increased haemolysis leads to expansion of the marrow into the shafts of the long bones. In children with severe congenital haemolytic anaemia, expansion of the marrow cavity may lead to changes in the cortical bone, producing clinical and radiological evidence of bone expansion. Hyperbilirubinaemia occurs because of increased haemoglobin breakdown. Pigment gallstones are commonly found in chronic haemolysis and splenomegaly occurs in many types of haemolytic anaemia.

Table 11.6. Causes of haemolytic anaemia

Congenital red cell defects

Membrane defects
  Hereditary spherocytosis
  Hereditary elliptocytosis (severe haemolysis rare)
Enzyme defects
  Pyruvate kinase (PK) deficiency
  Glucose-6-phosphate dehydrogenase (G6PD) deficiency
Haemoglobin defects
  Structural abnormalities: sickle cell disease
  Abnormal chain synthesis: thalassaemia

Acquired haemolytic anaemia

Immune
  Autoimmune haemolytic anaemia (AIHA)
  Isoimmune—incompatible blood transfusions
  Haemolytic disease of the newborn
Infections
  Malaria
  Septicaemia (especially *Staphylococcus, Clostridium welchii*)
Drugs and chemicals (usually overdose or industrial exposure)
Membrane disorders
  Paroxysmal nocturnal haemoglobinuria (PNH)
Mechanical
  Microangiopathic haemolytic anaemia
  Cardiac valve prosthesis
  March haemoglobinuria
Hypersplenism
Miscellaneous (usually several causes for anaemia)
  Liver disease
  Malignancy
  Uraemia

Symptoms and signs

Usually the only symptoms are those of anaemia. Upper abdominal pain may be caused by gallstones.

The principal signs are of anaemia and jaundice. Splenomegaly is common and, rarely, leg ulcers may be present.

Investigations

See Table 11.7.

Treatment

Treatment should be directed at the elimination of the cause, if possible. Folic acid should be given to all patients with chronic haemolysis. Splenectomy may be indicated in some cases.

Specific causes of haemolysis

Hereditary spherocytosis

This disorder, inherited as an autosomal dominant of incomplete penetrance, is a membrane defect causing the formation of spherocytic red cells which are sequestered in the spleen.

Many patients are asymptomatic. The commonest clinical picture is of recurrent episodes of anaemia and jaundice in childhood caused by a

Table 11.7. Investigation of haemolytic anaemia

Haemoglobin concentration	Reduced, depending on the degree of compensation
Reticulocyte count	Raised
Red cell size and appearance	Increased MCV and polychromasia (cytoplasmic staining from residual RNA) due to reticulocytosis Nucleated red cells Spherocytosis, elliptocytosis Fragmented red cells
Coombs' test	Test for antibody adherent to red cell surface (direct antiglobulin test)
Serum bilirubin	Increased unconjugated bilirubin (production exceeds conjugating capacity of liver)
Urinalysis	Increased urobilinogen (colourless metabolite of bilirubin made in the gut). No increase in urinary bilirubin (unconjugated form is water-insoluble) Increased urinary haemosiderin
Serum haptoglobin	Decrease in intravascular haemolysis
Survival of ^{51}Cr-labelled red cells	Decreased Surface scanning may show selective splenic sequestration

temporarily increased rate of haemolysis and/or bone marrow suppression, usually caused by infection.

Severe cases may present at birth as haemolytic disease of the newborn. Other modes of presentation include gallstones and intractable leg ulcers.

The diagnosis is made clinically, from family and blood studies, and by exclusion of autoimmune haemolytic anaemia.

Treatment is splenectomy if there are recurrent crises or gallstones.

Glucose-6-phosphate dehydrogenase (G6PD) deficiency

This is a widespread sex-linked abnormality occurring in Blacks and certain Mediterranean and Oriental groups. The red cells are unusually susceptible to oxidative stress, caused by drugs, particularly antimalarials (primaquine), phenacetin, sulphonamides, dapsone, nitrofurantoin and vitamin K in the newborn. Severe self-limiting haemolysis may occur following exposure to these drugs.

Patients with the Mediterranean variety ('Favism') may be susceptible to the broad bean (*Vicia faba*), usually seen in childhood and adolescence.

Diagnosis is made by G6PD assay.

Autoimmune haemolytic anaemia (AIHA)

AIHA results from the destruction of red cells by autoantibodies. The two main types depend on the nature of the antibody, i.e. IgG (warm) and IgM (cold) antibodies. The causes of AIHA are shown in Table 11.8.

Warm-antibody AIHA causes extravascular haemolysis and the symptoms are principally those of anaemia. The blood film shows spherocytosis and the diagnosis is confirmed by a positive Coombs' test. A search for a primary cause, particularly systemic lupus erythematosus (SLE) or lymphoma, should be made.

Treatment is with steroids starting at a high dose, e.g. prednisolone 60 mg per 24 hours, reduced as the haemolysis comes under control. Most cases of idiopathic AIHA become chronic. If the disease cannot be controlled by a minimal dose of steroids, then splenectomy is the next choice.

Table 11.8. Causes of autoimmune haemolytic anaemia

'Warm' antibody	IgG, occasionally with complement, Coombs' positive
Primary	Idiopathic
Secondary	Lymphoma, chronic lymphatic leukaemia (CLL)
	Autoimmune disease, e.g. systemic lupus erythematosus
	Viral infections, e.g. infectious mononucleosis
	Drugs, e.g. methyldopa
'Cold' antibody	IgM, usually with complement, Coombs' weakly positive or negative
Primary	The cold haemagglutination syndrome (CHAD)
Secondary	Lymphoma
	Infections—mycoplasma, infectious mononucleosis
	Paroxysmal cold haemoglobinuria (PCH)

Cold-antibody AIHA causes intravascular haemolysis. The symptoms are due to cold-induced red cell agglutination causing Raynaud's phenomenon and to intravascular haemolysis causing haemoglobinuria. Most cases respond to avoidance of cold but if this is ineffective, alkylating agents (e.g. chlorambucil) should be used. Steroids have no place in the treatment of cold-antibody AIHA.

Microangiopathic haemolytic anaemia

Microangiopathic haemolytic anaemia is caused by the destruction of red cells by a fibrin meshwork laid down within small blood vessels. It is characterised by the presence of fragmented red cells of bizarre shapes in the blood film.

It may occur in a wide variety of conditions as a result of either disease of the vessels themselves or as a part of the disseminated intravascular coagulation (DIC) syndrome, e.g. malignant hypertension, glomerulonephritis and malignant invasion of small vessels, especially by mucin-secreting carcinomas. It is usually associated with thrombocytopenia.

Haemolytic uraemic syndrome (HUS) and thrombotic thrombocytopenic purpura (TTP). These diseases are caused by endothelial damage, often as a result of bacterial toxins, e.g. the verotoxin produced by *E. Coli* 0157. Thrombocytopenia and red cell fragmentation occur. In HUS, renal damage predominates: it is more common in children but may occur at any age. TTP is characterised by neurological involvement due to multiple thrombotic lesions.

Miscellaneous causes of haemolysis

See Table 11.9.

Table 11.9. Miscellaneous causes of haemolysis

Type	Cause	Effects/diagnosis	Therapy
Hereditary elliptocytosis	Membrane defect	Elliptocytes Variable haemolytic anaemia	Usually none
Pyruvate kinase deficiency	Enzyme defect	'Prickle cells' Haemolytic anaemia, may be severe	Splenectomy
Paroxysmal nocturnal haemoglobinuria	Acquired inability to resist complement-mediated lysis	Haemolytic episodes Haemoglobinuria Thrombotic episodes Positive Ham's test	Blood transfusion (washed red cells) Anticoagulants if thromboses
March haemoglobinuria	Mechanical damage to red cells caused by running	Haemoglobinuria following exercise	Run in trainers with spongy soles
Paroxysmal cold haemoglobinuria	Cold antibody usually related to viral infection, especially in children	Acute intravascular haemolysis with haemoglobinuria	Usually self limiting. Keep patient warm

Disorders of haemoglobin

Haemoglobin is a tetramer of four chains. In the normal adult, most of the haemoglobin is haemoglobin A (alpha 2, beta 2) and the remainder haemoglobin A_2, (alpha 2, delta 2). In the fetus, most of the haemoglobin is haemoglobin F (alpha 2, gamma 2). Disorders of haemoglobin are of two types: the structural variants, in which an abnormal form of haemoglobin is produced; and the thalassaemias, in which there is failure to produce haemoglobin chains at the required rate (Table 11.10).

Sickle cell disease

Sickle cell disease is due to an abnormal beta haemoglobin chain, haemoglobin S. In the homozygous state (SS), virtually all the haemoglobin is in the form of haemoglobin S. In the heterozygous state, sickle cell trait (SA), about 40% is haemoglobin S, the remainder being haemoglobin A.

Table 11.10. Disorders of haemoglobin

	Haemoglobin	Haematology	Clinical effects
Normal adult	A 97%, A_2 3%		
Fetus	F 85%		
Sickle cell disease	S 80–100%	Sickle cells Target cells	Sickle crises, anaemia
Sickle cell trait	S 40%, A 60%	Target cells	Usually none
Hb SC disease	S C	Target cells	Mild anaemia, sickle crises
Hb C disease	C 90%	Target cells +	Mild anaemia, Splenomegaly
Sickle thalassaemia	β^0 S 85–90% β + 55–75%	Hypochromic Microcytic Target cells	Sickle crises, anaemia Usually asymptomatic
β Thalassaemia major	F 70–100% A_2	Hypochromic Microcytic + Target cells	Severe anaemia
β Thalassaemia minor	A_2 3.5–7%	Hypochromic Microcytic Target cells	Normal or mild anaemia, asymptomatic
α Thalassaemia	Barts (Fetus)	Hypochromic	Stillbirth
Hb H disease	H 5–40%	Microcytic 'H' bodies Target cells	Moderate anaemia, splenomegaly
Hb H trait	H trace	Mild hypochromia 'H' bodies	None
Unstable haemoglobins	e.g. Hb Köln	Heinz bodies Heat-unstable haemoglobin	Mild haemolytic anaemia, often precipitated by oxidant drugs

In the deoxygenated state, haemoglobin S molecules can link to form chains which distort the red cell, making it inflexible, leading to entrapment of the red cells in small vessels causing infarction and haemolysis. Infarction occurs in many tissues including bones, muscles, the gut, the spleen, the kidney and the retina. Precipitating factors are *hypoxia, infection, dehydration and cold.*

Sickle cell disease occurs principally in Blacks of African origin and is therefore common in Afro-Caribbeans. Amongst this population, 10% carry the haemoglobin S gene and 0.25% have sickle cell disease. There are smaller pockets in Greece, the Middle East and India. Sickle cell trait protects against *P. falciparum* malaria.

Symptoms and signs. The symptoms are mainly due to infarction, which causes acute pain—sickle cell 'crisis'. Gut infarcts may mimic an acute abdomen and bone infarcts may be confused with acute arthritis or osteomyelitis.

Two particularly dangerous complications are the acute chest syndrome, which presents with dyspnoea and severe chest pain, and acute splenic sequestration, which occurs in children causing rapid splenic enlargement and severe anaemia.

Patients with sickle cell trait are usually asymptomatic.

Investigations. Patients with sickle cell disease are invariably anaemic (haemoglobin 8–9 g/dl). Sickle cells are usually present in the blood film, especially in crises.

Screening tests are available to detect the presence of haemoglobin S but the definitive diagnosis is made by haemoglobin electrophoresis.

Patients with sickle cell trait are usually not anaemic.

Treatment. Prevention of sickle crises is important. The management of a crisis depends on ensuring adequate oxygenation, rehydration and treatment of infection. *Sickle crises are extremely painful and adequate analgesia is essential.* Severe crises, particularly the acute chest syndrome, may require exchange transfusion.

Other sickling syndromes

Another form of abnormal haemoglobin also found in Africa is haemoglobin C. Homozygous C disease (CC) gives rise to mild anaemia and splenomegaly but without crises. The combination of haemoglobin S and C disease causes mild anaemia and sickle crises, particularly affecting the retina and kidney. In some populations where the genes for sickle cell disease and thalassaemia co-exist, sickle thalassaemia may occur. In most cases, this is asymptomatic, although in some, where the level of haemoglobin S is high, sickle crises may occur.

Thalassaemia

Background. In the thalassaemias, there is defective synthesis of one of the chains needed to form adult haemoglobin. The most common variety is *beta thalassaemia* in which there is restriction of beta chain synthesis resulting in defective formation of haemoglobin A. In the homozygous condition, *thalassaemia major*, there is little or no haemoglobin A synthesis resulting in severe anaemia. In the heterozygous condition, *thalassaemia trait*, although there is restriction of haemoglobin A synthesis, the degree of anaemia is not severe.

In *alpha thalassaemia*, there is a restriction of alpha chain synthesis. As a compensation, tetramers are formed of gamma chains (haemoglobin Barts) in the fetus, and beta chains (haemoglobin H) in the adult.

Thalassaemia is widespread, occurring around the Mediterranean and into the Middle East, India and the Far East, where alpha thalassaemia predominates. Thalassaemia is protective against severe malaria, although the mechanism for this protection is uncertain.

Symptoms and signs. Beta thalassaemia major causes severe anaemia a few months after birth. It is associated with skeletal abnormalities and gross hepatosplenomegaly due to ineffective erythropoiesis.

The severest form of alpha thalassaemia is not compatible with life, and death occurs in utero. An intermediate form, known as haemoglobin H disease, causes moderate anaemia and splenomegaly. Less severe forms resemble thalassaemia minor and are symptomless.

Investigations. Beta thalassaemia major causes gross anaemia with microcytosis and hypochromia. Electrophoresis shows the almost complete absence of haemoglobin A.

In beta thalassaemia minor, there is a microcytic, hypochromic blood picture with a normal or slightly reduced haemoglobin which has to be distinguished from iron deficiency. This is achieved by demonstrating a normal ferritin level and an increased level of haemoglobin A_2.

Alpha thalassaemia is diagnosed by finding the presence of haemoglobin Barts in the fetus and haemoglobin H in the adult. Haemoglobin H can be detected by a special stain which shows inclusions in the red cells (H bodies).

Treatment. Children with thalassaemia major will die unless regularly transfused. Hypertransfusion prevents the development of skeletal abnormalities and hepatosplenomegaly. Nevertheless, death will occur in adolescence unless chelation therapy with desferrioxamine is started early to prevent iron overload. This must be given by slow s.c. infusion on at least 5 days per week. Bone marrow transplantation offers the chance of permanent cure for a few patients.

Patients with thalassaemia minor require no treatment. It is important that the condition is diagnosed so that repeated investigation and treatment of non-existent iron deficiency is avoided.

Other abnormal haemoglobins

Many of these are known but most produce no clinical effects. One important group are the unstable haemoglobins, e.g. haemoglobin Koln in which haemolytic anaemia can be precipitated by oxidant drugs (as in G6PD deficiency).

DISORDERS OF WHITE CELLS

The normal total white blood cell (WBC) count is $4-11 \times 10^9/1$ in adults, but note that Blacks have a constitutionally lower, and children a higher, WBC count. Variations in the number and distribution of WBC occur in many diseases and is a useful aid to diagnosis.

MAJOR VARIATIONS IN WHITE CELLS

Neutrophil leukocytosis ($>7.5 \times 10^9/1$)
An increased neutrophil count may be seen in:

1. physiological states; considerable variation in neutrophil count occurs during the day, the influencing factors being exercise, food and stress
2. late pregnancy
3. infections (especially pyogenic infections)
4. tissue necrosis
5. haemorrhage
6. malignant neoplasms
7. metabolic disorders (e.g. diabetic ketoacidosis)
8. myeloproliferative disorders (e.g. primary polycythaemia, chronic granulocytic leukaemia)
9. corticosteroid treatment.

Eosinophilia ($>0.4 \times 10^9/1$)
Causes of an increased eosinophil count include:

1. allergy, asthma, drug sensitivity
2. parasitic infestation (usually with tissue invasion), e.g. filarial and helminth infection; may be associated with eosinophilic pulmonary infiltrates
3. bronchopulmonary aspergillosis
4. skin diseases, e.g. pemphigoid, exfoliative dermatitis
5. malignancy, particularly Hodgkin's disease
6. Churg–Strauss vasculitis
7. hypoadrenalism (Addison's disease)
8. sarcoidosis.

Lymphocytosis ($>3.5 \times 10^9/1$)
An increased lymphocyte count is seen in:

1. viral infections, especially in children—infectious hepatitis and infectious mononucleosis
2. leukaemia—acute and especially chronic lymphatic leukaemia
3. 'atypical lymphocytosis' in many viral diseases, especially infectious mononucleosis.

Monocytosis ($>0.8 \times 10^9/1$)
An increased monocyte count occurs with:

1. infections, especially chronic (e.g. tuberculosis, subacute bacterial endocarditis), protozoal infections, and infectious mononucleosis
2. malignant disease—monocytic leukaemia, carcinoma
3. chronic inflammatory intestinal disease, e.g. Crohn's disease.

Neutropenia (<2.5 × 10⁹/1)

Neutropenia ($<2.5 \times 10^9/1$)

A decreased neutrophil count occurs with:

1. Blacks (physiological)
2. aplastic anaemia
3. bone marrow infiltration, e.g. leukaemia, carcinoma, etc.
4. viral or overwhelming bacterial infections
5. hypersplenism, particularly Felty's syndrome (depression of neutrophil production may be a factor in this condition)
6. immune disorders, e.g. SLE
7. chronic idiopathic neutropenia and 'cyclic neutropenia', a rare condition with a cyclic change in the neutrophil count.

Drug-induced agranulocytosis

Several drugs are known to cause agranulocytosis either as part of the aplastic anaemia syndrome or selectively, e.g. gold, antithyroid drugs and clozapine. Great care should be taken over the prescription of all drugs known to cause agranulocytosis and regular blood counts should be performed.

MALIGNANT AND PROLIFERATIVE DISEASES OF HAEMOPOIETIC TISSUE

These diseases are confusing because they are difficult to classify and overlap occurs between them. Several basic concepts need to be borne in mind.

1. Most of these diseases are clonal, i.e. they arise from an abnormality affecting one cell line which has the biological advantages to outgrow normal marrow cells.
2. Most affect stem cells and the transformation may cause either uncontrolled but orderly proliferation of end cells, as in polycythaemia, or uncontrolled proliferation of stem cells without differentiation, as in acute leukaemia.
3. It is likely that a series of events occurs that transforms a normal cell into a malignant cell. Consequently, the disease may show evolution from a benign proliferative process to an aggressive malignant one.
4. The nature of the events that cause transformation is unknown but postulated factors include viruses, drugs and radiation.
5. Improved technology has allowed identification of the cell of origin by analysis of surface markers, leading to a greater understanding of these diseases.

A simple division may be made between diseases of the *myeloid cells*, i.e. those giving rise to red cells, granulocytes and platelets, and diseases of the *lymphoid system*.

Clinically, it is convenient to consider these diseases under the following headings:

1. myeloproliferative disease
2. acute leukaemia and myelodysplasia
3. lymphoproliferative disease.

THE MYELOPROLIFERATIVE DISORDERS (Fig. 11.2)

This group of disorders arises from an aberration of myeloid stem cells, characterised by an initial benign phase, followed by transformation to a more aggressive malignant phase. There are common features and transition from one form to another may occur. All may terminate as acute myeloid leukaemia. The diseases involved are primary polycythaemia (polycythaemia rubra vera), essential thrombocythaemia, myelofibrosis and chronic granulocytic leukaemia.

PRIMARY POLYCYTHAEMIA

Polycythaemia, i.e. an increase in haemoglobin and haematocrit, may be either true or relative. True polycythaemia is due to an increase in circulating red cell mass. Relative polycythaemia is due to a decrease in plasma volume. True polycythaemia may be either primary or secondary. Secondary polycythaemia is caused by increased erythropoietin, which may be either appropriate, as in hypoxia, or inappropriate, as in erythropoietin-secreting tumours.

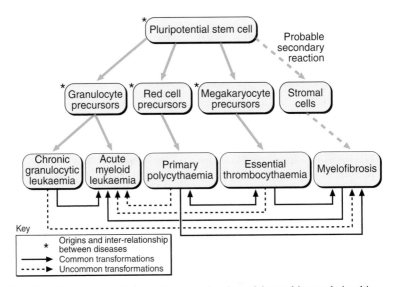

Fig. 11.2 The myeloproliferative disorders showing origins and inter-relationship between diseases.

Symptoms and signs

These may be due to:

1. raised blood viscosity—headache, confusion, arterial and venous thromboses, congestive cardiac failure, stroke
2. abnormal bleeding, particularly gastrointestinal, often leading to iron deficiency because of abnormal platelet function
3. pruritus (especially after hot baths), possibly caused by histamine over-production
4. gout because of hyperuricaemia from increased cell turnover.

These patients often show a ruddy cyanosis and 70% of cases have splenomegaly.

Investigations

The haemoglobin level and haematocrit are above the upper limit of normal. In 70% of cases, the white cell count and platelet count are elevated. The absolute red cell mass is increased.

Differential diagnosis

Secondary and relative polycythaemia (Table 11.11).

Treatment

The cardinal rule of treatment is to keep the haematocrit within the normal range. The simplest method is venesection. If this is unacceptable or if there is thrombocytosis, a myelosuppressive agent must be used. ^{32}P is simple but leukaemogenic and should be reserved for older patients. In younger patients, hydroxyurea is the treatment of choice.

Table 11.11. Differential diagnosis of polycythaemia

Type	Primary	Anoxic	Renal	Other secondary causes	'Pseudopolycythaemia' (relative polycythaemias)	
PCV	↑	↑	↑	↑	↑	
WBC	N or ↑	N	N	N	N	
Platelets	N or ↑	N	N	N	N	
Red cell mass	↑	↑	↑	↑	N	
Plasma volume	N or ↑	N	N	N	↓	
PO$_2$	N	↓	N	N	N	
Renal imaging	N	N	Abnormal	N	N	N
Erythropoietin	N or ↓	↑	↑	↑	N	

PCV = packed cell volume; WBC = white blood cells.

Provided that thrombosis is avoided, the prognosis is very good. Transition to myelofibrosis or acute leukaemia may occur but usually only after several decades.

Essential thrombocythaemia

This myeloproliferative disorder principally affects the committed platelet stem cell causing a high platelet count. Overlap with polycythaemia occurs. It is mainly seen in middle-aged or elderly patients but may occur in younger people.

Symptoms and signs
Essential thrombocythaemia may be asymptomatic, especially in younger patients.

Microthrombotic lesions, particularly in digital vessels in the feet, are caused by abnormal platelet aggregation. There may be digital ischaemia. Defective platelet function leads to abnormal bruising and bleeding.

Splenomegaly may become marked as the disease progresses to myelofibrosis.

Investigations
The platelet count is usually markedly raised, often in excess of $1000 \times 10^9/1$. Abnormal platelet morphology and function may be present.

Differential diagnosis
Other causes of reactive thrombocytosis are haemorrhage, infection, malignant disease and chronic inflammatory disease. (Platelet function and morphology may help to discriminate.)

Treatment
The aim is to reduce the platelet count to normal using hydroxyurea, busulphan or ^{32}P. Younger patients may require no treatment.

Prognosis is usually excellent. Long remissions may occur after treatment although eventual transition to myelofibrosis or acute leukaemia may be seen.

Myelofibrosis

Replacement of bone marrow by fibrous tissue and new bone formation is often the terminal stage of polycythaemia or thrombocythaemia but may be seen de novo. Extramedullary haemopoiesis with massive splenomegaly occurs.

Symptoms and signs
These are caused by anaemia. Splenomegaly (often massive) leads to abdominal discomfort and splenic infarction to acute pain (see Table 11.12). Sweating and weight loss result from a raised metabolic rate.

Investigations
The blood film usually shows a leukoerythroblastic anaemia with immature

Table 11.12. Causes of splenomegaly

Infections	
Bacterial	Septicaemia
	Subacute bacterial endocarditis (SBE)
	Typhoid
	Tuberculosis (TB)
	Brucellosis
Viral	Acute viral illness, especially in children
	Infectious mononucleosis
	HIV
Parasitic	Acute malaria
	Chronic malaria (tropical splenomegaly)*
	Leishmaniasis (kala-azar)*
	Schistosomiasis (portal hypertension)
Haemolytic anaemia	Hereditary spherocytosis
	Autoimmune haemolytic anaemia
	Sickle cell disease (children; in adults, often splenic atrophy)
	Other haemoglobinopathies
	Thalassaemia*
Haematological malignancy	
Myeloproliferative disease	Primary polycythaemia
	Myelofibrosis*
	Chronic myeloid leukaemia*
Acute leukaemia	Mainly ALL in children
Lymphoproliferative disease	Hodgkin's disease
	Non-Hodgkin's lymphoma*
	Chronic lymphatic leukaemia
	Hairy cell leukaemia*
Miscellaneous	
Anaemia (usually only minor enlargement)	Iron deficiency
	Megaloblastic anaemia
Idiopathic	Primary hypersplenism (? lymphoma)
Congestive	Portal hypertension
	Cirrhosis
	Splenic or portal vein thrombosis
Connective tissue disease	Systemic lupus erythematosus (SLE)
	Rheumatoid arthritis (Felty's syndrome)
Storage disease	Gaucher's*
	Niemann-Pick disease
	Histiocytosis X (children usually)
Other	Amyloid (often associated with hyposplenic blood picture)
	Sarcoid
	Cysts
	Tumours (rare)

*Enlargement may be massive

red and white cells. Tear drop poikilocytes are characteristic. White cell and platelet counts are variable, usually normal or low, but they may be high.

Bone marrow aspiration yields a dry tap. Trephine biopsy shows increased fibrosis and new bone formation.

Differential diagnosis
From other causes of leukoerythroblastic anaemia, principally infiltration by carcinoma.

Treatment
There is no effective treatment other than blood transfusion if indicated symptomatically. Splenectomy may be helpful in reducing transfusion requirements, and should preferably be performed before the spleen becomes massive. Patients usually survive several years from diagnosis although termination as acute leukaemia is common.

Chronic myeloid (granulocytic) leukaemia (CML)

CML is a malignant disease of either a totipotential or a committed myeloid stem cell. Peak incidence is in middle age and a juvenile form exists. It characteristically progresses through three stages:

1. a benign phase which is responsive to treatment
2. an accelerated phase unresponsive to treatment
3. a terminal phase resembling acute leukaemia.

Exposure to radiation is a known aetiological factor. A unique feature is the presence of a specific chromosomal abnormality, the Philadelphia chromosome, in the majority of cases. This is a reciprocal translocation between chromosomes 9 and 22, resulting in the activation of the oncogene, c-*abl*.

Symptoms and signs
CML is usually of insidious onset with weakness and weight loss or symptoms of anaemia. Splenomegaly may be massive. Gout is caused by hyperuricaemia.

Investigations
The white cell count is invariably raised and usually $> 100 \times 10^9/1$. Some asymptomatic cases may be picked up before this on routine blood count. The differential white cell count shows a neutrophilia with immature forms, i.e. bands, metamyelocytes, myelocytes (left shift). There may be a basophilia.

Anaemia is usual. The platelet count is usually normal or raised with abnormal forms. It often falls as the disease progresses.

The neutrophil alkaline phosphatase (NAP) is low or absent. Cytogenetic studies usually show the Philadelphia chromosome.

Differential diagnosis
Advanced cases present little difficulty but cases detected by chance with a white cell count of around $50 \times 10^9/1$ need to be distinguished from a myeloid

leukaemoid reaction, e.g. severe infection, malignancy. The NAP and cytogenetic studies are useful in these cases.

Treatment

This remains disappointing. Bone marrow transplantation offers the only hope of a permanent cure and should be considered the treatment of choice for younger patients.

Although the disease in the benign phase may be readily controllable with hydroxyurea or busulphan, this does not eliminate the Philadelphia clone and does not significantly prolong survival. Recent work suggests that alpha-interferon may eliminate the clone in some cases and prolong the duration of the benign phase and this is now regarded as the treatment of choice. Once transformation to the accelerated phase or acute leukaemia has occurred, treatment is very unsuccessful.

Prognosis

Conventional treatment gives a median survival of less than 4 years and virtually all patients are dead by 10 years. Interferon may significantly improve survival.

ACUTE LEUKAEMIA

The acute leukaemias are disorders of primitive stem cells which proliferate showing little or no differentiation. Two main varieties are recognised, *myeloid* and *lymphoid*, each being further subdivided into several types (Table 11.13). Correct diagnosis depends on analysis of surface markers and, increasingly,

---

Table 11.13. Classification of acute leukaemia and myelodysplasia

Acute leukaemia
Lymphoblastic (ALL)
    Common ALL, mainly children
    T cell ALL (poor prognosis)
    B cell ALL (resembles Burkitt's lymphoma)
    'Lymphosarcoma' leukaemia (elderly)
Myeloblastic (AML)
    Myeloid (with or without differentiation)
    Promyelocytic (often associated with DIC)
    Myelomonocytic
    Monocytic
    Erythroleukaemia
    Megakaryocytic

Myelodysplasia
    Refractory anaemia (RA)
    Refractory anaemia with ring sideroblasts (RAS)
    Refractory anaemia with excess blasts (RAEB)
    RAEB in transformation (RAEB-t)
    Chronic myelomonocytic leukaemia (CMMoL)

on DNA studies. Chromosome abnormalities are common and some have predictive value. Correct diagnosis is important because treatment and prognosis may depend on it. Acute lymphoblastic leukaemia (ALL) has its peak incidence in early childhood. Acute myeloid leukaemia (AML) is predominantly a disease of the elderly.

The aetiology is unknown but several factors have been postulated. These include viruses, genetic abnormalities, e.g. Down syndrome, drugs and ionising irradiation. The importance of exposure to naturally occurring radiation, particularly radon, is becoming increasingly recognised.

Symptoms and signs

Acute leukaemia usually has a short history although some cases, particularly in the elderly, may have a more gradual onset.

The symptoms and signs are principally due to bone marrow failure from replacement of normal haemopoietic tissue by leukaemic blast cells. They include anaemia, infection (due to neutropenia), shock (due to septicaemia), mouth ulceration (neutropenia) and gingival overgrowth (especially in monocytic leukaemia). Skin lesions (infection, infiltration or miscellaneous, e.g. pyoderma gangrenosum) are seen. Bleeding into skin and mucous membranes is caused by thrombocytopenia.

Other symptoms include bone pain, particularly in children, and joint pain due to hyperuricaemia.

Signs include tonsillar enlargement or splenomegaly (usually ALL).

Investigations

Most patients are pancytopenic, often severely so. The white cell count is variable but usually raised with a predominance of blast cells. Some cases have a low white cell count with no blast cells (aleukaemic leukaemia) and diagnosis depends on bone marrow examination.

Accurate typing of the blast cells and cytogenetic studies should be carried out in all younger patients.

Treatment

The treatment of acute leukaemia is complicated, usually unpleasant for the patient, and expensive. It should only be practised in specialist centres. The mainstay of treatment is chemotherapy but equally important is supportive therapy with platelet transfusions and antibiotics.

The principal of therapy is to induce remission with cytotoxic drugs, that is, elimination of all visible leukaemic cells and restoration of normal marrow function. This is followed by more intensive chemotherapy aimed at eliminating any residual leukaemic cells.

In ALL, maintenance therapy is usually given for several years. There is no evidence that maintenance therapy is beneficial in AML. Also, in ALL, CNS prophylaxis is essential to prevent meningeal relapse.

Bone marrow transplantation, particularly if there is an HLA-compatible sibling, should be considered in all younger patients with AML in first remission and in patients with ALL with poor prognostic features.

The role of autotransplantation is still to be established.

Treatment of AML in the over 60 age group is very unrewarding. Even though remissions may be obtained, they are usually short lived. It is doubtful whether most of these patients should be subjected to intensive chemotherapy.

Prognosis

The prognosis in common ALL in childhood has improved dramatically with over 90% achieving remission and over 50% having long-term survival and probable cure.

The prognosis of AML and ALL in adults remains poor. Although remission rates of over 80% can be expected, the problem of relapse remains and 5-year survival is around 30% with conventional chemotherapy. The results are particularly poor in the elderly with the majority relapsing within 2 years. In some elderly patients, the disease runs a chronic course and reasonable quality survival for several years may be achieved with supportive therapy only.

At the moment, allogeneic bone marrow transplantation seems to offer the best hope for younger patients.

Myelodysplastic syndromes (MDS) (see Table 11.13)

This term is applied to a miscellaneous group of disorders characterised by progressive cytopenias with a cellular marrow and morphological changes affecting all cell lines. At the most benign end of the spectrum is refractory anaemia which affects red cells only. In many cases, all three cells lines are affected, giving rise to pancytopenia. Other cases show a progressive increase in the number of blast cells and eventually terminate as acute leukaemia. The interest in MDS is that it provides a model for the development of acute leukaemia. Many cases are associated with chromosomal abnormalities and are thought to be clonal in origin.

There is no effective treatment other than blood transfusion and the prognosis is variable. Patients with refractory anaemia may survive for 5 years or more with regular transfusions. Those who have an excess of blasts rarely survive longer than 1 year.

LYMPHOPROLIFERATIVE DISEASE

These diseases arise from malignant transformation of lymphoid cells at some stage of their development (Fig. 11.3). Clinically, they may be divided into the following groups:

1. chronic lymphatic leukaemia
2. lymphoma
   (a) Hodgkin's disease
   (b) non-Hodgkin's lymphoma
   (c) T cell lymphoma
3. immunoproliferative disease
   (a) myeloma
   (b) macroglobulinaemia.

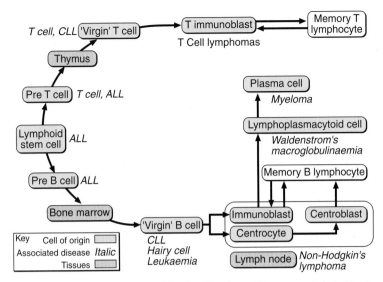

Fig. 11.3 The origin of lymphoproliferative disorders. ALL = acute lymphoblastic leukaemia; CLL = chronic lymphatic leukaemia.

Chronic lymphatic leukaemia (CLL)

CLL is a common form of leukaemia occurring principally in elderly patients. There is progressive proliferation of lymphocytes (usually B cells) with infiltration of the bone marrow causing a peripheral blood lymphocytosis. These may be lymph node enlargement and/or splenomegaly.

Normal lymphocyte function is impaired and immune paresis develops. Autoimmune phenomena, i.e. anaemia and thrombocytopenia, may occur.

Symptoms and signs

Often there are no symptoms and the disease is discovered by chance. Anaemia and thrombocytopenia may be due to marrow infiltration or autoimmunity. There is lymph node enlargement and splenomegaly. Occasionally, there is skin infiltration or salivary gland enlargement. Recurrent infection, particularly chest infection due to hypogammaglobulinaemia, occurs.

Investigations

Lymphocytosis ($> 5 \times 10^9/1$) is invariable. The lymphocyte count may exceed $500 \times 10^9/1$. 'Smear cells' (disintegrated lymphocytes) are seen in the blood film.

The bone marrow is infiltrated by lymphocytes with variable reduction in normal haemopoietic tissue.

Lymph node biopsy is rarely needed but shows replacement of normal structure by small lymphocytes. Reduction of serum immunoglobulin is common. The Coombs' test may be positive.

Differential diagnosis

CLL has to be distinguished from hairy cell leukaemia, prolymphocytic leukaemia and exfoliative lymphoma.

Treatment

Patients with lymphocytosis only require no treatment.

Indications for treatment are marrow failure, progressive lymph node enlargement or autoimmune phenomena. Intermittent chlorambucil and prednisolone are the mainstays of treatment. Localised lymph node masses may be treated with radiotherapy. Vigorous treatment of infection is needed and patients with recurrent infection may benefit from immunoglobulin replacement.

Many patients with CLL survive for many years without treatment but marrow failure is a bad sign and the survival is usually under 5 years.

Lymphoma

Hodgkin's disease

This form of lymphoma is separated from the others because of its histology and natural history. It has a peak incidence in early adulthood. Epidemiological evidence suggests that it has an infective origin and there is increasing evidence to link it with Epstein-Barr virus (EBV) infection.

Pathology. The hallmark of the disease is the Reed-Sternberg cell, which is a large cell with two or more nuclei with prominent nucleoli. It is accompanied by reactive cells, lymphocytes, histiocytes and eosinophils. It is unusual amongst tumours in that the malignant cell is in the minority. The origin of the Reed-Sternberg cell is uncertain but it is now thought that it can be of either B or T cell origin. Various histological grades are recognised. The greater the lymphocyte proliferation, the better the prognosis.

The disease spreads in an orderly fashion from one group of lymph nodes to another. Extranodal involvement is rare. Characteristically there is early loss of cellular immunity, leading to infections with opportunistic organisms.

Symptoms and signs. The most common presentation is painless enlargement of cervical nodes. In more advanced disease, other lymph node areas may be involved.

Systemic symptoms (B symptoms) include undulating fever, night sweats and weight loss. Pruritus and alcohol-induced pain are uncommon symptoms of uncertain aetiology. Splenomegaly may occur.

Investigations. Lymph node biopsy is essential for histological diagnosis.

The blood count is usually normal although anaemia, eosinophilia and raised plasma viscosity or ESR may occur. Bone marrow involvement is uncommon.

It is important to delineate the extent of the disease. This is most easily done by CT scanning.

Differential diagnosis. Other causes of lymphadenopathy (Table 11.14).

Table 11.14. Causes of lymphadenopathy

Generalised	Localised
Infectious mononucleosis	Local infection (pyogenic, tuberculosis, pediculosis)
HIV infection, AIDS	
Chronic lymphatic leukaemia	Cat scratch fever
Acute lymphoblastic leukaemia	Rubella (occipital)
Lymphoma	Lymphoma—non-Hodgkin's lymphoma or Hodgkin's disease
Rheumatoid arthritis (and Still's disease)	
	Secondary carcinoma
Sarcoidosis	
Tuberculosis	
Toxoplasmosis—cytomegalovirus	
Drug therapy, e.g. Phenytoin, PAS	
Secondary syphilis	

PAS = para-aminosalicylic acid.

Treatment. Stage 1 disease, i.e. that limited to one group of lymph glands, is treatable by radiotherapy. All other stages, particularly if B symptoms are present, should be treated with combination chemotherapy. With modern treatment, the prognosis is excellent. With localised disease, the cure rate is in the order of 80%. Even advanced disease with extranodal spread has the possibility of long remission and even cure.

Non-Hodgkin's lymphoma (NHL)

This is a heterogeneous group of disorders which may affect any age group although the most common incidence is in the elderly. The aetiology is unknown but a viral cause is suspected in some cases, notably Burkitt's lymphoma (EBV) and T cell leukaemia lymphoma syndrome (HTLV1).

Pathology. Most NHLs are of B cell origin, particularly the follicular centre cells; some are of T cell origin. True histiocytic lymphomas are exceedingly rare.

Modern classifications try to identify the cell of origin but, clinically, they can be divided into three groups:

1. low grade—predominantly small lymphocytes or cells arranged in a follicular pattern
2. intermediate grade—usually a mixture of follicular cells, centrocytes and centroblasts
3. high grade—predominance of centroblasts or immunoblasts with total destruction of nodal architecture.

Unlike Hodgkin's disease, blood-borne spread is common and the disease may be widespread at presentation even if only microscopically. Extranodal involvement is much more common.

T cell diseases frequently involve the skin and CNS. Two cutaneous T cell lymphomas are *mycosis fungoides* and *Sezary's syndrome.*

Symptoms and signs. Lymphadenopathy, either localised or generalised, is the most common presentation. Splenomegaly, often massive, may occur and, in some cases, the disease may be localised to the spleen.

B symptoms are as for Hodgkin's disease. Lymphoma should be suspected in any case of pyrexia of unknown origin (PUO). The presentation of NHL may be very varied and almost every organ may be affected. Marrow involvement may cause pancytopenia.

Investigations. Histological diagnosis is essential. Staging is less important as treatment depends more on histological grade.

Differential diagnosis. Other causes of lymphadenopathy and other causes of PUO. Marrow and blood involvement may resemble leukaemia.

Treatment. Low-grade disease, particularly in the elderly, may require no treatment for several years. Localised disease may be treated with radiotherapy. Low-grade NHL is not curable and eventually transforms to aggressive disease. The mean survival is approximately 7 years.

High-grade disease, particularly in younger patients, requires intensive combination chemotherapy and usually responds well to treatment but relapse is frequent. Long-term survival is around 30%, most of these cases being permanently cured. The role of autotransplantation still needs to be defined.

Myeloma

This disease is the result of malignant proliferation of plasma cells. It occurs principally in the elderly.

Pathology

Low-grade proliferation of a single clone of plasma cells results in increased production of a single immunoglobulin molecule. This can be detected as a discrete 'monoclonal' band on serum electrophoresis. Immunoglobulin light chains may be produced in excess of heavy chains and appear in the urine as 'Bence-Jones' protein. Light chains may be toxic to renal tubules and may also polymerise to form amyloid proteins. Secretion of osteoclast activating factor causes lytic bone lesions and osteopenia. Bone marrow infiltration causes suppression of normal immunoglobulin production and, terminally, bone marrow failure.

Symptoms and signs

Bone pain, particularly back pain, is the most common symptom and is caused by vertebral collapse and nerve entrapment. Pathological fractures of ribs or long bones are common, as is bone tenderness. Spinal cord compression may also lead to neurological complications.

Symptomatic hypercalcaemia results from bone destruction. Renal failure may result from light chain toxicity, hypercalcaemia, amyloidosis or sepsis. Amyloid deposits can also occur in the skin, mucous membranes, tongue, gut, liver, spleen, adrenals, nerves, and heart and may cause dysfunction of any of these organs, including bleeding, neuropathy, and cardiomyopathy.

Infections are frequent because of immune paresis.

Occasionally, excess of paraprotein may result in the hyperviscosity syndrome which is characterised by weakness, visual disturbance, bleeding and, in severe cases, coma.

Investigations

The diagnosis is confirmed by detection of a monoclonal protein (usually IgG or IgA) in serum or urine, lytic lesions or radiological skeletal survey, and excess plasma cells in the bone marrow. Anaemia or pancytopenia may occur. Plasma viscosity or ESR is often raised. Detection of urinary light chains requires specific tests; dipstick tests for protein are insensitive to light chains.

Biochemical tests for hypercalcaemia and renal failure are essential. The alkaline phosphatase activity is usually normal, allowing differentiation from metastatic carcinoma involving bone.

Radiology may also show diffuse osteopenia: isotope bone scans are often normal, even when there are multiple lytic lesions.

Differential diagnosis

Distinguishing features of other causes of paraproteinaemia, particularly benign monoclonal gammopathy, are absence of immunosuppression, lack of plasmacytosis and skeletal changes. Follow-up shows little change in the paraprotein level with time.

Treatment

Melphalan and prednisolone are the mainstay of treatment, particularly in the elderly. Younger patients may benefit from combination chemotherapy. Localised bone lesions causing pain can be treated with radiotherapy.

Correction of metabolic abnormalities, e.g. hypercalcaemia, is essential. Occasionally, the hyperviscosity syndrome may require plasmapheresis.

Prognosis

For most patients, the mean survival is around 3 years. Renal failure often indicates a high tumour burden, and is associated with decreased survival.

Waldenstrom's macroglobulinaemia

This is an uncommon disorder in which the paraprotein is IgM. Unlike myeloma, bone lesions do not occur but lymphadenopathy and splenomegaly may. The main symptoms are due to hyperviscosity or marrow failure.

Plasmapheresis may be needed, otherwise the treatment is with chlorambucil.

BLEEDING DISORDERS

The arrest of haemorrhage is a complicated process and depends on the interaction between the vessel wall, platelets, coagulation system and fibrinolytic system (Figs 11.4 and 11.5). The key factor is damage to vascular endothelium which causes platelet adhesion and activation of the coagulation mechanism. These result in the formation of a platelet plug which is reinforced by a fibrin clot.

Failure of haemostasis results from vascular disorders, thrombocytopenia, platelet functional disorders (thrombocytopathy), coagulation disorders and excessive fibrinolysis.

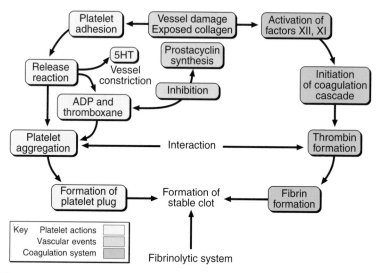

Fig. 11.4 Mechanism of haemostasis.

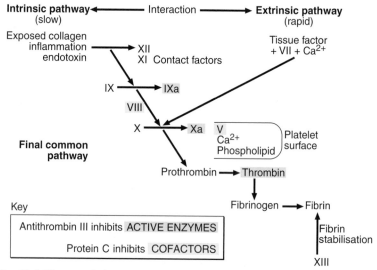

Fig. 11.5 The coagulation system.

Symptoms

Platelet disorders give rise to bleeding into the skin and mucous membranes whereas coagulation disorders cause bleeding into joints and muscles.

Investigations

The type, extent and onset of bleeding, and past history, particularly surgical operations and dental extractions, are important points. Other points to note are family history, other medical conditions and drug therapy.

Measurement of bleeding time after a standardised skin incision may be used to detect platelet dysfunction.

Diagnosis depends upon laboratory investigation. Essential investigations are a full blood count and screening test of blood coagulation. The most useful are (Fig. 11.6):

1. *The prothrombin time* (PT), a test of the extrinsic system, is useful in the diagnosis of coagulation defects secondary to liver disease, or to monitor warfarin therapy.
2. *Activated partial thromboplastin time* (APTT), a test of the intrinsic system, is used to diagnose haemophilia A and B and monitor heparin therapy.
3. *Thrombin clotting time (TCT)* detects fibrinogen deficiency and inhibitors including heparin and fibrin degradation products (FDPs). Its main use is in the diagnosis of DIC.

Other useful investigations include factor assays and platelet function tests. Tests of fibrinolytic activity are difficult and rarely useful clinically.

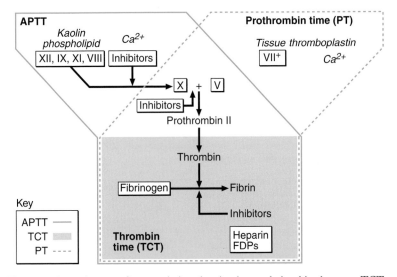

Fig. 11.6 Screening tests for coagulation showing inter-relationships between TCT, APTT and PT.

VASCULAR DISORDERS

These are congenital or acquired and characterised by bleeding into the skin and from mucous membranes. They are caused by inflammatory damage to small vessels or changes in the supporting matrix (Table 11.15)

Hereditary haemorrhagic telangiectasia (Osler–Rendu–Weber disease)

This is inherited as an autosomal dominant and is characterised by multiple telangiectases in the skin and mucous membranes, particularly in the nose and GI tract. Arteriovenous shunts may develop in the lungs and elsewhere.

Symptoms and signs

Epistaxis, haemoptysis and GI tract bleeding, leading to anaemia, are more noticeable with ageing.

There are multiple telangiectases in the mouth, lips and finger tips. Bruits are present over the skull, chest or abdomen if there are arteriovenous fistulae.

Investigations

Essentially, the diagnosis is clinical although endoscopy may be necessary.

Differential diagnosis

Other vascular abnormalities include Campbell De Morgan's spots and purpura. Note: telangiectases blanch on pressure.

Table 11.15. Vascular causes of abnormal bleeding

Congenital
Hereditary haemorrhagic telangiectasia (Osler–Rendu–Weber disease)
Ehlers–Danlos disease (loose skin, joint hypermobility)

Acquired
  Simple, easy bruising (young women, normal clotting studies)
  Thin skin (geographic lesions on extensor surface),
  e.g. senile purpura, steroids, Cushing's syndrome
  Scurvy (perifollicular haemorrhage)

Damage to blood vessels (non-thrombocytopenic purpura)
  Drugs–penicillin, sulphonamides
  Infections
  Henoch–Schönlein purpura
  Systemic lupus erythematosus
  Rheumatoid arthritis
  Amyloid

Dysglobulinaemia
  Benign hyperglobulinaemia
  Cryoglobulinaemia
  Macroglobulinaemia

Treatment

Repeated bleeding usually requires iron. Repeated epistaxis may be helped by oestrogen therapy and antifibrinolytic agents, e.g. tranexamic acid.

GI lesions may respond to endoscopic laser therapy.

Small vessel vasculitis

Inflammation of cutaneous capillaries and small arterioles (p. 379) causes bleeding into the skin which may be confused for purpura due to thrombocytopenia. In vasculitis the purpura are palpable, and skin infarction may be present in the centre of the lesions. The most common example is Henoch–Schonlein purpura. Platelet count and coagulation tests are normal.

THROMBOCYTOPENIA (see Table 11.16)

Idiopathic thrombocytopenic purpura (ITP)

This is an autoimmune disease, although in children it may be post-viral. There is bleeding into skin and mucous membranes. The most serious complication is CNS haemorrhage. Splenomegaly does not occur; if it is present, an alternative diagnosis should be considered.

Table 11.16. Causes of thrombocytopenia

A Impaired platelet production (decreased megakaryocytes in bone marrow)
Hereditary congenital hypoplasia (rare), e.g. Wiskott–Aldrich syndrome, May–Hegglin anomaly
Megaloblastic anaemia
Marrow replacement, e.g. carcinoma, leukaemia
Viral infections
Aplastic anaemia caused by drug, chemicals, alcohol, radiation

B Excessive platelet destruction or use (increased megakaryocytes in bone marrow)
Immune mediated
Autoimmune idiopathic thrombocytopenic purpura, systemic lupus erythematosus, lymphoproliferative diseases
Drug induced (thiazides, quinine)
Evans syndrome (autoimmune haemolysis and autoimmune thrombocytopenia)
Heparin-associated thrombocytopenia, AIDS, other viral infections
Excessive consumption
Disseminated intravascular coagulation (DIC)
Giant haemangioma
Hypersplenism
Cardiac bypass operations
Massive transfusion (dilution effect and possible DIC)

Investigations

The blood count is normal other than the thrombocytopenia. Increased megakaryocytes are seen in the bone marrow. Antiplatelet antibodies are rarely demonstrable in the serum but are found on platelets (platelet-associated IgG).

Screening tests for SLE should be performed.

Differential diagnosis

ITP must be distinguished from drug-induced thrombocytopenia, SLE and immune thrombocytopenia complicating lymphoproliferative disease.

Treatment

The basis of treatment is steroids starting at a high dose, e.g. prednisolone 60 mg per 24 hours. Relapse usually occurs when steroids are withdrawn and a small maintenance dose may be needed. If a high maintenance dose of steroids is necessary to control the platelet count, splenectomy may be needed.

Immunosuppressive agents such as azathioprine or vincristine may help to reduce steroid dosage.

High-dose intravenous immunoglobulin will raise the platelet count quickly in an emergency although its effect is temporary and it is very expensive.

In children, the disease is usually self-limiting but in adults it is usually chronic.

FUNCTIONAL PLATELET DEFECTS (THROMBOCYTOPATHY)

The clinical picture is similar to that of thrombocytopenia but the platelet count is normal. Congenital platelet defects are extremely rare. The most common causes are drugs, particularly aspirin and NSAIDs. Other causes include uraemia, paraproteinaemia and myeloproliferative disease.

COAGULATION DISORDERS (see Table 11.17)

Haemophilia

There are two main types, haemophilia A (factor VIII deficiency) and haemophilia B (factor IX deficiency). Both are inherited as sex-linked characters and have a similar clinical picture. An abnormal protein which retains some functional activity is produced. The severity depends upon the level of functional activity: < 2% is severe, 2–10% moderate, and 10–25% mild.

Patients with severe haemophilia suffer spontaneous bleeds into joints, muscles and soft tissues. Repeated haemarthroses lead to synovial overgrowth and eventually to joint destruction (haemophiliac arthropathy). Bleeding from mucous membranes is rare and purpura does not occur. Mild haemophilia only leads to bleeds in response to trauma or surgery.

Symptoms and signs

Acute, painful joints are caused by haemarthrosis. There is chronic arthropathy. Retroperitoneal haemorrhage may mimic an acute abdomen.

Table 11.17. Coagulation disorders

Inherited factor deficiencies
  VIII Haemophilia A
  IX Haemophilia B (Christmas disease)
  VIII Related antigen Von Willebrand's disease
  Other rare deficiencies: I, II, V, VII, X, XI, XII, XIII.
Acquired factor deficiencies
  Prothrombin complex deficiency (II, VII, IX, X)
  Prolonged PT and APTT
  Oral anticoagulants
  Severe vitamin K deficiency
Liver disease
  Prothrombin complex plus V and fibrinogen deficiency
  PT and APTT prolonged
Intravascular coagulation syndrome (DIC)
  Fibrinogen, V, VIII and platelet deficiency
  PT and APTT and TCT may be prolonged
  Fibrin degradation products (FDPs) raised
Factor VIII inhibitor
  Haemophiliacs (mostly severe)
  Pregnancy
  Malignancy
  Autoimmune disease

Severe bleeding post-surgery, particularly dental extraction, may be the first manifestation in mild haemophilia.

Investigations
The APTT is prolonged. Specific factor assays confirm the diagnosis, and DNA studies are useful in detecting carriers.

Differential diagnosis
Other congenital bleeding disorders. Mild haemophilia must be distinguished from Von Willebrand's disease. In older patients, acquired haemophilia, caused by inhibitor formation, must be considered.

Treatment
The treatment of acute episodes is by intravenous factor replacement, given as freeze-dried concentrate. It is usually necessary to raise the factor level to around 30% for spontaneous haemarthroses, and to maintain a level above 50% for surgery until healing has occurred.

Most haemophiliacs can now be taught to treat themselves.

DDAVP (vasopressin) raises the factor VIII level. It may be all that is required for treatment in mild haemophilia. A test dose should be given first.

The management of the haemophiliac patient as a whole is very important. A team approach, consisting of physician, orthopaedic surgeon, dentist, physiotherapist, geneticist and social worker, is best and all haemophiliacs should be under the care of a haemophilia centre.

Modern factor concentrates are virtually free of the risk of viral contamination, but in the past HIV infection and virus B and C hepatitis have been serious side-effects of infused factor VIII.

With proper care and treatment, there is no reason why haemophiliacs should not have a normal lifestyle and life expectancy.

Von Willebrand's disease

This disease may be confused with mild haemophilia. It is inherited as an autosomal character and therefore women may be affected. There is defective synthesis of the carrier part of the factor VIII molecule, resulting in defective platelet function as well as a reduction in factor VIII activity. Von Willebrand's disease varies widely in severity. Common symptoms include epistaxis, menorrhagia or abnormal bleeding following surgery or dental extraction. Haemarthrosis is uncommon.

Most patients can be treated with DDAVP although more severely affected patients may need factor VIII concentrate.

Bleeding caused by multiple factor deficiency

This is usually caused by defective synthesis of factors in the liver, particularly those that are vitamin K dependent (factors II, VII, IX and X).

Aetiological conditions include liver disease, obstructive jaundice, severe malabsorption and oral anticoagulant overdose. Excessive bruising, GI tract bleeding and haematuria may occur and treatment is with fresh frozen plasma 10–15 ml per kg.

Disseminated intravascular coagulation (DIC)

Intravascular coagulation occurs in many conditions (Table 11.18). The clinical picture and laboratory findings vary widely depending upon the cause, extent and speed of the onset and, as a consequence, several seemingly different syndromes exist. They all have in common the formation of fibrin within the vascular tree, the consumption of clotting factors (including platelets) to a variable degree and the stimulation of fibrinolysis.

Factors that may trigger DIC include:

1. The release of thromboplastin into the bloodstream, e.g. obstetric accidents, carcinoma and leukaemia.
2. Activation of factor XII by contact with foreign surfaces, endotoxin and complement components.
3. Platelet aggregation by endotoxin, immune complexes or contact with a foreign surface.
4. Endothelial damage, e.g. malignant hypertension, renal disease, acute hepatic necrosis. This activates factor XII and stimulates platelet aggregation.

Activation of the clotting mechanism causes fibrin formation with consumption of some of the clotting factors, particularly platelets, fibrinogen and

Table 11.18. The intravascular coagulation syndromes

Acute

Obstetric complications
    Placental abruption
    Amniotic fluid embolism
    Eclampsia
    Retained products of dead fetus
    Septic abortion

Infections
    Septicaemia, especially gram-negative, meningococcal
    Malaria

Surgery
    Especially on the lungs and prostate
    Extracorporeal circulation

Trauma and burns

Shock

Snake bites, e.g. vipers

Incompatible blood transfusions, especially ABO

Chronic

Neoplasms, e.g. lung, stomach, colon

Leukaemia, especially promyelocytic

Thrombotic thrombocytopenic purpura

Haemolytic–uraemic syndrome

Giant haemangiomas

Miscellaneous causes, e.g. collagen disorders, amyloid, allergic vasculitis

---

factors V and VIII. In chronic DIC, increased synthesis may balance excessive consumption and their level may be normal or even raised. DIC activates the fibrinolytic system causing the production of fibrin degradation products (FDPs). These have an anticoagulant effect by inhibiting fibrin formation and thus may potentiate the bleeding tendency. Fibrin formation in small vessels may lead to microthrombi and micro-infarcts, which may be responsible for the clinical picture. They may also cause microangiopathic haemolytic anaemia.

Symptoms and signs

1. Acute cases, e.g. obstetric complications, cause severe bleeding because of the rapid depletion of clotting factors.
2. In chronic DIC, e.g. that associated with disseminated malignancy, thrombocytopenia is the principal manifestation.
3. Where microthrombus formation predominates, widespread symptoms affecting many organs may occur. This is particularly so in TTP, where neurological complications are prominent.

Investigations

Full blood count. Results are variable. Thrombocytopenia is usual. Features of microangiopathic haemolytic anaemia may be present.

Clotting tests. In severe cases, depletion of fibrinogen and factors V and VIII leads to prolongation of the TCT, PT and APTT.

Prolongation of the TCT may be caused by hypofibrinogenaemia or the presence of FDPs. Fibrinogen assay and tests for FDPs are essential.

In chronic cases, the clotting tests may be normal or even shortened because of circulating activated clotting factors. In such cases, the presence of raised FDPs is diagnostic.

Treatment

The cardinal rules of the treatment of DIC are to treat the cause, if possible, and to replace missing factors and platelets.

There is little place for heparin except in some chronic conditions where it may block the process and stop microangiopathic haemolytic anaemia.

Antifibrinolytic drugs may give rise to generalised fibrin deposition and are therefore not suitable.

DIC is often a marker of serious disease and the prognosis reflects the underlying state. TTP has a high mortality.

Bleeding caused by excessive fibrinolysis

Primary fibrinolytic disorders are very rare; usually, excessive fibrinolysis is secondary to intravascular coagulation. Primary fibrinolysis may occur in some neoplasms, especially prostatic carcinoma, and during some operations, especially prostatic and pulmonary.

Excessive fibrinolysis may be blocked by antifibrinolytic drugs such as tranexamic acid. These should be used with care but have a part to play in the management of postoperative bleeding.

THROMBOPHILIA

The term thrombophilia is applied to familial or acquired abnormalities of the haemostatic mechanism that predispose to venous thromboembolic disease. The causes of thrombophilia are given in Table 11.19.

The importance of thrombophilia screening has been highlighted in recent years with the discovery of several inherited factors. Deficiency of these factors predisposes to thrombosis, mainly venous. Thrombosis may occur without any precipitating cause and often in unusual sites such as the axillary vein or mesenteric vein. The tendency to thrombosis is increased if other risk factors are present, such as pregnancy or oral contraceptives.

Antithrombin III (ATIII) is a serine protease inhibitor which neutralises many activated clotting factors. Women with ATIII deficiency are particularly susceptible to thrombosis during pregnancy and the post-partum period.

Protein C inhibits activated factors V and VIII, and protein S acts as a co-factor. Deficiency of both increases the risk of thrombosis, including superficial thrombophlebitis. They are both vitamin K-dependent proteins and are reduced by warfarin. When warfarin therapy is commenced, there

Table 11.19. Causes of thrombophilia

Inherited factors
Activated protein C resistance (factor V Leiden)
Antithrombin III deficiency
Protein C deficiency
Protein S deficiency
Homocystinuria
Dysfibrinogenaemia
Raised factor VIII level
Raised fibrinogen level

Acquired factors
Antiphospholipid syndrome
Pregnancy
Oestrogen therapy (oral contraceptives)
Obesity
Surgery
Immobility
Malignancy (Trousseau's syndrome)
Myeloproliferative syndromes
Hyperviscosity syndromes
Heparin-induced thrombocytopenia
Paroxysmal nocturnal haemoglobinuria

is a period of dramatically increased thrombotic risk, which may be manifest as coumarin-induced skin necrosis. This period must be covered by heparin. Neonates who are homozygous for protein C or S develop neonatal purpura fulminans.

Activated protein C resistance (APCR) is the most common thrombo-philic abnormality, occurring in approximately 5% of the population. It is due to an abnormality of factor V known as factor V Leiden, which is resistant to the action of protein C. Approximately 40% of patients with otherwise unexplained thrombosis possess this abnormality. Homozygotes are more likely to develop thrombosis than heterozygotes. Women on oestrogen-containing oral contraceptives are particularly at risk.

Antiphospholipid antibodies, formerly known as the lupus anticoagulant, are found in a wide range of conditions other than SLE. They cause a prolongation of the APTT in vitro, but the clinical picture is of venous thromboembolism and recurrent miscarriages.

A full thrombophilia screen is expensive and should not be undertaken without adequate indication (Table 11.20).

Thrombophilia is not a predictor for arterial thrombosis except in patients under the age of 30 years. A case could be made for screening for APCR in young women wishing to take an oestrogen-containing oral contraceptive.

Thrombophilia tests need to be interpreted with care. Pregnancy and

Table 11.20. Indications for thrombophilia screening

Venous thrombosis in young patients
Recurrent venous thrombosis or thrombophlebitis
Thrombosis in an unusual site
Skin necrosis if on coumarin
Relatives of patients with known thrombophilia
Recurrent miscarriages (antiphospholipid antibody)

oestrogen can lower protein S levels, and low protein S levels may be found in patients with factor V Leiden. Falsely low levels may also be found in patients who have had a recent thrombotic event.

The presence of a thrombophilic abnormality is not an indication for lifelong anticoagulation unless there has been a history of thrombosis. All patients suspected of having a thrombophilic abnormality should be referred to a specialist clinic for advice and management.

12

RHEUMATOLOGY
Peter Hollingworth

Many rheumatic disorders are mediated through the immune system, so a better understanding of their pathogenesis and major advances in therapy are promised by pharmacological manipulation of the immune system.

Contrary to popular misconceptions, the more serious rheumatic diseases commonly begin in young adults and they become chronic as the joint has little capacity for repair. Much can be done to alleviate pain and maintain function, although cure is still rarely possible.

Rheumatic diseases are a major health burden; they account for one-fifth of GP consultations and for one-third of the disabled population.

The principal rheumatic diseases are listed in Table 12.1. Connective tissue diseases are described in Chapter 13. Many general medical diseases have rheumatological manifestations and many rheumatic diseases have extra-articular manifestations that may present to other specialists.

Table 12.1. The principal rheumatic diseases

Rheumatoid arthritis
Spondyloarthritides
   Ankylosing spondylitis
   Reiter's disease
   Arthritis of inflammatory bowel disease
   Psoriatic arthritis
Connective tissue diseases
Osteoarthritis
Back pain
Crystal deposition diseases
Septic arthritis
Shoulder pain
Polymyalgia rheumatica

Terminology

'Arthritis' applies specifically to joint inflammation, and 'arthrosis' or 'arthropathy' apply to non-inflammatory joint diseases. 'Arthralgia' indicates joint pain with no particular connotations. 'Rheumatism' and 'rheumatic' have no medical use except in general terms such as 'soft tissue rheumatism' or 'rheumatic disorders'.

SYMPTOMS OF JOINT DISEASE

Pain

This is the most common presenting symptom. Joint pain worse after rest suggests joint inflammation. Joint pain better after rest, or worsening with activity and as the day goes on, suggests osteoarthritis. Night pain which prevents sleep is a major burden. By enhancing pain perception, depression and anxiety make management difficult.

As pain fibres arising from central joints enter the spinal cord at several levels, pain from these joints is perceived over a wide area: glenohumeral pain radiates down the outer upper arm to the elbow; lumbar spinal pain to the buttock and posterior thigh; hip pain from the groin to the anterior thigh and, sometimes exclusively, the knee. In contrast, the patient accurately localises pain arising from a distal interphalangeal joint (DIPJ).

Never assume that pain felt in a joint arises from that joint; always exclude pain arising from juxta-articular or distant structures (Table 12.2).

Immobility stiffness

A cardinal sign of joint inflammation is prolonged joint stiffness, lasting from

Table 12.2. Joint pain arising from juxta-articular structures

Structures	Signs
Bone destruction: stress fracture, sepsis, metastases	Tenderness away from the joint line, abnormal radiograph
Sprain of ligament or tendon	Point tenderness away from joint line Worse on passive stretching—ligamentous Worse on resisted movement—tendinous
Bursa	Tenderness or swelling
Referred pain, e.g. shoulder pain may arise from cervical nerve irritation, thoracic or abdominal structures	Joint clinically normal, signs of distant disease
Diffuse limb pains	Consider—radiculopathy, spinal stenosis, peripheral neuropathy, polymyalgia rheumatica, bone disease, arterial or venous claudication, Parkinson's disease, depression

30 minutes to several hours, on getting up in the morning. It improves with activity and returns on resting and in the evening.

Loss of function

The consequences of unremitting inflammatory joint disease may be loss of leisure pursuits, loss of employment and, finally, loss of independence.

When assessing function, questions should be directed to practical difficulties relating to the patient's life—ambulation, personal toilet, housework, cooking, employment, sexual function, etc. Each impaired joint brings its own particular functional problem (Table 12.3).

SIGNS OF JOINT DISEASE

Examination can indicate the joint pathology (Table 12.4) and diagnosis. Pain felt in a clinically normal joint suggests that either it is referred pain or it has a psychological cause.

Look for diagnostic clues on the general examination, paying particular attention to the hands, skin, eyes and mucous membranes (Table 12.5, Figs 12.1 and 12.2).

DIAGNOSIS OF RHEUMATIC DISORDERS

Often the diagnosis is given by the history and examination alone, while investigations merely confirm it and assess the extent of joint damage. Additional clues are given by the age, sex and race of the patient, the family history, the time course of the disease, and the distribution of joints affected.

Age, sex and race

Certain diseases tend to strike specific groups. Rheumatoid arthritis and connective tissue diseases chiefly affect women while ankylosing spondylitis

Table 12.3. Functional problems peculiar to particular joints

Joint	Functional problems
Cervical spine	Reversing car
Shoulder	Reaching nape of the neck, perineal toilet, fastening brassiere or tucking in shirt tail
Elbow	Fastening top shirt button, reaching face for drinking, eating, blowing nose
Wrist	Taking change, weakness of the hand from collapse of the carpus slackening the flexor tendons
Hip	Lifting the leg high to climb stairs, alight a bus, get into a car, get out of a bath, dress lower half, sexual intercourse in women
Subtalar joint	Walking on uneven ground or sideways across a slope

Table 12.4. Signs of joint disease

Sign	Pathology	Diagnosis
Swelling		
Fluctuation (i.e. fluid)	Non-inflammatory synovial effusion: high viscosity, low WBC count	Osteoarthritis
	Inflammatory synovial effusion: low viscosity, high WBC count	Inflammatory joint disease
	Blood	Trauma, anticoagulants, haemophilia
	Pus: green or yellow	Septic arthritis
Bony	Osteophytes	Osteoarthritis
Synovial thickening	Synovitis	Inflammatory joint disease
Deformity		
Flexion	Periarticular contracture	Mainly inflammatory joint disease
Later: valgus/varus deformity	Cartilage or ligament damage	Any destructive joint disease
Redness	Intense synovitis	Acute crystal arthritis, septic arthritis, periarthritis
Crepitus	Cartilage damage	Usually osteoarthritis

Non-specific signs: muscle wasting, warmth, pain on movement, tenderness at the joint line, resticted movement

and primary gout affect men. Pyrophosphate arthropathy and polymyalgia rheumatica are diseases of the elderly, while Reiter's disease and gonococcal arthritis present in the young. Systemic lupus erythematosus (SLE) is more common in Blacks and Asians.

Family history

Spondyloarthritides, primary gout and psoriatic arthritis tend to run in families.

Time-course of the disease

Inflammatory joint disease may begin dramatically and fluctuate in severity, while osteoarthritis tends to progress slowly. Recurrent bouts of brief severe arthritis affecting one or a few joints at a time and resolving in hours or days is called palindromic arthritis. It occurs in gout, early rheumatoid arthritis, SLE and spondyloarthritides.

The distribution of joints affected

This is a most important diagnostic indicator (Fig. 12.3). The differential diagnosis of a monoarthritis is wholly different from a polyarthritis. When

Table 12.5. Skin and mucous membrane findings in rheumatic diseases

Clinical features	Diagnosis
Psoriasis	Psoriatic arthritis
Butterfly rash	Systemic lupus erythematosus (SLE)
Gottron's papules	Dermatomyositis
Vasculitis	Vasculitic syndromes
Erythema nodosum	Acute sarcoidosis and inflammatory bowel disease
Pustular psoriasis	Reiter's disease
Livedo reticularis	Antiphospholipid syndrome
Raynaud's syndrome or acrocyanosis	Rheumatoid arthritis and connective tissue diseases, especially scleroderma, SLE and mixed connective tissue disease
Subcutaneous tophi	Tophaceous gout
Rheumatoid nodules	Rheumatoid arthritis
Thickened tethered skin	Scleroderma
Diffuse or scarring alopecia	SLE
Mouth and genitourinary ulceration	Painless: Reiter's disease; painful: Behçet's disease
Dry eyes and mouth	Sjögren's syndrome

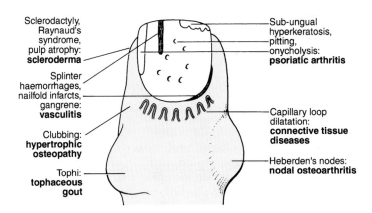

Sclerodactyly, Raynaud's syndrome, pulp atrophy: **scleroderma**

Splinter haemorrhages, nailfold infarcts, gangrene: **vasculitis**

Clubbing: **hypertrophic osteopathy**

Tophi: **tophaceous gout**

Sub-ungual hyperkeratosis, pitting, onycholysis: **psoriatic arthritis**

Capillary loop dilatation: **connective tissue diseases**

Heberden's nodes: **nodal osteoarthritis**

Fig. 12.1 The fingertips in rheumatic diseases.

acute, it suggests a crystal arthropathy or bacterial sepsis, and when chronic, osteoarthritis.

INVESTIGATIONS

Imaging techniques
Plain radiographs are most important in the investigation and monitoring

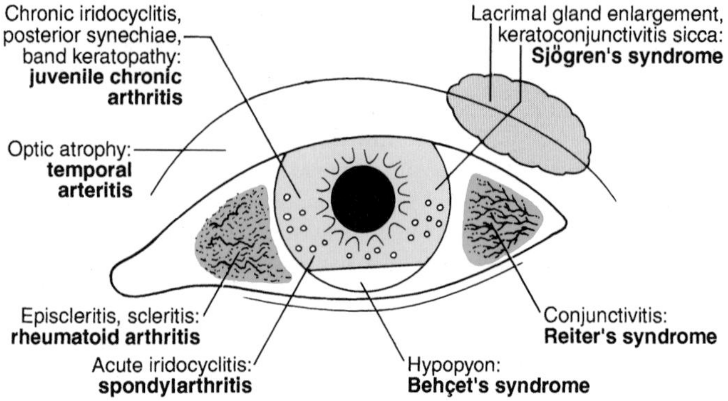

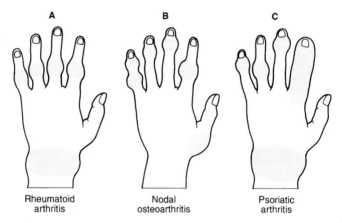

Chronic iridocyclitis,
posterior synechiae,
band keratopathy:
**juvenile chronic
arthritis**

Lacrimal gland enlargement,
keratoconjunctivitis sicca:
Sjögren's syndrome

Optic atrophy:
**temporal
arteritis**

Episcleritis, scleritis:
rheumatoid arthritis

Acute iridocyclitis:
spondylarthritis

Hypopyon:
Behçet's syndrome

Conjunctivitis:
Reiter's syndrome

Fig. 12.2 The eye in rheumatic diseases.

A

B

C

Rheumatoid
arthritis

Nodal
osteoarthritis

Psoriatic
arthritis

Fig. 12.3 Characteristic distribution of polyarticular disease.

of joint disease. For monitoring, single views only of appropriate sites no more frequently than 6-monthly are indicated.

Bone scintigraphy scanning soon after injection of radiolabelled technetium diphosphonate detects synovitis; late scans detect bone disease—metastases, Paget's disease and osteomyelitis.

Computed tomography is useful in the assessment of spinal stenosis. Magnetic resonance imaging is used in the detection of spinal and disc disease, osteonecrosis and internal joint derangement.

Blood investigations

Non-specific indices of inflammation are elevation of the ESR, plasma viscosity, C-reactive protein and complement levels.

IgM rheumatoid factor (RF) is found in high titre in rheumatoid arthritis. The latex test for RF is so sensitive it tends to give false positive results. The Rose Waaler test is less sensitive but more specific.

Some antinuclear and extractable nuclear antibodies are strongly associated with certain disease features in connective tissue disease (Ch. 13).

Complement consumption occurs in active connective tissue diseases, notably SLE and systemic rheumatoid arthritis.

Immune complexes are usually elevated in rheumatoid arthritis and connective tissue diseases but only crudely reflect disease activity.

Analysis of synovial fluid detects infection or crystal arthropathies.

Other investigations include arthroscopy, synovial biopsy and arthrography, and are used in the diagnosis of monoarticular disease.

PRINCIPLES OF MANAGEMENT OF JOINT DISEASE

Arthritis may disrupt all aspects of the patient's life, so management is of the whole person, not just of the joints, and involves the combined facilities of physiotherapy, occupational therapy, surgery, drugs, psychological and social support. With regular evaluation, problems are anticipated and corrected early.

Explanation of the probable disease course, self-help and the use of drugs allay unnecessary fears.

Bedrest is rarely indicated. Individual joints should be rested with splinting. Special shoes accommodate deformed feet. Shoe inserts correct or support painful foot deformities.

Physiotherapy
A combination of active, passive and resisted exercises maintain or correct joint position, joint movement and muscle strength.

Occupational therapy
Functional problems are overcome by exploitation of residual function, mechanical devices, or altering the patient's environment.

Drugs
The principles are: (a) prescribe the minimum number; and (b) use the least toxic first, at the minimum therapeutically effective dose.

Several groups of drugs are available. Some drugs for specific conditions are mentioned later.

Analgesics. Paracetamol and co-proxamol.

Non-steroidal anti-inflammatory drugs (NSAIDs). Used principally for inflammatory joint disease to alleviate pain, stiffness and swelling, many are available and the response individualistic. Side-effects are common, particularly in the elderly, and include gastrointestinal ulceration, renal impairment and fluid retention.

Slow-acting antirheumatic drugs (SAARDs). These appear to modify the course of rheumatoid arthritis and other inflammatory joint diseases. Indications for use include failure to respond to NSAIDs, progressive joint damage, serious extra-articular complications and reduction of steroid dosage. The disease may appear to remit and the rate of joint destruction decrease. The trend is to introduce SAARDs early in the course of the disease.

The dosage is slowly increased. No benefit is seen for weeks or months. Regular monitoring detects side-effects early, which are common but rarely irreversible.

The principal SAARDs and their side-effects are shown in Table 12.6.

Prednisolone. This is reserved for severe synovitis in inflammatory joint diseases or serious extra-articular complications. A dose lower than 7.5 mg per 24 hours carries minimal risk, perhaps less than that for NSAIDs in the elderly.

Intra-articular steroids. These are used for relieving symptoms from synovitis, where one or a few joints are particularly affected. The benefit may last weeks. Post-injection 'flares' are common. The risk of infection is small.

Intra-articular radioactive colloids. These give longer relief than steroid injections by giving a 'chemical synovectomy'.

Surgery

The inflamed synovium may be removed, sometimes arthroscopically, and destroyed joints excised, fused, realigned or replaced by prostheses.

RHEUMATOID ARTHRITIS

Rheumatoid arthritis (RA) is the most common serious rheumatic disorder and affects 1% of people worldwide. The six-fold greater prevalence in women halves after the menopause. All ages after puberty are affected, it is rare in adolescence, peaks between the third and fifth decades and tends to be more severe in the elderly.

Its exact cause is unknown. Reports implicating various triggering infectious agents remain unconfirmed. The risk is increased with HLA-DR4 (four-fold), particularly for severe disease, with female sex and with multiparity. Oral contraceptives may be protective. Remission occurs in pregnancy.

Table 12.6. Slow-acting anti-rheumatic drugs and their side-effects

Sulphasalazine	Neutropenia, headaches, intestinal disturbance, male subfertility
Methotrexate	Marrow suppression, pulmonary and hepatic fibrosis
Azathioprine	Marrow suppression, hepatitis
Penicillamine	Rashes, thrombocytopenia, proteinuria
Gold salts (oral and injectable)	As for penicillamine
Hydroxychloroquine	Retinopathy

Pathology

The disease starts in the synovium, but all organs except the brain may eventually be affected.

The immunopathology commences with antigen-presenting cells in the synovium activating T helper cells to induce B cell production of RF. This spills out from the synovium and forms immune complexes with IgG in the synovial fluid, cartilage and blood. Activation of the complement pathway and other inflammatory mediators causes the synovitis. and some of the extra-articular complications. In an attempt to eradicate immune complexes in cartilage, the pluripotential cells at the chondrosynovial junction metamorphose to granulation tissue which creeps centripetally over the cartilage, secreting enzymes that destroy the underlying cartilage and bone.

Symptoms

The onset of RA is usually subacute with a symmetrical arthritis of the hands and feet causing pain, prolonged morning stiffness, and swelling. Involvement of more proximal joints follows, potentially affecting all synovial structures—joints, bursae and tendon sheaths.

Less common presentations include systemic onset (fever, weight loss, anaemia), palindromic, monoarthritis and polymyalgic, particularly in the elderly.

Extra-articular features

These occur in 75% of patients. The most common are the least severe.

1. Subcutaneous nodules over pressure points, notably the olecranon and in the finger pulp.
2. Eye problems: episcleritis, scleritis and keratoconjunctivitis sicca (dry eye).
3. Vasculitis. Nailfold infarcts are common. Fevers, weight loss, night sweats and falling haemoglobin, associated with complement consumption and high levels of immune complexes, suggests systemic (widespread) vasculitis. Vasculitic leg ulcers are large, deep and develop rapidly. Rarely, digital vasculitis causes gangrene of toes.
4. Neurological complications: erosion of the odontoid peg or cruciate ligament causes atlantoaxial subluxation which can compress the cervical cord and result in a quadriparesis. Pressure by deformed or swollen joints on peripheral nerves can cause an entrapment neuropathy, such as carpal tunnel syndrome (see p. 161). A mild sensory neuropathy is common. Mononeuritis multiplex is a serious complication of systemic vasculitis.
5. Kidney: amyloidosis; drug-induced glomerulonephritis; analgesic nephropathy.
6. Felty's syndrome: neutropenia, splenomegaly, recurrent sepsis and leg ulcers.

Signs

In the early stages there is symmetrical synovitis of the metacarpophalangeal joints (MCPJs), proximal interphalangeal joints (PIPJs) and the wrists, notably over the ulnar styloid. A complete fist cannot be made. The late deformities are: ulnar deviation of the fingers at the MCPJs; hyperextension of the PIPJs (Boutonnière deformity); hyperextension of the PIPJs (swan-necking); a Z-shaped thumb (hyperflexion of the MCPJ and hyperextension of the inter-phalangeal joint); subluxation of the wrist (Figs 12.4 and 12.5). Shoulders lose abduction and external rotation. Elbows and knees flex. Hind-feet slip into valgus. The toes deviate laterally and cock-up, pulling the fibrous fatty cushion forwards from under the metatarsal heads.

Investigations

Blood shows normochromic and normocytic anaemia, and elevation of the ESR or plasma viscosity. RF is present in 80%.

Early radiographs show juxta-articular osteoporosis and soft-tissue swelling. Later, marginal erosions, loss of joint space and deformity are seen, and eventually there is complete joint destruction with secondary osteoarthritis.

Before anaesthesia or where there is an unexplained functional decline, a lateral radiograph of the cervical spine in flexion should be examined for atlantoaxial subluxation.

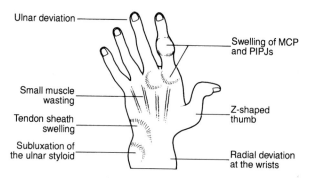

Fig. 12.4 The hand in rheumatoid arthritis.

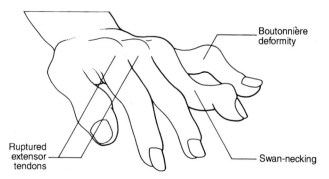

Fig. 12.5 Finger deformities in rheumatoid arthritis.

Differential diagnosis

The diagnosis of RA is definite with the combination of a peripheral symmetrical arthritis, serum RF, radiographic erosions and extra-articular features, particularly nodules.

When the diagnosis is not definite, Reiter's disease, psoriatic arthritis, SLE, nodal osteoarthritis, crystal arthropathies and viral arthritis should be considered.

Treatment

Treatment should be tailored to the stage of the disease: paracetamol for mild disease; NSAIDs for relief of pain and stiffness; SAARDs where NSAIDs fail, erosions or deformities develop, for troublesome extra-articular features, or to reduce steroid requirements; prednisolone for severe resistant synovitis or major extra-articular complications; surgery for destroyed joints.

Prognosis

Ten per cent of patients remit altogether, 10% run a remittent course, and the remainder have persistent, fluctuating disease with slow deterioration. The presence of RF, early marginal erosions, and late age of onset suggest a worse prognosis. Most joint damage occurs in the first 2 years with a slower deterioration subsequently.

Ten per cent of patients become severely disabled and the remainder have mild or moderate disability. Mortality is increased, particularly in older patients, from infection, extra-articular disease and complications of therapy, notably NSAID-induced peptic ulceration.

SERONEGATIVE SPONDYLOARTHRITIDES

The principal members of this group are ankylosing spondylitis, Reiter's disease/reactive arthritis, arthritis of chronic inflammatory bowel disease and psoriatic arthritis. These are considered together as they share characteristics that suggest a similar pathogenesis, notably a strong association with HLA-B27 and the implication of infection as a trigger (Table 12.7). The term seronegative spondyloarthritis (spondyloarthropathy) emphasises the distinction from RA (negative serum test for RF), the spinal (spondylos = vertebra), and the peripheral joint involvement.

Infection is a proven trigger in Reiter's disease and suspected in the others. The immune response against the infecting organism appears to be misdirected against structures bearing the HLA-B27 molecule. Why the enthesis is attacked is unknown. The spine is particularly involved as it is rich in entheses (hence spondylitis) notably in the sacroiliac joint (hence sacroiliitis) which is bridged by a large ligament. Involvement of the entheses of the plantar fascia and Achilles tendon into the calcaneum commonly causes heel pain.

Table 12.7. Characteristic features of the spondyloarthritides

- Strong association with HLA-B27: family history common
- Infection implicated as a triggering factor
- Primary lesion at the enthesis (the site of insertion of ligament, joint capsule, tendon or fascia into bone)
- Peripheral arthritis: often asymmetrical and lower limb
- Mucocutaneous manifestations: psoriasis, genital and mouth ulcers, conjunctivitis
- Actue iritis: independently associated with HLA-B27
- Absent rheumatoid factor

The early enthesopathy is tender and may show radiographically as an erosion. It heals with a spur of new bone, so forming a new enthesis at its tip. If the process continues the ligament may be entirely replaced by bone and fuse the joint it bridges, leaving a rigid painless joint.

The peripheral arthritis is a synovitis, and is often asymmetrical.

Mucocutaneous manifestations include psoriasis, genital and mouth ulcers and conjunctivitis.

ANKYLOSING SPONDYLITIS (AS)

Ninety-five per cent of patients carry HLA-B27. The geographic distribution reflects the racial gene frequency of HLA-B27, which is found in 10% of Whites, 0.5% of whom develop AS, rarely in Blacks or Japanese, and up to 50% of certain North American Indian tribes.

Males predominate eight-fold with the classical disease, but when atypical disease is included the sex ratio equalises. The age of onset is usually about 20 and rarely over 45. One-third give a family history of a spondyloarthritis.

Klebsiella infections and occult inflammatory bowel disease have been implicated.

Symptoms and signs

Presentation is with low back pain from sacroiliitis or spondylitis. Sacroiliitis causes buttock pain radiating to the posterior thigh.

Spondylitic pain is typical; it disturbs sleep, is worse in the morning, when the back is stiff, and it improves with activity to return with rest.

Early, the normal lumbar lordosis is flattened. If the disease progresses, a lumbar kyphosis develops, lumbar spinal movements are lost, chest expansion is diminished (from costovertebral joint involvement) and the cervical spine is craned forward and restricted.

One-fifth have large joint disease, chiefly involving the hip. Heel pain is common. Twenty per cent suffer from recurrent acute iritis. Aortic regurgitation and pulmonary fibrosis are rare complications.

Women tend to present with neck pain and peripheral arthritis.

Investigations

Radiographs show symmetrical sacroiliitis: cortical erosions, sub-articular sclerosis with fusion later. Lateral radiographs of the lumbar spine show enthesopathic new bone bridging the disc spaces (syndesmophytes).

Differential diagnosis

This includes all causes of back pain (Table 12.8).

Treatment

A daily exercise regime will maintain spinal position and movement, and chest expansion. NSAIDs, hip arthroplasty and genetic counselling will all need to be considered.

Prognosis

Ninety per cent of patients have mild disease settling in the fourth decade; 10% have severe spinal restriction, often with hip disease, within 10 years.

REITER'S DISEASE

The 15-fold excess in young men may be an overestimate as the genitourinary features are easily missed in women; 90% of patients carry HLA-B27.

Table 12.8. Specific causes of back pain

Diagnosis	Clinical features
Spondylitis: Ankylosing spondylitis Psoriatic or Reiter's disease Complicating inflammatory bowel disease	Prolonged morning stiffness, radiographic sacroiliitis
Malignancy or infection	Unremitting pain, often thoracic, unrelieved by rest, weight loss and fever, elevated ESR and alkaline phosphatase level, destructive changes on radiograph
Osteoporotic collapse	Recurrent bouts of sudden back pain in postmenopausal women, radiographic osteoporosis and vertebral collapse
Lumbar disc prolapse	Dermatomal pain radiating below the knee worse on coughing or sneezing, limited straight leg raising, motor or sensory deficit in one leg
Back pain referred from retroperitoneal structures	Spine clinically normal, evidence of abdominal disease
Psychogenic back pain	Normal spine, psychological disturbance

The triggering organisms are *Salmonella*, some *Shigella* species, *Yersinia* and *Campylobacter* which present with diarrhoea, and *Chlamydia trachomatis*, contracted venereally and presenting with urethritis.

Symptoms and signs

The disease starts 1–3 weeks after the infection, which may be subclinical. Reiter's disease refers to a triad of arthritis, urethritis and conjunctivitis, but incomplete forms are common, and the term 'reactive arthritis' is used when arthritis is the sole feature. The manifestations of Reiter's disease include:

1. arthritis (100%): lower limb, principally the foot, acute, asymmetrical and migratory
2. conjunctivitis (60%): usually bilateral and often severe
3. urethritis (90%): dysuria and urethral discharge distinct from chlamydial urethritis as it is sterile and an integral feature of the disease
4. enthesopathy: one-third have sacroiliitis or spondylitis at the onset and two-thirds have heel pain. Painful, red, swollen 'sausage toes' may be caused by periostitis
5. balanitis—coalescing around the corona of the glans penis
6. pustular psoriasis of the soles—keratoderma blenorrhagica
7. painless buccal ulceration
8. recurrent acute iritis.

Investigations

Testing for HLA-B27 is not helpful. Early, there may be evidence of the triggering infection. Later, radiographs may show sacroiliitis or spondylitis, but unlike AS, these are asymmetrical and the syndesmophytes are coarse.

Differential diagnosis

Psoriatic arthritis, RA, gout, gonococcal arthritis.

Prognosis

Half improve over several months, the remainder have repeated episodes of arthritis or mucocutaneous manifestations over many years. One-third develop spondylitis.

Treatment

The triggering infection is treated with antibiotics, both in the patient and any sexual partner. NSAIDs usually control joint pain. Sulphasalazine, azathioprine or methotrexate may be required.

ARTHRITIS OF INFLAMMATORY BOWEL DISEASE

Spondylitis, clinically and radiographically identical to AS, occurs in one-fifth of patients, two-thirds of whom carry HLA-B27, and progresses regardless of the activity of the bowel disease.

Twenty per cent of patients with ulcerative colitis and 10% with Crohn's disease develop a peripheral arthritis, probably mediated by immune complex deposition and unassociated with HLA-B27. It usually affects the large joints, parallels the bowel disease and resolves completely.

PSORIATIC ARTHRITIS

Five per cent of patients with psoriasis develop arthritis; 90% of these have psoriatic nail changes. The sex incidence is equal and the peak age of onset 30–50 years. The arthritis usually presents with or after the rash. Several forms are recognised (Table 12.9).

Investigations

RF is absent. The radiographic features are typical: predilection for DIPJs, a combination of erosions and new bone formation at the joint margins, tendency to bony fusion, heel spurs, sacroiliitis and spondylitis.

Treatment

Sulphasalazine, methotrexate or azathioprine are indicated for the few with severe destructive disease.

OSTEOARTHRITIS

Osteoarthritis (OA, osteoarthrosis, degenerative joint disease) is a major cause of disability. Radiographically it is universally evident after the age of 60 years and symptomatic in 10% of the population.

Table 12.9. Patterns of psoriatic arthritis

70% (1) Predominantly hands and feet; asymmetrical; DIPJs; all the joints and the flexor tendon in one finger	5% (3) Arthritis mutilans: Resorption of the ends of the phalanges causing flail fingers
Sausage toes / Heel pain	5% (4) Isolated DIPJ involvement in the hands: drumstick fingers
15% (2) Peripheral, symmetrical arthritis distinguished from RA only by the presence of psoriasis and the absence of RF or rheumatoid extra-articular features	5% (5) Spondylitis, clinically identical to AS, but radiographically resembling Reiter's syndrome—90% carry HLA-B27
One-third of those with peripheral arthritis also have sacroiliitis	

Normal use and ageing alone do not cause OA. It is not a single disease, but a final common pathway following various insults to the cartilage. It should be regarded as an attempt at healing which becomes symptomatic only when it fails.

In the early stages, the virtually inert chondrocytes increase the turnover of cartilage matrix, which swells, fibrillates and is eventually lost. The underlying bone becomes vascular and sclerotic, and remodels at the margins (osteophyte formation).

The hips or knees are most commonly affected. Mild hip dysplasia may predispose to the former. Occasionally previous cartilage damage from joint inflammation, incongruity of joint surfaces following orthopaedic problems or metabolic abnormalities are identifiable causes.

Nodal OA is a polyarticular variant affecting chiefly middle-aged women, often with a family history (see below).

Symptoms and signs

The main problem is pain, which tends to improve with rest and worsen with activity. Exacerbations may follow trauma. Night pain results from interosseus venous hypertension. Morning stiffness is brief. Progression is slow, and serious loss of function occurs only after many years.

Nodal OA in the hand causes bony enlargement of the DIPJs and PIPJs (Heberden's and Bouchard's nodes) and at the base of the thumb.

The hip loses rotation, flexes up and may develop an adduction deformity.

The knee develops effusions, periarticular thickening with tender points, crepitus, a flexion deformity with loss of free flexion, quadriceps wasting and, later, varus or valgus deformities as the medial tibiofemoral compartment is affected first.

Investigations

Blood tests are normal. Radiographs show loss of joint space, marginal osteophyte formation with remodelling, and subchondral sclerosis with cysts.

Differential diagnosis

Avoid attributing symptoms to radiographically evident OA, which is a common incidental finding. Mono-articular onset of a polyarthritis, pyrophosphate arthropathy or chronic infection must be considered. Gouty tophi and psoriatic arthritis of the DIPJs may mimic Heberden's nodes.

Treatment

Nothing has been proved to alter disease progression. Pain may be alleviated by strengthening the quadriceps, weight loss and walking aids. Avoid NSAIDs in the elderly. Peri- or intra-articular steroid injections help acute exacerbations. Prosthetic replacement is needed for incapacitating symptoms.

BACK PAIN

Few escape back pain; 4% of the adult population consult their family doctors for it annually, half are better within 1 week. Two-thirds have 'non-specific' back pain which is postural or occupational, and no specific cause can be found: lumbar osteoarthritis is a common incidental finding.

One-fifth of the cases of back pain have a specific cause, requiring a specific treatment (Table 12.8). A prolapsed lumbar disc accounts for most of these. Warnings of a specific cause of back pain are onset before age 20 or after age 55, symptoms persisting beyond 2 months, thoracic pain and marked restriction of spinal movements.

CRYSTAL ARTHROPATHIES

Joints and periarticular tissues are susceptible to crystal deposition. Several kinds occur which manifest either as a recurrent acute monoarthritis or destructive chronic arthritis (Table 12.10). The former is initiated by crystal activation of inflammatory mediators, and release of lysosmal enzymes from neutrophils phagocytosing the crystals. The latter results from the physical effects of the crystals and synovial release of destructive enzymes.

GOUT

Hyperuricaemia predisposes to the crystallisation of sodium urate. Most of the body pool of urate derives from endogenous purine breakdown from nucleic acids, and the dietary contribution is small. Excretion is principally by the renal tubule. Obesity and excess alcohol intake accelerate urate production. Hyperuricaemia is associated with hypertension and hyper-triglyceridaemia, which predispose to atherosclerosis.

Urate levels are lower in women than in men until the menopause, when they equalise. Hence, gout is eight times more common in men, with a prevalence of 0.1%, and presents at a mean age of 40, compared with 70 in women.

In practice, gout in men is commonly 'primary': obese, hypertensive, middle-aged men with a high alcohol intake and a family history (one-third)

Table 12.10. Crystal arthropathies

Crystal	Acute arthritis	Chronic destructive arthritis
Sodium urate	Gout	Tophaceous gout
Calcium pyrophosphate	Pseudogout	Chronic pyrophosphate arthropathy

who are under-secretors of urate. In women, it presents after the age of 70 and results from diuretic inhibition of urate excretion from the renal tubules. Less common is gout from overproduction from a myeloproliferative disorder, especially during treatment. Occasionally, a young man with severe gout and marked overproduction will be found to have an inherited partial deficiency of hypoxanthine-guanine-phosphoribosyl-transferase.

Urate slowly crystallises on the cartilage surface. Crystal shedding initiates acute attacks. Further accumulation of solid deposits of urate eventually damages the joints: tophaceous gout. Uric acid crystallisation within the renal collecting ducts causes stones in 10% of gout sufferers.

Symptoms and signs

Acute gout

Hyperuricaemia may be present years before the first attack. This is precipitated by trauma, including surgery, intercurrent illness, dietary or alcohol excess. Typically, the attack is monarticular in a lower limb joint, notably at the base of the great toe. Within hours the joint is very painful, swollen, red and shiny. It resolves completely within days on NSAIDs and 2 weeks if untreated, often with skin desquamation. Ninety per cent of patients have recurrent attacks.

Tophaceous gout

This is usually associated with diuretic intake. After recurrent acute gout, solid deposits of urate develop around the IPJs of the fingers and great toe, the pinna and olecranon. They shine white through the overlying skin which may ulcerate or become infected. Untreated, tophi eventually destroy joints.

Diagnosis and differential diagnosis

Patients are hyperuricaemic even between attacks. Only 20% of individuals with hyperuricaemia ever develop gout, which is diagnosed too frequently. Hence, it is important to confirm the diagnosis by identification of urate crystals from synovial fluid or tophi, which have a characteristic appearance on polarised light microscopy. Early radiographs are normal. Later, tophi produce periarticular erosions with a sclerotic margin.

Other causes of acute monoarthritis are septic arthritis, pseudogout, Reiter's disease, psoriatic and palindromic arthritis. Tophi in the hands may be mistaken for nodal OA or psoriatic arthritis.

Treatment

Asymptomatic hyperuricaemia should not be treated. Gout often points to more serious problems: alcohol abuse, obesity, atherosclerosis, hypertriglyceridemia and hypertension.

High-dose NSAIDs or colchicine are effective in acute attacks.

Further acute attacks may be prevented by reducing weight or alcoholic intake, or stopping diuretics.

The urate-lowering drug allopurinol is indicated for life when there are frequent attacks, tophi, joint damage or renal calculi. Frequent acute attacks may be triggered for 3 months after starting allopurinol and are prevented by concomitant NSAIDs.

PYROPHOSPHATE ARTHROPATHY

Pyrophosphate is formed in many metabolic reactions and its calcium salt may be deposited in cartilage, particularly fibrocartilage; it is identified radiographically as chondrocalcinosis (age 40: 1%, age 90: 40%). Pyrophosphate arthropathy is chiefly a disease of elderly women. Other associations are joint instability (hypermobility, following meniscectomy), metabolic (hypothyroidism, hyperparathyroidism) and rare inherited forms.

The distribution of joints affected reflects the presence of intra-articular fibrocartilaginous structures. In order of frequency are the knees, with particular patellofemoral joint involvement, wrists, shoulders, hips and ankles.

Pseudogout

This is the most common cause of acute monoarthritis in the elderly.

The joint, usually the knee or the wrist, rapidly becomes severely inflamed and swollen, sometimes with marked systemic features. Resolution may take weeks and attacks tend to recur.

Diagnosis is by demonstration of pyrophosphate crystals in synovial fluid by polarised light microscopy.

Treatment is with an intra-articular steroid injection or NSAIDs.

Chronic pyrophosphate arthropathy

The clinical picture resembles OA, affecting particularly the knees, but there are important differences: joints are involved that are rarely affected by OA—shoulders, elbows or wrists; a history suggesting pseudogout; radiographs show chondrocalcinosis, exuberant osteophyte formation, and greater joint destruction; pyrophosphate crystals are present in the synovial fluid.

Treatment is as for OA (see p. 368).

POLYMYALGIA RHEUMATICA

This is a common disease of the elderly. The onset is usually after the age of 60, and women are affected twice as frequently. It is strongly associated with temporal arteritis. The cause is unknown.

Severe, symmetrical pain, stiffness and tenderness in the muscles of the neck, shoulder and hip girdle develop, over days or weeks. Characteristically, sleep is disturbed by pain and with difficulty in rolling over in bed, getting up and dressing in the morning. Fever, weight loss, night sweats and anaemia may be marked. The girdle muscles may be tender. The ESR is markedly raised, and the response to prednisolone dramatic.

A similar picture may be seen in the onset of RA, bacterial endocarditis, occult malignancy and hypothyroidism.

Prednisolone is slowly withdrawn over about 2 years. Giant cell (temporal) arteritis occasionally develops.

RHEUMATOLOGICAL EMERGENCIES

There are five warning signs: fever, neurological symptoms, acute mono-arthritis, renal impairment and collapse. The principal emergencies are:

1. Septic arthritis: a severe monoarthritis with fever. Misleadingly mild features are found in patients who are debilitated, taking immunosuppressive drugs, or who have arthritis.
2. Atlantoaxial subluxation: complicating RA, this may cause a general functional decline.
3. Acute cerebral lupus: fits, focal neurological signs or impaired consciousness.
4. Rapidly progressive renal failure may result from NSAIDs, SLE, polyarteritis nodosa or scleroderma.
5. Mononeuritis multiplex: RA, SLE and polyarteritis nodosa.
6. Temporal arteritis: sudden blindness.
7. Collapse: gut bleeding or perforation from NSAIDs.

13

CONNECTIVE TISSUE DISEASES AND IMMUNOLOGY

John R. Kirwan

CONNECTIVE TISSUE DISEASES

A group of disorders sharing many clinical characteristics enter into the differential diagnosis in most patients presenting with multisystem inflammatory disease. These conditions are often referred to as 'collagen vascular diseases' or '(systemic) connective tissue diseases' (Table 13.1). These names are historical and not related to our current understanding of the diseases. There is evidence that these conditions share pathogenetic and even aetiological factors, including multisystem involvement, arthritis and vasculitis, the presence of antibodies against 'self' antigens and evidence of immune complex deposition. Furthermore, many patients either present with a mixture of features that overlap two or more diagnostic categories, or are clearly in one category but gradually change their clinical picture to that of another. These features all raise the possibility of a common underlying pathology which is modulated by genetic and environmental factors so as to be expressed in a particular way in each patient. Much evidence points to abnormalities in immune function as this common pathology.

Immune system function and connective tissue disease

Immunity is usually concerned with the disposal of foreign or 'non-self'

Table 13.1. Systemic connective tissue diseases

Systemic lupus erythematosus (SLE)
Systemic sclerosis (Scleroderma)
Vasculitis (e.g. polyarteritis nodosa, Wegener's granulomatosis)
Polymyositis and dermatomyositis
Sjögren's syndrome
Raynaud's disease
Mixed connective tissue disease (MCTD)

material. This involves recognition of the material, intracellular processing and stimulation of natural (usually non-specific) or adaptive (specific) responses, priming the system for future specific responses, and controlling or suppressing the response when it is no longer required (Fig. 13.1). The 'final common pathway' is the initiation of inflammation (Fig. 13.2). These processes are amplified at each step, producing an increasing cascade of response. Uncontrolled, this positive feedback system would continue to generate tissue damage after the initiating event had been dealt with, but most of the mechanisms by which the immune system 'switches off' inflammation are not understood. In connective tissue diseases immune stimulation and inflammation become chronic. This could result from a persisting stimulus from either non-self or self antigens, or from a failure in the feedback control of inflammation.

Autoantibodies

Autoantibodies are immunoglobulins that react with 'self' antigens. Low levels of autoantibodies are frequently found in normal individuals. In the connective tissue diseases, autoantibodies reach high titres and account for a large proportion of the circulating immunoglobulin. Of all the possible

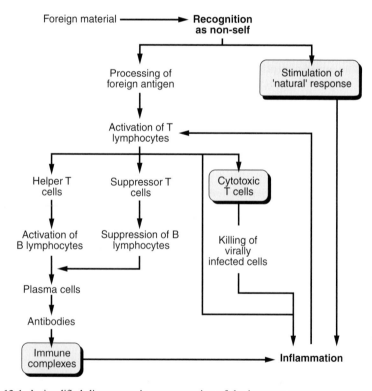

Fig. 13.1 A simplified diagrammatic representation of the immune system.

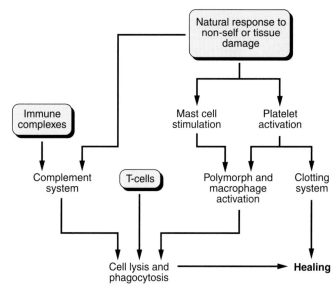

Fig. 13.2 The process of inflammation.

antibodies that might be produced, only a few are synthesised in excess in any one condition. In rheumatoid arthritis, IgM autoantibodies are directed against the Fc portion of IgG molecules and are called rheumatoid factors. They can be detected by their ability to stick together sheep red blood cells coated with human IgG (the sheep cell agglutination test) or similarly coated latex beads (the latex test). Other autoantibodies may be detected by enzyme linked immunosorbent assay (ELISA) while antibodies against tissue components are frequently identified by immunofluorescent staining.

Many of the antigens have been identified. A few are nucleic acids but most are proteins, often ones that form macromolecular complexes with other proteins and nucleic acids. Scl-70, for example, is the enzyme topoisomerase I, which unwinds the supercoiled structure of DNA prior to replication or transcription.

It may be that the function of each antigen is not relevant to the pathogenesis of autoimmune disease because there is little evidence that antibodies enter cells, but these functions may throw light on aetiology. One current hypothesis is that the autoantibodies are made to react with bacterial or viral material and, almost by chance, cross-react also with various cellular components. Another postulates viral infection which renders cellular replication systems antigenic when they are complexed with viral, 'non-self' material.

SYSTEMIC LUPUS ERYTHEMATOSUS (SLE)

SLE is an uncommon disorder (Table 13.2), predominantly affecting females of child-bearing age. It is more common in Black and Chinese races, and

Table 13.2. Characteristics of some connective tissue diseases

	Approximate prevalence (per 1000)	Sex ratio (F : M)	Usual age of onset	Common autoantibodies*
Rheumatoid arthritis	20	3:1	30–50	RF 75%, ANA 10%
Systemic lupus erythematosus	1	10:1	15–30	ANA 90%, dsDNA 30%, Others 25%
Systemic sclerosis	0.1	3:1	30–50	Scl-70 20%
Wegener's granulomatosis	< 0.1	2:1	50–70	ANCA 80%
Sjögren's syndrome	10	9:1	40–50	Anti-Ro 85%, Anti-La 60%
Mixed connective tissue disease	0.1	9:1	15–30	RNP 100%

*RF = Rheumatoid factor; ANA = antinuclear antibody; dsDNA = double-stranded DNA antibodies; ANCA = anti-neutrophil cytoplasmic antibodies; RNP = ribonucleoprotein antibodies.

Table 13.3. Systemic effects of SLE

Organ system	Effects	Organ system	Effects
Joints	Flitting arthralgia	Blood	Leucopenia
	Persistent arthralgia		Anaemia
	Synovitis		Thrombocytopenia
	Joint destruction		Autoimmune haemolytic
Skin	Photosensitivity		anaemia
	Hair loss	CVS	Raynaud's phenomenon
	Cutaneous vasculitis		Vasculitis
	Nailfold capillary changes		Myocarditis
	Butterfly rash		Endocarditis
Kidney	Proteinuria	RS	Pleurisy
	Microscopic haematuria		Pulmonary effusion
	Hypertension		Pulmonary fibrosis
	Chronic renal failure	Nervous	Headache
	Acute renal failure	system	Psychosis
	Nephrotic syndrome		Epilepsy
Muscles	Myositis		Hemiplegia
	Myopathy		Peripheral neuropathy

in patients with inherited complement deficiency. There is polyclonal B-lymphocyte activation and widespread tissue deposition of immune complexes, with a very wide range of clinical presentations (Table 13.3).

Nephritis occurs when immune complexes in the glomerular basement membrane activate complement and initiate inflammation. Deposition in blood vessel walls leads to vasculitis, which may underlie most manifestations of the disease. SLE is episodic and may be life-threatening at times. Because any organ or tissue may be involved, SLE may mimic many other diseases.

Symptoms and signs

Joint involvement (pain and/or inflammation) occurs in over 90% of cases, although joint destruction is rare. A wide variety of skin rashes and photosensitivity are common. Raynaud's phenomenon (Fig. 13.3) (intermittent digital artery spasm) and hair loss are also characteristic.

One of the important clinical complications is renal disease, manifest by proteinuria and microscopic haematuria. This may progress to hypertension, nephrotic syndrome or renal failure.

Other serious developments that warrant urgent treatment include cerebral vasculitis, retinal vasculitis and autoimmune haemolytic anaemia.

Investigations

The diagnosis of SLE usually requires identification of antinuclear antibodies and clinical differentiation from other connective tissue diseases. During active episodes serum complement may be reduced because of complement consumption at inflammatory sites, and complement breakdown products may be increased. Skin vasculitis may be confirmed by biopsy. Plasma viscosity or ESR increase in active disease, but monitoring complement levels

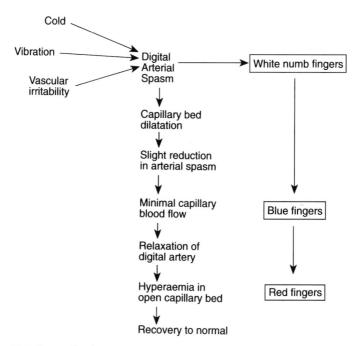

Fig. 13.3 Raynaud's phenomenon.

is more useful for monitoring activity. C-reactive protein remains normal unless there is infection.

Treatment
Treatment of acute episodes requires large doses (perhaps 80 mg per 24 hours) of prednisolone and sometimes immunosuppressive drugs such as cyclophosphamide or azathioprine. In between acute episodes patients may require only analgesics or anti-inflammatory drugs, although some who have evidence of persisting disease activity may require low doses of glucocorticoids.

Prognosis
Immunosuppressive therapy has transformed the prognosis of patients with renal and widespread systemic disease and about 90% of patients seen in hospitals survive more than 10 years after diagnosis. As increasingly milder cases are now being identified this figure may increase.

SYSTEMIC SCLEROSIS (SCLERODERMA)

Systemic sclerosis (SS) is a rare disease in which there is excessive collagen deposition and fibrosis of interstitial tissues, particularly in the skin and in small arterioles where vasculitis may also develop. The nature of the underlying stimulus for excessive fibrosis is unknown. Skin lesions may be localised ('morphea') confined to the extremities (especially when SS overlaps with other conditions), or generalised.

Symptoms and signs
Skin changes vary from a mild thickening and induration of the fingertips (sclerodactyly) to extensive involvement of the arms, face, trunk and sometimes the legs with taut, hidebound thickened skin (scleroderma), loss of skin appendages, telangiectasia, oedema, altered pigmentation, atrophy of the finger pulps and calcinosis (calcification within soft tissues).

Facial involvement may produce microstomia. Loss of oesophageal motility may cause difficulty in swallowing or symptoms of heartburn while pulmonary fibrosis may lead to slowly progressive dyspnoea.

Raynaud's phenomenon (Fig. 13.3), which may occur with any of the connective tissue diseases, is particularly common in SS. Renal arteriolar involvement may lead to accelerated hypertension and renal failure. Small bowel bacterial invasion in the immobile gut leads to malabsorption.

Investigations
There are no specific diagnostic tests for systemic sclerosis but autoantibodies against nucleolar antigens are found in up to 80%. Anti-centromere antibodies are highly specific for limited disease and anti-Scl 70 highly specific for diffuse disease.

Treatment and prognosis
There is no treatment available that can halt this process, although long periods with little deterioration or even some improvement may occur. Com-

plications (Raynaud's, hypertension, organ failure) are managed as they occur. ACE inhibitors are the best agents for controlling hypertension. About half of the patients survive more than 5 years after diagnosis. Renal lesions are the most common cause of death.

SYSTEMIC VASCULITIS

Inflammation of blood vessels caused by autoimmune disease may be secondary to diseases such as SLE and rheumatoid arthritis, but may occur as a primary phenomenon. The clinical manifestations depend on the size and location of vessels involved. All are associated with an acute inflammatory response, with raised viscosity, ESR and C-reactive protein, and normochromic anaemia.

Large vessel vasculitis comprises giant cell arteritis (temporal arteritis) (pp. 41, 127), which may cause headache, scalp tenderness, ocular nerve palsies and blindness, and frequently occurs in association with polymyalgia rheumatica (p. 371); and Takayasu's arteritis (p. 42). The former is a disease of the elderly; the latter usually occurs in adults of less than 50 years.

Medium vessel vasculitis includes classical polyarteritis nodosa and Kawasaki syndrome. Classical polyarteritis nodosa involves muscle (causing painful myopathy), nerves (causing mononeuritis multiplex), skin (causing ischaemic changes, livedo reticularis, ulcers), CNS (ischaemic stroke), coronary arteries (myocardial infarction) and arteries in the coeliac, hepatic and renal circulations. The renal involvement causes hypertension and renal impairment, but not glomerulonephritis (which would indicate small vessel involvement, which by definition is absent). There is an association with asthma. The diagnosis may be made by biopsy of affected muscle or nerve, showing necrotising arteriolar lesions, or by demonstration of aneurysms on coeliac or renal angiography. Polyarteritis nodosa is treated with corticosteroids and cyclophosphamide.

Kawasaki syndrome (mucocutaneous lymph node syndrome) affects children aged under 15, and usually under the age of 5. There is an acute onset of fever, inflammation of the mucous membranes, conjunctivae and skin (causing an erythematous rash), and cervical lymphadenopathy. Involvement of the coronary arteries may cause myocardial infarction and coronary artery aneurysms, and is fatal in up to 10% of cases. Diagnosis is based on the clinical findings and on imaging of the coronary arteries with angiography. Treatment is with high-dose aspirin and intravenous human immunoglobulin; corticosteroids are ineffective.

Small vessel vasculitis includes Wegener's granulomatosis, microscopic polyangiitis, Henoch–Schönlein purpura, and Churg–Strauss syndrome. The first three may cause a vasculitic rash, with palpable purpura (p. 345, plate 7), glomerulonephritis, which may be rapidly progressive (p. 22), and arthritis due to synovial involvement. Small arterioles, venules and capillaries are involved. Similar appearances may be caused by some infections and hypersensitivity reactions to drugs.

Wegener's granulomatosis and microscopic polyangiitis have similar presenting features, pathology and treatment. Both are associated with the presence of circulating antibodies to enzymes found in neutrophil cytoplasm (anti-neutrophil cytoplasmic antibodies, ANCA), and are often referred to as ANCA-positive vasculitides. Although it is not yet known whether these antibodies are the cause or the result of vasculitis, their concentration is a reliable indicator of disease activity. In addition to glomerulonephritis, arthritis and rash, pulmonary involvement may occur in both diseases causing interstitial pulmonary inflammation with fluffy chest X-ray shadowing and hypoxia. Wegener's granulomatosis may have a much wider tissue distribution, including the sinuses, middle ear and nasal cartilage, sclerae, glottis and genitalia, and may affect larger vessels as well. Wegener's granulomatosis is usually associated with a 'cytoplasmic' ANCA staining pattern, reflecting antibodies to proteinase 3, whereas microscopic polyangiitis is associated more commonly with antibodies to myeloperoxidase, which is dispersed towards the nucleus when neutrophils are fixed, resulting in a 'perinuclear' pattern of ANCA staining. However, as with the clinical manifestations, there is overlap between the two diseases in staining pattern and antigen specificity. Treatment of both diseases is similar, with prednisolone and cyclophosphamide.

Henoch–Schönlein purpura is most common in childhood, and often follows respiratory infections or drug treatment. It causes a purpuric rash, especially over the buttocks and lower limbs. Arthritis, affecting the knees, ankles and wrists, is common. Glomerular involvement is variable. Involvement of the gut is a distinctive feature, causing colicky abdominal pain, gastrointestinal bleeding and, occasionally, intussusception. The diagnosis is usually made on the clinical findings, after exclusion of thrombocytopenia (which can cause a similar purpuric rash), and may be confirmed by skin biopsy (showing a leucocytoclastic vasculitis) or, if there is evidence of renal involvement, renal biopsy (which shows mesangial proliferative glomerulonephritis with IgA deposition).

Churg–Strauss syndrome (p. 93) is a small and medium vessel vasculitis associated with asthma and eosinophilia.

POLYMYOSITIS (Table 13.4)

Diffuse skeletal muscle inflammation causing weakness and pain may occur in many of the connective tissue diseases. When it predominates (which is rare) it is called 'pure' polymyositis and this may occur with particular skin changes (dermatomyositis). The pattern of progress is extremely variable ranging from rapid deterioration producing myoglobinuria and death within a few weeks to such gradual development that the patient may not notice the weakness coming on.

Diagnosis is based on muscle weakness, increased serum levels of muscle breakdown enzymes (especially creatine phosphokinase), electromyographical evidence of muscle cell destruction and muscle biopsy. There is an increased frequency of polymyositis in patients with malignancy but most cases will not suffer from neoplasia and investigations should depend upon and be guided by other clinical evidence of malignancy.

Table 13.4. Systemic effects of polymyositis (dermatomyositis)

Skin	Various skin rashes
	Characteristically violaceous rash and oedema of eyelids. Red patches over heads of metacarpals, elbows and knees
Muscles	Proximal muscle weakness and tenderness
	Bulbar neck and respiratory weakness
	Atrophy of muscles/calcification
Lungs	Aspiration pneumonia
	Fibrosing alveolitis
Heart	Heart failure/cardiac arrythmias
General	In older patients there may be underlying cancer(s)

SJÖGREN'S SYNDROME

Defective tear secretion (xerophthalmia) and salivary secretion (xerostomia) are the most obvious signs of a more general exocrine failure in some patients with a connective tissue disease or rheumatoid arthritis. This condition is called Sjögren's syndrome and is mediated by cellular inflammatory infiltrates which invade and destroy exocrine glands.

'OVERLAP' DISEASES

Mixed connective tissue disease (MCTD). This 'overlap' syndrome combines features of SLE, scleroderma and polymyositis and has been proposed as a separate entity because of the very frequent occurrence of a particular autoantibody (against ribonucleoprotein) which is relatively rare in other conditions. It is not yet clear whether this really does represent a separate disease.

Antiphospholipid syndrome. Autoantibodies to phospholipids (anti-cardiolipin antibodies) cause *in vitro* prolongation of the APTT but, *in vivo*, cause arterial and venous thrombosis, resulting in recurrent abortion, stroke and livedo reticularis. They may occur in SLE or independently.

HIV infection. Some patients with AIDS develop a variety of rheumatological conditions, but it is not yet clear if HIV is directly responsible or if they represent the chance occurrence of AIDS and arthritis.

IMMUNODEFICIENCY

Immunodeficiency diseases are principally manifest by deficient antibody production by B cells, deficient cellular response by T cells, or a combination of the two (Table 13.5). They cause recurrent infections and severe combined immunodeficiency usually leads to death within the first or second year of life. The genetic basis for many types of hereditary immunodeficiency has now been identified and this increased understanding of the molecular

Table 13.5. Immune deficiency syndromes
These may be primary or secondary to factors such as cancer, drugs, X-ray therapy or AIDS

Syndrome	Clinical effects	Cause
Hypogammaglobulinaemia Selective IgA deficiency, IgM deficiency Brutons disease (X-linked) (congenital)	Bacterial infections	Deficient antibody production by B cells
Di George syndrome Ataxia telangiectasia Wiscott-Aldrich syndrome	Viral infections	T cell deficiency
Common variable immune deficiency	Childhood infections	T and B cell deficiency
Chronic granulomatous disease	Abscesses Chronic granulomatous infections	Neutrophil dysfunction

and cellular basis of immune system function is leading to the development of inhibitors and modifiers. These are potential treatments for many illnesses, which, like the connective tissue diseases, are driven by the immune system.

14

DERMATOLOGY

Clive B. Archer

The number of different diseases in dermatology has been estimated at nearly 2000. Commonly seen skin disorders include inflammatory dermatoses (psoriasis, the eczemas and urticaria), acne, and benign and malignant skin tumours. Most rashes are recognised by the pattern of the eruption, the history being used for fine tuning (e.g. in deciding on the distinction between an endogenous or exogenous eczema). Redness, or erythema, can be helpful in identifying inflammatory diseases but this sign may be difficult to assess in pigmented skin. If the diagnosis is not obvious it can be useful to consider which level of the skin is involved (e.g. is this an epidermal or dermal problem?) (Fig. 14.1). Table 14.1 shows a classification of skin diseases according to the main site of pathology within the skin, although in some disorders more than one level will be involved. A list of commonly used dermatological terms is shown in Table 14.2.

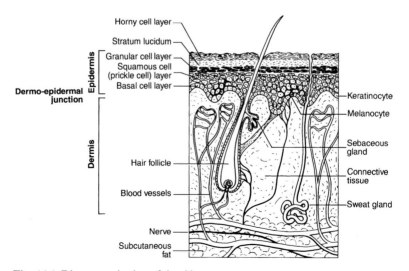

Fig. 14.1 Diagrammatic view of the skin.

Table 14.1. Dermatoses according to the level of pathology within the skin

Predominant change/ site of pathology	Disease
Epidermal changes (e.g. scaling, hyperkeratosis, crusting)	Psoriasis, eczema/dermatitis, superficial fungal infections, the ichthyoses
Epidermal appendages	Acne vulgaris, rosacea, hidradenitis suppurativa (apocrine glands in axillae and groin), alopecia areata
Dermo–epidermal interface and dermis	Pityriasis rosea, lichen planus, lupus erythematosus, erythema multiforme
Epidermal and dermo–epidermal cohesion (blistering disorders)	Pemphigus (e.g. vulgaris/foliaceus), pemphigoid, dermatitis herpetiformis, epidermolysis bullosa
Dermis	The urticarias, granuloma annulare, morphoea/scleroderma, dermatomyositis, xanthoma/xanthelasma, lymphoma (e.g. T cell lymphoma/mycosis fungoides)
Subcutaneous tissue	Erythema nodosum and other forms of panniculitis

PSORIASIS

Psoriasis is an inflammatory, hyperproliferative disorder characterised by red scaly plaques (see Plate 1). It affects 1–2% of the population with equal sex incidence, occurs at any age (peak incidence 18–25 years) and tends to run a chronic course. It has a multifactorial inheritance, often skipping generations, and has been associated with several HLA-specific antigens, particularly the HLA-CW6 antigen. Trigger factors in genetically primed individuals include streptococcal infections, trauma and probably stress. Altered cell regulatory mechanisms in the epidermis may account for the increase in the mitotic rate and reduced epidermal cell transit time from the basal layer to the stratum corneum in active lesions. Research has focused on altered lymphocyte–keratinocyte interactions, with associated release of various inflammatory mediators (e.g. leukotriene B_4, platelet activating factor, PAF) and cytokines (e.g. interleukins 1 and 8).

Pathology

Inflammation in the dermis with a particular pattern of epidermal changes (elongation of rete ridges) and sometimes epidermal collections of neutrophils (microabscesses) are seen.

Symptoms and signs

The most common pattern is plaque psoriasis, usually affecting the elbows,

Table 14.2. Dermatological terminology

Lesion	Any single small area of skin pathology
Macule	A flat area of colour change
Papule	A small* elevated (palpable) lesion
Weal (wheal)	An oedematous slightly raised lesion, often with a pale centre and reddish margin
Nodule	A large* elevated spherical lesion, often extending deeply into the skin
Plaque	A flat-topped palpable lesion
Vesicle	A small fluid-filled blister
Pustule	A small blister filled with neutrophils (pus)
Bulla	A large fluid-filled blister
Purpura	A visible collection of free red blood cells in the skin
Scale	Thickened fragments of the outermost layer of the epidermis, the stratum corneum
Crust	Dried plasma exudate
Excoriation	An abrasion caused by scratching
Lichenification	Area of increased epidermal thickness and increased skin markings as a result of chronic rubbing
Erosion	An absence of the epithelial surface
Ulcer	An absence of the epithelial surface with dermal damage (i.e. deeper than an erosion)
Scar	A permanent lesion resulting from repair by replacement with connective tissue
Telangiectasia	Dilated blood vessels visible on the skin surface

*It is not usually helpful to be dogmatic about precise measurements

knees, extensor aspects of the limbs and the scalp. Other patterns include guttate (frequently following a streptococcal sore throat in young individuals), flexural (moist red patches), pustular (localised to the hands and feet or generalised) and erythrodermic psoriasis.

In generalised pustular or erythrodermic psoriasis, sometimes occurring after erroneous administration of systemic corticosteroids, the patient may be very ill.

Nail changes include pitting, thickening and onycholysis, and in about 10% of cases there is an associated seronegative arthritis. Some patients with psoriasis complain of itching.

Investigations

Histology is not usually required to confirm the diagnosis. A throat swab, antistreptolysin O (ASO) titre, rheumatoid factor (RF) and X-rays of painful joints may be helpful.

Differential diagnosis

Common possibilities include eczema, pityriasis rosea and drug eruptions.

Treatment

Psoriasis can be actively and successfully treated in several ways, depending on its severity, persistence and the distribution of skin involvement.

Topical agents include moisturisers and emollients, vitamin D analogues (e.g. calcipotriol), appropriate corticosteroid ointments or creams, dithranol (anthralin) preparations and tar compounds.

Ultraviolet light can be helpful in the form of sunlight, UVB or PUVA therapy (in which the skin is sensitised by the administration of an oral or topical psoralen).

Antibiotics are used for the treatment of streptococcal infections and, in severe cases, systemic drugs such as acitretin, methotrexate, hydroxyurea or cyclosporin A, with careful monitoring for side-effects, can be very beneficial.

Prognosis

Guttate psoriasis often clears spontaneously whereas plaque psoriasis is usually a chronic problem. There is a small mortality rate associated with generalised pustular or erythrodermic psoriasis, particularly in the elderly.

ECZEMA/DERMATITIS

These terms are often used synonymously. There are several types of eczema, characterised by the clinical appearance of itchy, red, scaly skin, sometimes with vesicles, exudation and crusting (Table 14.3).

Atopic dermatitis (atopic eczema) occurs in 2–3% of children, with onset of the disease in the first year of life in 60%, and is frequently seen in patients with a personal or family history of atopic diseases (i.e. asthma, allergic rhinitis or atopic dermatitis). A gene defect has been established in atopy.

Table 14.3. A classification of the eczemas

Endogenous	Exogenous
Atopic dermatitis	Irritant dermatitis
Discoid eczema	Allergic contact dermatitis
Asteatotic eczema	Seborrhoeic dermatitis
Pompholyx	Photo-dermatitis
Varicose (venous) eczema	Drug-induced eczema

This may underlie several reported cell regulatory abnormalities in mononuclear leucocytes (monocytes and lymphocytes) in atopic dermatitis which may, in turn, lead to an exaggerated response of the skin to trigger factors in the environment, such as irritants (e.g. detergents, house dust) and antigens (e.g. cow's milk, house dust mite).

Seborrhoeic dermatitis is common and yeasts on the skin play an important causative role. Exogenous factors can worsen all types of eczema and may be causative in primary irritant or allergic contact dermatitis. Common sensitisers include nickel (as in costume jewellery), chromium, rubber, medicaments (including topical neomycin and preservatives), plants and pre-polymerised plastics and glues in industry.

Pathology

Oedema is present in the epidermis (spongiosis) with dilatation of blood vessels and infiltration with mononuclear cells in the dermis. Chronic changes include epidermal thickening (acanthosis).

Symptoms and signs

In atopic dermatitis the skin is often dry and extremely itchy. Scratching makes the eczema worse and produces lichenification (see Plate 2). The severity fluctuates with time and secondary bacterial infection, usually with *Staphylococcus aureus*, can be recognised by exudation and crusting.

Any part of the body can be affected, often symmetrically; in infancy, the face and extensor aspects of the limbs are usually involved whereas in older children and adults eczema tends to affect the flexures (e.g. antecubital and popliteal fossae), the periocular regions and the nape of the neck.

Seborrhoeic dermatitis in infants affects the scalp and flexures (napkin dermatitis), frequently allowing the distinction from atopic dermatitis. Feaures of seborrhoeic dermatitis in adults include dandruff, paranasal and eyebrow scaling, and sometimes eczema in the presternal, interscapular, axillary and groin regions.

The circular lesions of discoid eczema usually occur on the extensor aspects of the limbs in adults. In pompholyx, patients often have large painful blisters on the palms and soles, with smaller itchy vesicles along the side of the fingers.

In the elderly, varicose eczema is common, affecting the lower legs and sometimes accompanied by venous ulcers.

Asteatotic eczema, associated with drying of the skin (e.g. following admission to hospital) usually affects the shins and the scaling takes on a 'crazy paving' appearance.

Contact dermatitis often involves the hands where it can be difficult to be sure of the aetiology based on the pattern of eczema alone. However, primary irritant dermatitis may initially involve the finger webs and the flexor aspects of the wrists, where the epidermis is thinner than on the palms.

Investigations

Patch testing to a standard battery of allergens and sometimes other potential sensitisers will often confirm a clinical diagnosis of allergic contact dermatitis. The distinction between allergic and irritant responses can be difficult and, to minimise false positive results, patch tests should be performed.

Skin and nasal swabs (before antibiotic therapy), can help to direct treatment, particularly in atopic dermatitis. Patients with atopic dermatitis usually have raised serum IgE levels with multiple positive prick test or radio-allergosorbent test (RAST) responses to common antigens. However, these tests are not performed routinely since they are of limited diagnostic use, and patients (or their parents) may overinterpret the significance of an individual positive result, assuming for example that the eczema is 'caused' by the house dust mite, which may be one of many trigger factors.

A skin biopsy is not usually required.

Differential diagnosis

Psoriasis, pityriasis rosea, fungal infections (which are often unilateral) and drug eruptions.

Treatment

Eczema can be dramatically improved by the use of a combination of the following measures: moisturisers/emollients, topical corticosteroids ('the weakest that works'; 1% hydrocortisone is safe and can be obtained without a doctor's prescription), antihistamines (especially at night) for control of itching, and treatment of secondary infection.

In atopic dermatitis, additional measures include trial of a diet avoiding cow's milk and eggs (important in only 10–15% of children), avoidance of house dust (an irritant) and house dust mites (an antigen), excessive drying of the skin, excessive heat and sweating, clothes that can irritate (e.g. wool and nylon) and close contact with 'cold sore' (herpes simplex) sufferers.

Seborrhoeic dermatitis responds well to the continued use of combined topical antifungal/corticosteroid preparations.

In contact dermatitis, strict avoidance of irritant and/or allergic factors is essential.

Prognosis

Atopic dermatitis improves with age, around 50% of those presenting in infancy resolving by the age of 10 years. Seborrhoeic dermatitis is usually responsive to therapy but tends to recur if treatment is stopped. The tendency to develop discoid eczema and pompholyx often resolves over a period of 2 years, whereas varicose eczema usually persists. Contact dermatitis can resolve completely on avoidance of exogenous factors, although this may not be so for certain sensitisers (e.g. chromate in cement workers).

ACNE

Acne vulgaris is a common disorder of the pilosebaceous units, affecting up to 90% of adolescents, in which hyperactivity of the sebaceous glands leads to seborrhoea (greasy skin) with blockage of follicular openings and the formation of comedones (blackheads and whiteheads), inflammatory papules, pustules, nodules and cysts. Within the blocked follicle, normal skin bacteria (*Propionibacterium acnes* and *Staph. albus*) produce lipases causing the breakdown of triglycerides to irritant fatty acids which are thought to induce the clinical lesions.

Genetic factors may be important and the sebaceous glands seem to be hyperresponsive to circulating androgens. Acne can also be produced by drugs such as bromides, iodides, systemic corticosteroids and phenytoin.

Pathology

The pilosebaceous unit is distended and surrounded by inflammatory cells comprising neutrophils and lymphocytes, sometimes with foreign body giant cells, granulation tissue and fibrosis.

Symptoms and signs

Adolescents may present with blackheads (open comedones) in which the colour is caused by melanin pigmentation, whiteheads (closed comedones), papules, pustules, nodules, cysts and varying degrees of scarring, usually on the face, chest and back.

Differential diagnosis

Rosacea, perioral dermatitis (as induced by application of a fluorinated corticosteroid to the face), milia (small epidermal cysts), sarcoidosis or plane warts.

Treatment

Acne should be treated actively in order to avoid unnecessary scarring and psychological distress. Combinations of the following treatments are used:

1. simple desquamating agents or creams
2. topical or systemic antibiotics (e.g. oxytetracycline or erythromycin, 500 mg twice daily, usually for 6 months each, sometimes in rotation)
3. UVB light/sunlight (in moderation)
4. systemic antiandrogen drugs in females (e.g. Dianette)
5. isotretinoin therapy (teratogenic in females), with appropriate monitoring for side-effects, for severe cases with nodulocystic acne or those failing to respond to adequate dose of antibiotics
6. aspiration and injection of a corticosteroid for cysts.

The treatment of scarring by, for example, chemical peel or dermabrasion, is often unsatisfactory.

Prognosis

In most patients, acne resolves during the teenage years so that, in addition to providing active therapy, one can be reassuring. In some cases, acne persists into the mid-twenties or beyond; this was particularly common before the availability of isotretinoin.

ROSACEA AND PERIORAL DERMATITIS

Rosacea usually occurs between 30 and 50 years of age, with a female : male ratio of 3 : 1. Intermittent flushing of the cheeks, nose, forehead and chin is triggered by being in a hot room, alcohol, spicy foods and, in some, exposure to sunlight. The redness may become persistent with telangiectasia, papules, pustules and lymphoedema. Rhinophyma (enlargement of the nose, usually in men) may occur and ocular effects include blepharitis, conjunctivitis and keratitis.

The differential diagnosis includes perioral dermatitis, which may complicate rosacea if a fluorinated corticosteroid has been applied. Treatment includes oxytetracycline (e.g. 500 mg twice daily for 2–3 months), topical metronidazole and avoidance of trigger factors.

Perioral dermatitis responds to similar therapy. Other potential side-effects of potent fluorinated topical corticosteroids are thinning of the skin (dermal atrophy) and systemic absorption.

OTHER SKIN DISEASES

Space does not allow a detailed account of the large number of other skin diseases. Tables 14.4–14.12 provide additional important information.

Table 14.4 lists the benign and malignant skin tumours that commonly present to the dermatologist. The role of sun exposure in the pathogenesis of basal cell epithelioma, squamous carcinoma and malignant melanoma is now more widely understood, following public information programmes aimed at producing early recognition and treatment.

Common infections and infestations are summarised in Tables 14.5–14.8. Skin lesions may be a manifestation of an underlying disease (as in acanthosis nigricans) or may be part of a systemic process (as occurs in lupus erythematosus) (Tables 14.9–14.11). In addition, it is important to be aware that there are several potential dermatological emergencies (Table 14.12).

Table 14.4. Benign and malignant skin tumours

Lesion	Clinical features/diagnosis	Treatment options
Melanocytic naevus	Brown or skin coloured, sometimes hair-bearing, usually regular shape/colour	Reassurance, excision
Seborrhoeic keratosis (seborrhoeic wart, basal cell papilloma)	Brown hyperkeratotic/warty lesion on face and trunk, usually in the elderly Often multiple	Reassurance, cryotherapy, simple excision
Histiocytoma (dermatofibroma)	Firm pink or light brown dermal nodule, often on the leg	Reassurance, excision
Actinic (solar) keratosis	Red or light brown hyperkeratotic lesion(s) on sun-exposed skin (face, dorsa of hands) Small potential to become squamous cell carcinoma	Cryotherapy, topical 5-fluorouracil (5-FU), moisturiser
Keratoacanthoma (KA)	Domed lesion with central keratotic plug, growing rapidly (within 4 weeks) on sun-exposed skin; would spontaneously resolve over about 6 months Must distinguish from a squamous cell carcinoma	Excision (for histology and to avoid puckered scar)
Basal cell epithelioma/carcinoma (BCC, rodent ulcer)	Pearly papule with telangiectatic vessels, sometimes ulcerated with rolled edge, mainly on head and neck Potential for local erosion	Excision, curettage, radiotherapy
Squamous cell carcinoma (SCC)	Keratotic indurated lesion, usually growing over a few months Potential to metastasise	Excision
Bowen's disease (squamous cell carcinoma in-situ)	Red scaly plaque, often on the lower leg Diagnostic biopsy desirable	Excision, curettage, cryotherapy, topical 5-FU
Malignant melanoma (superficial spreading melanoma, nodular melanoma, acral lentiginous melanoma, lentigo maligna/ Hutchinson's freckle, lentigo maligna melanoma)	Often arises on normal-appearing skin but a benign naevus may enlarge, change colour (e.g. turn black), bleed spontaneously or become itchy or inflamed Some cases are familial (dysplastic naevus syndrome) Prognosis partly depends on depth of tumour so that early recognition is important	Wide excision (by a specialist)

Table 14.5. Superficial fungal infections

Disease	Cause
Dermatophyte infections	
Athlete's foot	*Trichophyton rubrum*
Nail infections	*Trichophyton interdigitale*
(tinea unguium)	*Epidermophyton flocosum*
Tinea corporis	*T. rubrum*
Scalp ringworm	*Trichophyton tonsurans*
(tinea capitis)	*Microsporum canis, T. rubrum,*
	T. verrucosum
Candidal infections	
Napkin candidiasis	*Candida albicans* infection,
Intertrigo (flexural)	often complicating an irritant
	dermatitis.
Candida paronychia	A hazard of regular immersion
	of the hands in water
Pityriasis versicolor	*Malassezia furfur* (pityriasis
	orbiculare in yeast-like form)

Table 14.6. Common bacterial infections of the skin

Disease	Cause
Impetigo	*Staphylococcus aureus* and
(plate 3)	group A streptococci
Erysipelas	Streptococcal infection (via
	minor abrasion) involving
	superficial lymphatic vessels
Cellulitis	Usually a streptococcal infection
	involving deeper layers of skin
	(distinction from erysipelas of
	little clinical importance)
Erythrasma	*Corynebacterium minutissimum*—

Clinical features/diagnosis	Therapy
Sore, itchy moist white fissures in toe webs Mycology + (skin scrapings)	Topical antifungal
Thickened discoloured powdery nails Mycology + (nail clippings)	Oral antifungal (e.g. terbinafine, griseofulvin)
Red scaly plaques, with an active red advancing edge and central clearing Often unilateral Mycology + (skin scrapings)	Topical ± oral antifungal
Hair loss, inflammation and scaling Mycology + (skin scrapings, hair roots) Wood's (UV) light fluorescence	Topical and oral antifungal (e.g. griseofulvin)
Red shiny patches with 'satellite' lesions Mycology + (swab)	Allow moist area to dry, topical antifungal
Boggy inflamed nail fold, with pus Mycology + (swab)	Topical and oral antifungal (e.g. itraconazole)
Pink asymptomatic coalescing lesions on trunk with fine scaling and hypo- or hyperpigmentation Mycology + (skin scrapings) Wood's light—pale yellow fluorescence	Topical selenium sulphide to whole trunk/arms

Clinical features/diagnosis	Therapy
Red, sometimes blistered, lesions develop into golden crusts May complicate atopic dermatitis Swab for micro-organisms and sensitivity	Topical (e.g. mupirocin) ± oral antibiotics (e.g. flucloxacillin, erythromycin)
Red oedematous area, often on a cheek or leg, with sharply demarcated border, and pyrexia and leucocytosis Organism often not isolated (swab, blood cultures), ASO titre	Systemic antibiotic (usually penicillin)
Red hot tender area of skin (e.g. surrounding a leg ulcer), accompanied by pyrexia and leucocytosis Palpable lymph nodes Swab and blood cultures (before antibiotics) may yield organism(s)	Systemic antibiotics (usually penicillin ± flucloxacillin)
Reddish patches in axillae or groin region with fine scaling Swab and Wood's light—coral red fluorescence	Oral erythromycin

Table 14.7. Common viral infections of the skin

Disease	Cause
Herpes simplex (e.g. cold sores herpetic whitlow, eczema herpeticum, genital herpes)	Herpes virus hominis type 1 (usually in cold sores), type 2 (usually in genital herpes)
Herpes zoster (shingles)	Herpes virus varicellae (reactivated chicken pox virus)
Warts	Human papilloma virus
Molluscum contagiosum	A pox virus
Pityriasis rosea	? viral
Acquired immune deficiency syndrome (AIDS)	Human immunodeficiency virus (HIV)

Table 14.8. Infestations

Disease	Cause
Scabies	Scabies mite (*Sarcoptes scabiei*) produces an allergic reaction
Lice	
Pedicularis capitis	Head louse
Pedicularis corporis	Body louse
Pedicularis pubis	Pubic louse

Clinical features/diagnosis	Therapy
Red vesicular sore then crusted lesions, often on lips or skin (e.g. finger or wrist) Eczema herpeticum may be a severe complication of atopic dermatitis May confirm diagnosis with a Tzanck smear or by electron microscopy of fluid	Symptomatic treatment ± topical acyclovir (systemic acyclovir for eczema herpeticum)
Dermatomal pain followed by linear red, macular, papular, vesicular then pustular eruption May be complicated by post-herpetic neuralgia	Symptomatic Systemic acyclovir in the elderly
Common warts (e.g. on hands), plane warts (often on face), plantar warts (verrucae), genital warts; usually self-limiting	Topical keratolytic agents, liquid nitrogen cryotherapy, podophyllin (for genital warts)
Reddish papules with umbilicated centre often on trunk or proximal limbs May be multiple Spontaneously remit	Expectant, sometimes topical phenol or cryotherapy (depending on age of child)
Red scaly asymptomatic oval macules on trunk, arms and upper thighs occurring a day after a solitary red 'herald patch' Spontaneous resolution in 6–8 weeks	Moisturisers ± weak topical corticosteroids
Kaposi's sarcoma: reddish-purple vascular nodules often multiple, associated with severe or persistent opportunistic infections	Excision or radiotherapy for Kaposi's sarcoma, if required Treatment of underlying disease

Clinical features/diagnosis	Treatment
Extremely itchy excoriated red papular rash particularly affecting finger webs, hands, wrists and pubic area Affected individuals may be asymptomatic Mite can be extracted from linear burrow	Permethrin cream ± cream rinse (for scalp) or malathion overnight (to all occupants of the home)
Lots of school children have nits (eggs) sometimes with excoriation and secondary infection	Permethrin or malathion Fine combing
Itching, excoriation and secondary infection usually in vagrants	Malathion
Itching and 'black dots' in pubic hair	Malathion

Table 14.9. Dermatological manifestations of systemic diseases

Disease/lesion	Clinical features/diagnosis/associated disorder
Acanthosis nigricans	Hyperpigmentation and hyperkeratosis of flexures (e.g. axillae) in absence of obesity Associated with adenocarcinoma, e.g. carcinoma of stomach
'Pseudo' acanthosis nigricans	Changes of acanthosis nigricans in an obese person Associated with hyperinsulinaemia ± overt diabetes mellitus
Dermatitis herpetiformis	Extremely itchy, excoriated vesicles on elbows, scalp, buttocks and lower back Associated gluten-sensitive enteropathy may be asymptomatic but jejunal histology usually shows some degree of subtotal villous atrophy. Skin biopsy for histology and direct immunofluorescence (IMF) (perilesional skin) Responds to dapsone ± gluten-free diet
Erythema nodosum (Plate 4)	Painful, red, circular, smooth-surfaced lesions on the shins, resolving over a few weeks to leave a bruise-like appearance. May be caused by streptococcal infection, sulphonamides, sarcoidosis or tuberculosis Investigations include a throat swab, ASO titre, Mantoux test (± Kveim test), viral titres
Generalised pruritus	In the absence of primary skin disease, generalised pruritus may be associated with iron deficiency anaemia, liver or renal failure, diabetes mellitus, primary biliary cirrhosis, hypo- or hyperthyroidism, polycythaemia vera and lymphoma
Granuloma annulare (Plate 5)	Reddish, annular, dermal lesions with palpable edge, often over knuckles and on elbows Resolves spontaneously in 6–18 months Skin biopsy for histology Exclude diabetes mellitus; occurs in only 5% cases
Necrobiosis lipoidica (Plate 6)	Reddish-yellow shiny plaques on shins, with atrophy and telangiectasia May ulcerate Skin biopsy for histology Usually (but not always) associated with diabetes mellitus
Pretibial myxoedema	Red raised dermal lesions, often on shins Skin biopsy for histology Associated with hyperthyroidism
Pyoderma gangrenosum (Plate 7)	Sometimes extensive, coalescing ulcers with undermined edge Skin biopsy may be helpful (not diagnostic) Associated with Crohn's disease, ulcerative colitis and rheumatoid arthritis Treated with prednisolone

Table 14.9 *cont.* **Dermatological manifestations of systemic diseases**

Disease/lesion	Clinical features/diagnosis/associated disorder
Systemic vasculitis (Plate 8) (e.g. Henoch–Schönlein purpura, polyarteritis nodosa)	Purplish palpable purpura (sometimes necrotic, ulcerated lesions) on limbs and buttocks Skin biopsy for histology ± direct immunofluorescence (IMF; early lesion) Investigate for antigenic stimulus (e.g. streptococcal infection) and degree of systemic involvement
Xanthelasma/ xanthoma	Xanthelasmata are flat yellowish lesions on eyelids Various types of xanthomata, e.g. eruptive papules on buttocks or tuberous xanthomata over elbows and knees Exclude hyperlipoproteinaemia

Table 14.10. **Dermatological aspects of autoimmune/connective tissue diseases**

Disease	Clinical features/diagnosis
Autoimmune diseases	
Addison's disease (adrenal insufficiency)	Melanin pigmentation in palmar creases and buccal mucosa
Alopecia areata	One or more bald patches on scalp with normal underlying skin Hair loss may occur at other sites, occasionally complete
Vitiligo	Symmetrical depigmented areas of skin Vitiligo, alopecia areata and Addison's disease may be associated with each other and with other organ-specific autoimmune diseases, including pernicious anaemia and thyroiditis
Connective tissue diseases	
Lupus erythematosus (LE)	
Discoid LE (Plate 9)	Red, often atrophic, plaques on sun-exposed areas, especially the face (may cause scarring alopecia) Chronic tendency but only 5% progress to SLE Skin biopsy for histology and direct immunofluorescence (IMF-lesional skin) ANA +ve in 20%
Systemic LE (SLE)	Red, macular 'butterfly' rash* on nose and cheeks ± dorsa of hands and other sun-exposed areas, mainly in females. Provoked by sunlight and drugs (e.g. hydralazine, methyldopa, isoniazid, phenytoin)

Table 14.10 *cont.* Dermatological aspects of autoimmune/connective tissue diseases

Disease	Clinical features/diagnosis
	May also have rheumatological, renal, cardiac or haemopoietic symptoms and signs Skin biopsy for histology and direct IMF of lesional and non-lesional sun-exposed skin, e.g. on upper arm ('lupus band' test) ANA +ve, double-stranded DNA antibody +ve Investigate other systems
Subacute LE	Sun-induced red lesions on face ± upper arms and trunk, associated with joint pains Skin biopsy for histology and direct IMF (lesional skin) Cytoplasmic antibodies +ve
Morphoea	Usually localised firm white patches of skin, initially with an inflamed border Sometimes linear, occasionally generalised Skin biopsy for histological confirmation
Generalised scleroderma (systemic sclerosis)	Loss of mobility of the skin and other organs due to progressive fibrosis, leading to tight perioral skin with gastrointestinal and respiratory problems Females > males
CRST (CREST) syndrome	Hand features of CRST syndrome (calcinosis, Raynaud's phenomenon, sclerodactyly, telangiectasia) ± oesophageal dysfunction may occur alone or as part of generalised scleroderma Skin biopsy for histology, autoantibody screen, barium swallow
Dermatomyositis	Red, oedematous periocular rash (dorsa of hands sometimes affected) with proximal myopathy. CPK level elevated, characteristic EMG changes, skin biopsy ± muscle biopsy Chest X-ray and limited search for more common forms of malignancy in the elderly

*Distinguish from rosacea which also produces a 'butterfly' rash

Table 14.11. Drug eruptions and skin ulceration

Drug-induced rashes

	Patterns of drug eruptions include morbilliform erythema, urticaria, exfoliative dermatitis, erythema multiforme (Stevens–Johnson syndrome), lichenoid/lichen planus-like eruption (Plate 10) vasculitis/purpuric eruption, pigmentation, fixed drug eruption and erythema nodosum
	Common agents include penicillins, sulphonamides and non-steroidal anti-inflammatory drugs
	History important

Ulcers

Leg ulcer	Venous leg ulcers, typically affecting the medial malleolar region(s), account for up to 90% of leg ulcers
	Important aspects of management are elevation and compression (e.g. with an elastic bandage or shaped tubigrip)
	Must distinguish from arterial (often painful) ulcers in which such measures would be inappropriate
	Other causes of ulceration include: diabetes mellitus, infection, rheumatoid arthritis, vasculitis, sickle cell anaemia, haemolytic anaemia, pyoderma gangrenosum and malignancy
Decubitus ulcer (pressure sore)	Commonly occur over sacrum
	Prevention by good nursing care important

*The ampicillin-induced rash in infectious mononucleosis does not necessarily imply penicillin allergy.

Table 14.12. Potential dermatological emergencies*

Disease/lesion	Cause
Angio-oedema	C1 esterase inhibitor deficiency (hereditary angio-oedema), severe urticaria, ACE inhibitors
Extensive burns	Various types
Toxic epidermal necrolysis (TEN)	Drug allergy, e.g. a sulphonamide
Staphylococcal scalded skin syndrome (SSSS)	Toxin from *Staphylococcus aureus*
Erythema multiforme	Herpes simplex, drug allergy
Erythroderma/ exfoliative dermatitis	Psoriasis, atopic, seborrhoeic or allergic contact dermatitis, drug eruption
Generalised pustular Psoriasis	e.g. following systemic corticosteroids
Eczema herpeticum	Herpes simplex
Pemphigoid (bullous pemphigoid)	Autoimmune
Necrotising fasciitis	Deep infection, usually with beta-haemolytic streptococci Sometimes multiple organisms (bacterial synergistic gangrene)
Pemphigus (various types)	Autoimmune
Pemphigoid (bullous pemphigoid)	Autoimmune
Arterial insufficiency —gangrene/ulceration	Arteriosclerosis, emboli

*Other potential dermatological emergencies include SLE, dermatomyositis, systemic vasculitis and pyoderma gangrenosum (see Tables 14.9 and 14.10).

Clinical features/diagnosis	Therapy
Gross urticarial swellings with subcutaneous involvement, e.g. throat and tongue	i.m. adrenaline then i.v. hydrocortisone
Large areas of blistered, denuded skin	Intensive care (good nursing, fluid balance, treatment of infection)
Large areas of blistered, denuded skin Skin biopsy for histology	Intensive care (good nursing, fluid balance, treatment of infection) N.B. Systemic corticosteroids may increase mortality
Blistered, denuded skin Skin biopsy for histology (to distinguish from TEN)	Sytemic antibiotics
Annular 'target' lesions with blistering of skin and lips Eyes and mucosa involved when severe (Stevens–Johnson syndrome) Skin biopsy for histology	Topical ± oral corticosteroids
Large areas of erythema with variable desquamation	Bed rest, emollients/moisturisers, mild topical corticosteroids Treatment of fluid loss
Erythematous psoriasis with sterile pustules	As above ± oral etretinate
Excoriated vesicles in atopic dermatitis Occasionally encephalitis Confirm by Tzank smear or electron microscopy of vesicular fluid	Systemic acyclovir
Red spreading cellulitis with necrosis Swab ± skin biopsy for culture (including anaerobes) and sensitivity	Surgical debridement, systemic antibiotics
Erosion of skin and mucous membranes Skin biopsy for histology and direct IMF (perilesional skin) Autoantibody titre (indirect IMF)	Prednisolone, azathioprine
Tense blisters on skin, with red haemorrhagic base Skin biopsy for histology and direct IMF (perilesional skin)	Prednisolone, azathioprine
Necrotic digits; painful necrotic ulceration Ultrasound studies, arteriography	Surgery

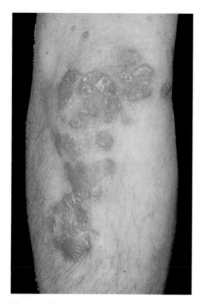

Plate 1 Psoriasis—red scaly plaques on the elbow.

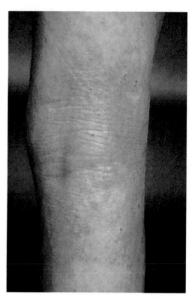

Plate 2 Atopic dermatitis—lichenified eczema affecting the popliteal fossa of a child.

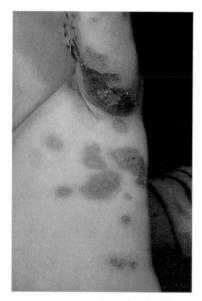

Plate 3 Impetigo—golden crusting and erosions in a baby.

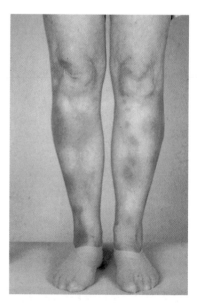

Plate 4 Erythema nodosum—painful red nodules on the shins, in this case associated with sarcoidosis.

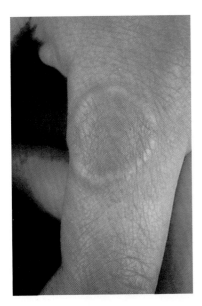

Plate 5 Granuloma annulare—a dermal circular lesion on the hand.

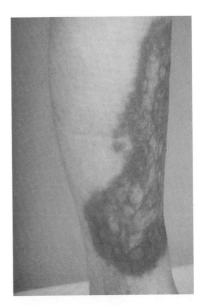

Plate 6 Necroblosis lipoidica—an extensive yellow-brown atrophic lesion on the shin of a patient with diabetes mellitus.

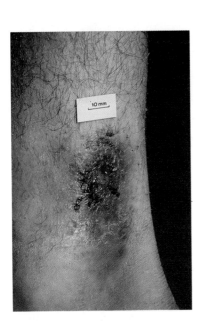

Plate 7 Pyoderma gangrenosum on the lower leg of a young man with Crohn's disease.

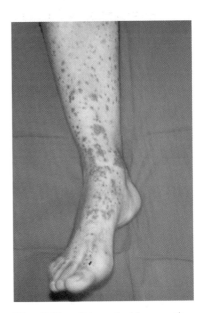

Plate 8 Vasculitis—palpable purpuric lesions on the lower legs.

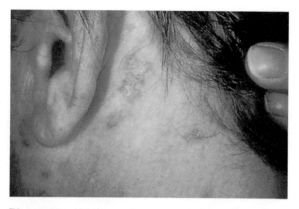

Plate 9 Discoid lupus erythematosus—red hyperkeratotic and atrophic plaques on a sun-exposed area.

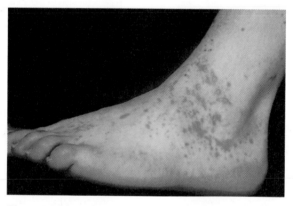

Plate 10 Lichen planus—reddish-brown (violaceous) flat-topped papules on the ankle.

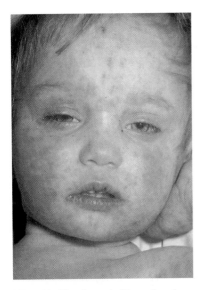

Plate 11 Measles rash. Reproduced with permission.

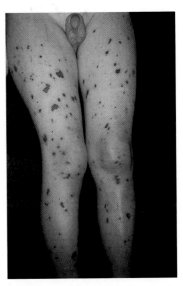

Plate 12 Meningococcal septicaemia causing 'purpura fulminans'.

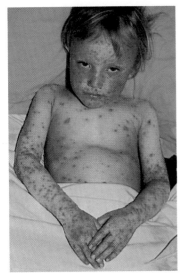

Plate 13 Varicella (chickenpox) rash. Reproduced with permission.

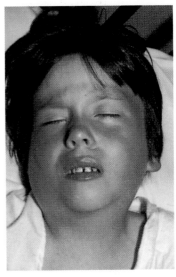

Plate 14 Mumps. Reproduced with permission.

15

INFECTIOUS DISEASES AND HIV

Stuart Glover

The pattern of infectious diseases has changed dramatically over the last 40 years in parallel with improvements in social and biomedical standards. Antibiotics have allowed better control of infection and immunisation has eradicated or reduced many common viral diseases. However, the 1980s have brought new diseases in the form of acquired immune deficiency syndrome (AIDS) while widespread international travel has introduced exotic infections.

GASTROINTESTINAL INFECTIONS

'Gastroenteritis' is a common cause of infant mortality in underdeveloped countries and a frequent cause of morbidity in the developed world. There are three clinical types:

1. food poisoning caused by the ingestion of preformed bacterial toxins and organic and inorganic chemicals
2. enteritis and enterocolitis caused by the multiplication of pathogenic microbes in the large and small bowel
3. dysentery caused by infection and mucosal invasion of the colon and rectum.

FOOD POISONING

There is rapid onset of vomiting, profuse watery diarrhoea and abdominal pain after eating contaminated food. It is often epidemic or institutional. Toxins may affect other organs, e.g. botulinum and the central nervous system (CNS); mycotoxins (mushrooms) and the liver; verotoxin from *Escherichia coli* 0157 and the endothelium.

The principal causative organisms are *Staphylococcus aureus*, *Clostridium perfringens* type A and *Bacillus cereus*.

Staphylococcus aureus

Heat-stable enterotoxins, types A, D and E. Infection arises from human nasal carriers. The onset is sudden after 1–6 hours' incubation with profuse salivation, vomiting, abdominal pain, and diarrhoea but no fever. It may result in severe salt and water deficiency and hypovolaemia. Treatment is supportive.

Clostridium perfringens type A

Heat-labile enterotoxin. The incubation period is 6–24 hours and there is cramping abdominal pain and diarrhoea but no fever. It is associated with reheated, previously cooked meat in institutional outbreaks.

Bacillus cereus

Two distinct toxins produce sudden onset of vomiting or a slightly delayed diarrhoea: the former is associated with reheated rice, the latter with many food products.

Other causes of food poisoning include enterotoxigenic *E. coli*. Other, non-microbial, causes of food poisoning include paralytic shellfish, neurotoxic shellfish, green potatoes (solanine), uncooked red kidney beans and monosodium glutamate (Chinese restaurant syndrome).

ENTERITIS/ENTEROCOLITIS

There are two major mechanisms of disease production:

1. Enteroinvasive: bacteria invade and damage the mucosa of the small intestine, e.g. *Shigella* spp, *Campylobacter jejuni*, *Salmonella* spp, enteroinvasive *E. coli* and *Yersinia enterocolitica*.
2. Damage to enterocytes and brush border, e.g. viruses (rotavirus, Norwalk, SRSV) and protozoa (*Giardia intestinalis*, *Cryptosporidium* spp).

Enteritis caused by invasive micro-organisms can be complicated by bacteraemia if the inoculum of micro-organisms is large, in patients with impaired gastric acid secretion (pernicious anaemia, post-gastrectomy, H_2-blocker therapy) and in neutropenia.

Symptoms

Enteroinvasive
The incubation period is 1–5 days. The patient is febrile and has colicky abdominal pain with diarrhoea containing blood and pus. The duration of the illness is 5–7 days.

Surface damage

1. Viral gastroenteritis occurs in children under 2 years of age with a winter onset. There is fever, vomiting, diarrhoea and upper respiratory tract symptoms.
2. Protozoal infestation leads to loose, offensive diarrhoea, steatorrhoea,

anorexia, weight loss and malabsorption. Abdominal pain occurs with distension and borborygmi, flatulence and eructation but no fever.

DYSENTERY

Microbial infection of the colon and rectum is characterised by frequent, small-volume stools containing blood and pus. Causative microbes include *Shigella* spp, *Campylobacter* spp, *Salmonella* spp, *Y. enterocolitica*, *E. coli* 0157, *Clostridium difficile*, *Entamoeba histolytica* and cytomegalovirus (CMV) in HIV disease.

Some of these micro-organisms also infect the small intestine and may produce enterotoxins in addition to infecting the colon and rectum.

Symptoms
There is fever, abdominal pain, small-volume but frequent stools that may contain blood, mucus and pus. Systemic invasion may occur in predisposed patients.

Investigation of gastroenteritis (see Table 15.1)
The epidemiology of gastroenteritis: type of food ingested, foreign travel, sexual orientation, occupation, animal exposure, contact history, recreational history, any predisposing medical conditions or recent antibiotic ingestion.

Table 15.1. Investigation of gastroenteritis

Stool sample	Leucocytes, ova, cysts, parasites and blood	Enteritis; dysentery Protozoans—*Giardia*, *Cryptosporidium*
	Modified acid-fast stain	*Cryptosporidium*
	Culture	Bacteria
	Cold enrichment	*Yersinia*
	Electron microscopy	Rotavirus
	ELISA	Rotavirus
	Toxin detection	*Clostridium difficile*
Sigmoidoscopy	Rectal biopsy	Amoebiasis cytomegalovirus, schistosomiasis, inflammatory bowel disease
Blood cultures		Systemic disease, e.g. salmonellosis
Serial serology		*Yersinia*, schistosomiasis
Radiology	Straight abdominal films	Toxic megacolon Colonic thumbprinting, ischaemic colitis, etc.
Duodenal aspiration		Protozoans—*Giardia*, *Cryptosporidium*, *Strongyloides*
Small bowel biopsy	Per-endoscope or Crosby capsule	Coeliac disease (not infective), Whipple's disease

NB. Barium enema studies are contraindicated in infective gastroenteritis.

Differential diagnosis (see Table 15.2)

Treatment
Rehydration is by mouth with the glucose electrolyte solution 'dioralyte' and by intravenous fluids: NaCl with K supplements.

Most infective gastroenteritis is self-limiting and requires no specific anti-microbial therapy. Predisposing factors require the early pre-emptive use of antibiotics (Table 15.3).

Anti-diarrhoeal agents are best avoided, and spread is prevented by hygienic disposal of faeces and by handwashing.

In the UK, the C.C.D.C. should be notified.

Prognosis
Toxin-induced diarrhoea is a major cause of infantile death in preschool children in the underdeveloped world. Death is caused by salt and water depletion.

Food poisoning rarely causes death. Botulism (see p. 151) and mushroom poisoning, although rare, have a very high mortality.

Enteritis and dysentery may be complicated by salt and water loss,

Table 15.2. The differential diagnosis of enteritis and dysentery

Enteritis	Dysentery
Early appendicitis Irritable bowel syndrome	Inflammatory bowel disease (Crohn's disease, ulcerative colitis)
Small bowel disease (coeliac disease, Whipple's disease)	Diverticular disease Colonic neoplasms
Chronic laxative abuse	Villous adenoma of rectum Ischaemic colitis

Table 15.3. Antibiotic treatment of gastroenteritis

Food poisoning	Not indicated
Toxin-induced diarrhoea	Not indicated
Vibrio cholerae	Tetracycline, ampicillin, quinolone
Shigella spp	Ampicillin, trimethoprim, quinolone
Salmonella spp	Quinolone, ampicillin, co-trimoxazole
Campylobacter jejuni	Quinolone, erythromycin
Yersinia spp	Chloramphenicol, quinolone, aminoglycoside, tetracycline, co-trimoxazole
Clostridium difficile	Vancomycin, metronidazole
Entamoeba histolytica	Metronidazole
Giardia intestinalis	Metronidazole

prerenal renal failure, acute tubular necrosis, septicaemia and metastatic abscesses, including mycotic aneurysms. Toxic dilatation of the colon and colonic perforation can occur. There may be reactive arthritis (Reiter's syndrome) especially after *Shigella, Salmonella, Yersinia* and occasionally *Campylobacter* infections.

FEVER AND RASH

A fever and skin rash often indicate an underlying infectious disease but may also be a sign of an important non-infective disease. Diagnosis is dependent on the type of skin lesions present, their number and distribution. Assessment of lymphadenopathy, respiratory signs and travel history add further clues.

ERYTHEMATOUS RASHES (sunburn, red skin, blanches on pressure)

Scarlet fever

An acute streptococcal infection caused by erythrotoxin-producing strains, scarlet fever is acquired from a carrier or a case of streptococcal infection. The primary site of infection is the oropharynx, wounds, burns or the female genital tract.

Symptoms and signs
The symptoms are sore throat, neck pain, fever, headache and myalgia.

The signs are exudative tonsillitis, cervical lymphadenopathy, a red tongue with large papillae (raspberry tongue) or a coated tongue with protruding papillae (strawberry tongue), erythematous rash and circumoral pallor.

The skin desquamates at the end of the first week.

Investigations
A throat or wound swab should be taken for culture. Serology will show raised anti-streptolysin O (ASO) and anti-deoxyribonuclease B (ADB) levels. White cell count will demonstrate leucocytosis and occasionally eosinophilia.

Treatment
Benzylpenicillin i.v. followed by phenoxymethylpenicillin to complete 10 days. Erythromycin is an alternative for those allergic to penicillins. The patient must be isolated at the outset.

Prognosis
The prognosis is excellent. Suppurative complications (peritonsillar abscess, retropharyngeal abscess, acute sinusitis, otitis media, pneumonia) are now rare.

Non-suppurative complications include acute rheumatic fever, acute post-streptococcal glomerulonephritis and erythema nodosum.

Differential diagnosis

Common conditions include viral pharyngitis (adenovirus, influenza, entero-viruses, EBV, CMV, measles), *Mycoplasma pneumoniae* and *Candida*.

Uncommon conditions are diphtheria, secondary syphilis, anginose agranulocytosis and gonorrhoea.

Erythema infectiosum (Fifth disease, slapped cheek syndrome)

This is caused by parvovirus B19 and is an epidemic febrile illness of school children and young adults. There is a maculopapular rash which may occur together with flushed cheeks. Large joint arthritis is found in 10% of children and > 50% of adults. Erythema infectiosum causes aplastic crises in chronic haemolytic disease, e.g. sickle cell disease. It mimics rubella. It is diagnosed serologically using radioimmunoassay or ELISA. There is no specific therapy. The prognosis is excellent but it may cause intrauterine infections leading to hydrops fetalis.

Erythema chronicum migrans (ECM)

ECM is the classic initial manifestation of Lyme disease, a systemic infection caused by the spirochaete *Borrelia burgdorferi*, which is transmitted by the tick *Ixodes*.

ECM is a large, erythematous, macular lesion spreading to 15–20 cm in diameter. The outer margin is bright and raised with central clearing. It spreads centrifugally and is associated with malaise, headache, myalgia, fever and lymphadenopathy. Later features of Lyme disease include neurological disease (meningitis, encephalitis, cranial neuropathies, motor and sensory radiculopathy), arthritis and cardiac disease (heart block).

Treatment is with tetracycline, penicillin or ceftriaxone.

Toxic shock syndrome

This is caused by the effects of an exotoxin produced by phage group 1 *Staphylococcus aureus*. It most often occurs in menstruating young women who are using tampons but can occur in either sex in association with focal staphylococcal sepsis. Onset is abrupt.

Symptoms and signs

Fever, with a temperature of 38.9°C or more, and diffuse macular erythema are the main manifestations. Desquamation, especially of the palms and soles, occurs 1–2 weeks after the onset of illness. Hypotension occurs, with a systolic blood pressure of < 90 mmHg.

Multisystem involvement includes vomiting, diarrhoea and raised bili-rubin, ALT and AST levels. There may be severe myalgia and a raised CPK level. The mucous membranes of the vagina, oropharynx and conjunctivae may be hyperaemic. Pyuria occurs and the urea and creatinine levels can be raised. Platelets are often < 100 000 and the patient may be disorientated or have altered consciousness without focal neurological signs.

Investigations
Swab or culture for *Staph. aureus* is necessary.

Differential diagnosis
Streptococcal toxic shock syndrome, measles, rubella, leptospirosis, rickettsial infections, scarlet fever.

Management
Supportive measures include the administration of i.v. fluids, removal of the tampon and drainage of focal sepsis. Parenteral flucloxacillin or vancomycin may be necessary.

Prognosis
The mortality rate is 3%, and there is a recurrence rate of 20% with subsequent menses.

MACULOPAPULAR RASHES AND FEVER

Measles

This is an acute febrile exanthematous disease of childhood caused by an RNA paramyxovirus. It is highly contagious and is spread by droplet inhalation. The incubation period is 10–17 days.

Symptoms and signs
In the prodromal phase, fever, malaise, coryza and cough are present.

A brick-red, confluent macular rash spreads from the head and face to the neck, trunk and limbs (see Plate 11). The skin may also be oedematous. It is followed by fine desquamation. Koplik spots are seen on the buccal mucosa and may occur before the skin rash.

Marked conjunctivitis, coryza and irritability occur.

Investigations
Viral culture of throat washings and paired serology are indicated.

Differential diagnosis
Scarlet fever, toxic shock syndrome and severe rubella should be considered.

Treatment
Antibiotics are used only if there is secondary bacterial infection.

Prevention. Active immunisation is with live attenuated measles vaccine, usually as part of MMR (measles, mumps, rubella vaccine). Passive immunisation in immunocompromised, non-immune patients is with human non-specific immunoglobulin.

Prognosis
Death from pneumonia and encephalitis is now rare but measles remains

a major contributory factor in the death of the malnourished. Here septic complications, e.g. otitis media, mastoiditis, pneumonia and bronchitis, are common. Measles may also cause obstructive laryngitis and croup. Acute measles post-infectious encephalitis is sometimes seen, as is subacute sclerosing panencephalitis (SSPE).

Rubella ('German measles')

This is an acute febrile exanthematous disease caused by an RNA togavirus. It is found worldwide causing mild febrile illness with a faint rash. Spread is by respiratory droplets and the incubation period is 14–23 days.

Symptoms and signs
There is a mild short-lived prodromal fever with occipital headache, sore throat and gritty eyes with conjunctivitis. Suboccipital and posterior auricular lymphadenopathy develop. The rash comprises pink macules on the face and trunk and fades within 3 days without desquamation.

Investigations
Paired serology: rubella haemagglutination inhibition test should be performed and rubella-specific IgM should be sought.

Differential diagnosis
Other viral infections, e.g. adenovirus, enteroviruses (Coxsackie and echoviruses), parvovirus B19, mild measles and scarlet fever.

Treatment
This is symptomatic only. Prevention is by active immunisation using a live attenuated vaccine (MMR).

Prognosis
The prognosis is usually excellent but complications include arthralgia and occasional large joint arthritis in adult females, thrombocytopenia and encephalitis in 1 in 6000.

Congenital rubella syndrome

Infection with rubella in the first trimester of pregnancy puts the fetus at risk of developing rubella syndrome. There can be multiple congenital defects, especially of the eyes and heart, together with deafness and psychomotor retardation. Viral infection of the liver, heart, lungs and brain may be persistent.

Enteroviral exanthem

These febrile rashes are caused by various members of the enterovirus group, e.g. Coxsackie A and B, and echoviruses. Enteroviral rashes are variable in extent and distribution, are non-pruritic, do not desquamate and heal without discoloration. Hand, foot and mouth disease is caused by both Coxsackie A and B viruses.

Other features include enanthem (herpangina, ulcers on fauces and palate) lymphadenopathy and lymphocytic ('aseptic') meningitis.

Investigations comprise isolation of the virus from the throat, stools and CSF, and also paired serology.

PETECHIAL AND PURPURIC RASHES

Meningococcaemia

Neisseria meningitidis can cause a transient bacteraemia or septicaemia, with or without meningitis. Chronic meningococcaemia may rarely occur in a relatively well patient. Meningococcaemia can be a rapid and fulminant infection characterised by a spreading purpuric rash (Plate 12), shock, disseminated intravascular coagulation (DIC) and adrenal haemorrhage with acute adrenal failure.

Symptoms and signs

There may be severe myalgia and chills of sudden onset. The rash has a centrifugal distribution affecting the wrists, palms, lower legs, ankles and the soles of the feet. It is initially petechial or macular but rapidly expands to become purpuric or ecchymotic.

The patients may be febrile or hypothermic and can be extremely ill with hypotension and oliguria.

Investigations

These include blood cultures, microscopy and culture of CSF and counterimmunoelectrophoresis (CIE) of serum for meningococcal antigen.

Differential diagnosis

This includes gonococcaemia, associated with tenosynovitis, acral pustular or papular rash and arthritis; bacteraemia caused by *Strep. pneumoniae* (asplenic patients), *Haemophilus influenzae* or *Staph. aureus*; and rickettsial infection. Infectious mononucleosis, rubella and measles with thrombocytopenia, infective endocarditis and fat embolism should also be excluded.

Treatment

Penicillin-G i.v. 1.2 g 3-hourly for 7–10 days or cefotaxime is appropriate, and if there is a history of penicillin allergy chloramphenicol should be given.

The patient should be isolated for the first 24 hours of treatment.

Prevention in contacts is with rifampicin, ciprofloxacin and meningococcal vaccine type A, C and W135.

Prognosis

Meningitis mortality is 2–10% but in septicaemia without meningitis it is 30%. Complications include cranial neuropathy, deafness, metastatic sepsis and immune-complex-mediated arthritis, iritis and pericarditis.

BULLOUS AND POX-LIKE RASHES

Varicella

The primary infection is chickenpox, a mild childhood illness but severe in immunocompromised patients and some adults, caused by the DNA-containing human (alpha) herpes virus 3 or varicella zoster virus (VZV). It is spread by droplets from human to human and the incubation period is 14–18 days. VZV becomes latent in the dorsal root ganglia of sensory nerves; reactivation presents as shingles in later life or if the patient becomes immunocompromised.

Symptoms and signs
There is a prodrome with fever, headache, malaise and a sore throat.

The rash comprises crops of rapidly evolving macules and papules which develop into vesicles and pustules with crusting (Plate 13). They first appear on the trunk, face and proximal limbs, and may be itchy. There may be mouth ulcers (enanthem).

Investigations
The diagnosis is usually clinically obvious and no investigations are required. However, electron microscopy of vesicle fluid may reveal the virus, and there is a complement fixation test for VZV.

Differential diagnosis
This includes Kaposi's varicelliform eruption (herpes simplex infection of eczematous skin), cow pox (cattle, cat contact) and monkey pox (West and Central Africa).

Treatment
Acyclovir is rarely indicated for chickenpox in children, being limited to complicated cases and the immunocompromised. Varicella zoster immune globulin (VZIG), given within 96 hours of exposure to varicella or zoster, may prevent or attenuate the disease in susceptible close contacts. It is indicated for newborn children of mothers who develop chickenpox 6 days prior to or within 48 hours of delivery.

Prognosis
Chickenpox is rarely fatal but visceral dissemination, including varicella pneumonia and lymphocytic meningitis, can occur, as can haemorrhagic chickenpox (in immunocompromised patients and in those with HIV disease). In children, Reye's disease may follow varicella.

OTHER INFECTIOUS DISEASES

Diphtheria

This is an acute infection by virulent *Corynebacterium diphtheriae* of the throat and upper respiratory tract. It is rare in countries such as Great Britain where children are usually immunised. The bacterium produces a toxin which can cause severe damage to the heart and nervous system.

Symptoms and signs

After an incubation period of 1–7 days, sore throat and malaise are the usual symptoms with dysphagia.

Signs include a greyish adherent membrane in the tonsillar area and pharynx. The membrane bleeds when attempts are made to remove it. There is often considerable oedema locally and of the neck.

Symptoms and signs are different when the nasal mucosa is affected; then there is usually a bloodstained nasal discharge only. Cutaneous diphtheria presents as an indolent leg ulcer.

Diagnosis

The disease must always be suspected when there is a membranous pharyngitis, and it can be confirmed by isolation of *C. diphtheriae* from the pharynx or nose. Growth on Löffler's medium produces satisfactory results.

Complications

An acute cardiomyopathy with tachycardia, hypotension and ECG changes may develop in the second week. This can be fatal.

Respiratory obstruction is caused by mechanical obstruction of the larynx by membrane, and it may require tracheostomy.

A neuropathy affecting the ocular, bulbar and peripheral nerves may occur 2–10 weeks after the onset of illness. Respiratory involvement may require assisted ventilation. Gradual recovery is the rule.

Treatment

Antitoxin is given if the disease is suspected, 10 000–80 000 units, provided there is no reaction to an initial subcutaneous dose of 0.2 ml.

Penicillin and erythromycin help to eradicate the infection and prevent toxin formation. Throat swabs should be taken from close contacts and their state of immunity to the disease assessed. Penicillin or erythromycin is given to non-immune subjects who should also be vaccinated.

Whooping cough (pertussis)

This highly infectious disease is due to *Bordetella pertussis*. It causes a lower respiratory tract infection in childhood. Epidemics occur every 4 years or so in the UK and are encountered in areas of poor uptake of protective immunisation. It is seen most commonly in the under 5-year-olds and is more serious in infants.

Symptoms and signs

After an incubation period of 7–10 days there is an initial coryza followed by a cough which becomes severe, paroxysmal and accompanied by vomiting. The coughing paroxysm is often worse nocturnally and causes cyanosis.

A whoop is the noise produced by inspiration following a paroxysm of coughing. The cough interrupts sleeping and eating and renders the affected child helpless.

Signs are few and are the result of pneumonia and pulmonary collapse. Occasionally subconjunctival haemorrhages or a frenal ulcer are found.

Investigations
A blood count shows a profound lymphocytosis. A bacteriological diagnosis can be obtained using nasal swabs.

Complications
These are serious and include pneumonia and lung collapse from secondary bacterial infection and mucus plugging, cerebral anoxia from prolonged coughing spasms which may cause fits and cerebral damage, and considerable weight loss because of vomiting and poor feeding.

Treatment
Careful nursing and frequent feeding are supplemented where necessary with antibiotic treatment of pneumonia using erythromycin. Cough suppressants may help to control paroxysms of coughing, but support and reassurance of the child are more helpful.

Prevention
A vaccine is protective (80%) but uptake has been impaired by problems arising from post-vaccination fits and occasional cases of encephalitis. The disease continues to be serious—400 deaths per year which could be prevented.

Mumps

This inflammatory disease is caused by a paramyxovirus infection leading to an acute painful inflammation of the parotid and occasionally other salivary glands.

Symptoms and signs
After an incubation period of 18–21 days there is severe malaise and fever, and tenderness in the neck and parotid glands (see Plate 14).

Signs include enlargement of parotid glands which obliterate the angle of the mandible, occasional painful enlargement of other salivary glands, e.g. submandibular, and a dry mouth with inflamed orifices of the parotid ducts.

Complications
Orchitis is seen in 20% of male sufferers. It may precede parotid involvement and lead to diagnostic confusion. Oophoritis in women is extremely rare.

CNS involvement (meningitis and encephalitis) is the most important complication. The former is much more common than the latter and encephalitis carries a mortality of 2–3%.

Pancreatitis (acute) is an occasional complication.

Diagnosis and treatment

The diagnosis is essentially clinical, but the virus can be isolated from throat washings and saliva, and antibody elevation can be detected. Treatment is supportive only, including oral hygiene and a soft diet.

Prevention

This is by vaccination, usually given with MMR at 18 months to 2 years.

Glandular fever (infectious mononucleosis)

This is a disease of predominantly young adults caused by the Epstein–Barr (EB) virus. Exact mode of transmission is uncertain but is probably by aerosol. Traditionally thought to be spread by kissing, there is little evidence to support this.

Symptoms and signs

Most infections are subclinical. In those with symptoms there may be fever, malaise, sore throat and cervical lymphadenopathy. A transient rash is seen in some patients and up to 50% have splenomegaly. Very rarely the spleen may rupture and cause death. Occasionally meningitis, encephalitis, myocarditis and pneumonitis occur but most patients recover fully in a few weeks.

Diagnosis

The clinical diagnosis is supported by atypical lymphocytosis, thrombocytopenia and screening tests for IgM antibodies (Monospot, Paul-Bunnell).

Treatment

Most cases pass off untreated. With systemic involvement steroids may be used. Amoxycillin and ampicillin cause a rash in 90% of patients with infectious mononucleosis and must be avoided.

In a few cases infectious mononucleosis persists as a debilitating illness for a year or more.

CHRONIC FATIGUE SYNDROME

This term refers to a syndrome of excessive fatigue, exacerbated by both mental and physical exertion. The syndrome may be triggered, particularly in subjects with pre-existing fatigue and psychological distress, by infections, in particular infectious mononucleosis, viral hepatitis and viral meningitis, but there is no convincing evidence of persisting viral infection or immune dysfunction. Less than 10% of patients with infectious mononucleosis develop chronic fatigue. Tests to exclude alternative diagnoses should include full blood count, ESR or CRP, tests of liver, renal and thyroid function, urinalysis and creatine kinase. Sufferers benefit from a sympathetic approach, from encouragement to engage in a graded exercise programme, and from cognitive behavioural therapy.

Leptospirosis

This occurs where people are exposed to infected rat or other urine or to contaminated stagnant or dirty water. The organisms *Leptospira icterohaemorrhagiae* (rat) and *L. canicola* (dog or pig) penetrate through the skin or mucous membranes.

Symptoms and signs

L. icterohaemorrhagiae causes Weil's disease with renal, hepatic and cardiac involvement, which can be fatal. *L. canicola* infection results in aseptic meningitis and is more benign. Overall, however, many infections are mild, may present as fevers of unknown origin and remit spontaneously or respond to treatment.

Diagnosis

This is made on the history of possible exposure, for example, farm workers, vets etc., and on positive blood cultures in the first week or urine cultures thereafter. Leptospira antibodies also appear in the blood.

Treatment

Appropriate antibiotic therapy (usually penicillin) and supportive measures, for example, of renal or hepatic failure.

HIV INFECTION AND AIDS

In 1981, the occurrence of *Pneumocystis carinii* pneumonia (PCP) and Kaposi's sarcoma (KS) in apparently immunocompetent homosexuals heralded the current pandemic of HIV infection and its ultimate sequela, acquired immune deficiency syndrome (AIDS). By 1983 the cause was identified as a human retrovirus, human immunodeficiency virus (HIV), which causes a progressive impairment of cell-mediated immunity. The resultant severe immunocompromise leads to many opportunistic infections, neoplastic growths and premature death.

HIV infection is pandemic but most prevalent in North, Central and South America, the Caribbean, Tropical Africa and South East Asia. It occurs in homosexual and bisexual males, i.v. drug abusers (IVDA), heterosexual contacts of infected patients, children born to infected females and recipients of infected blood and blood products, particularly haemophiliacs.

HIV infection is spread by the venereal route, blood and blood product infusions, close contact with body fluids, and by blood-contaminated needles and syringes. It is not spread by ordinary social or domestic contact.

The incubation period is variable. The time from infection to detection of the antibody to HIV is 1–3 months. The time from infection to development of an AIDS-defining infection or tumour is 2 months to more than 10 years. Patients are infectious to others throughout but may be more so in the acute early stage and in the terminal stages of AIDS.

Pathology

HIV preferentially infects cells expressing the CD4 epitope, the T helper cell identity molecule. CD4-positive macrophages and monocytes are also susceptible to HIV infection. The CD4-positive lymphocytes are gradually and progressively depleted (Fig. 15.1)

Clinical classification

The Center for Disease Control (CDC) classifies HIV infection as:

Group I   Acute HIV infection
Group II   Asymptomatic
Group III   Persistent generalised lymphadenopathy
Group IV   Other diseases
Subgroup A   Constitutional (AIDS-related complex or ARC)
         B   Neurologic
         C   Infectious diseases
         D   Secondary cancers
         E   Other conditions

Group I (acute HIV infection)

Acute illness may occur within 2–3 weeks of primary exposure to HIV,

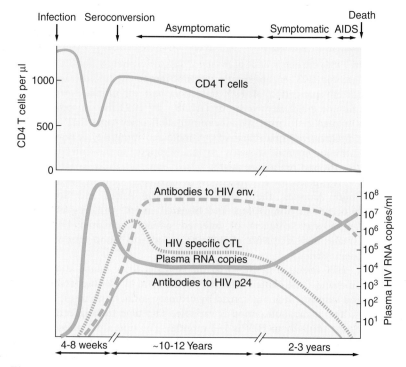

Fig. 15.1 The course of HIV-1 infection and disease.

presenting as either an acute infectious mononucleosis type illness or as an acute neurological disease (meningitis, meningoencephalitis, polyneuropathy).

Symptoms and signs
Fever, sweats, rigors, myalgia, arthralgia, headache, malaise, neck stiffness and sore throat may all be present as may lymphadenopathy, splenomegaly, pharyngeal erythema, palatal ulceration and a macular erythematous rash on the trunk.

Investigations
Measurement of 'viral load' by polymerase chain reaction (PCR) testing for HIV RNA is the investigation of choice but HIV antibodies remain the standard screening test. Lymphopenia, thrombocytopenia, atypical lymphocytes in blood film, mild liver dysfunction and CSF lymphocytosis may be present.

Differential diagnosis
EBV, CMV, toxoplasmosis, *Treponema pallidum*, rubella, HSV, hepatitis B and other causes of lymphocytic meningitis.

Treatment
Treatment is symptomatic.

Prognosis
Resolution is within 2–3 weeks. Lymphadenopathy, splenomegaly, lethargy, myalgia and fever may last several months. Patients remain HIV-infected for life, ultimately with the development of AIDS.

Group II (asymptomatic HIV-seropositive)

This group is characterised by the absence of symptoms and signs of HIV infection. However, identifiable leucopenia, thrombocytopenia and diminished CD4 count may be present.

Group III (persistent generalised lymphadenopathy)

This group is defined as the presence of palpable lymphadenopathy at two or more extra-inguinal sites, persisting for more than 3 months, in the absence of other illness or condition which could explain the findings.

Pathology
Follicular hyperplasia develops early in HIV infection, often within months of seroconversion.

Differential diagnosis
Lymphadenopathic KS, Hodgkin's lymphoma, non-Hodgkin's lymphoma, toxoplasmosis, *Mycobacterium avium* complex infection, angioimmunoblastic lymphadenopathy.

Group IV

This is subdivided into:

Subgroup A (constitutional symptoms (ARC)). One or more of the following will be present: fever for > 1 month, weight loss of more than 10% of initial bodyweight, diarrhoea for > 1 month, the absence of a concurrent illness or condition other than HIV infection.

Subgroup B (neurologic disease). For the CDC classification the indicated diseases are dementia, myelopathy and peripheral neuropathy.

Subgroup C1 (secondary infectious diseases). PCP, cryptosporidiosis, toxoplasmosis, extraintestinal strongyloidiasis, isosporiasis, candidiasis (oesophageal, bronchial, pulmonary), cryptococcosis, histoplasmosis, mycobacterial infection (*MAC, M. Kansasii*), CMV, severe HSV infection, progressive multifocal leucoencephalopathy (polyoma JC virus).

Subgroup C2. Oral hairy leukoplakia, polydermatomal HVZ, recurrent *Salmonella* bacteraemia, nocardiosis, tuberculosis, oral candidiasis.

Subgroup D (secondary cancers). Kaposi's sarcoma, non-Hodgkin's lymphoma, primary lymphoma of the brain.

Subgroup E (other conditions). Chronic lymphoid interstitial pneumonitis, infectious diseases and neoplasms not listed in subgroups C and D, respectively.

Treatment of HIV infection and its complications (see Tables 15.4 and 15.5)

Specific anti-HIV therapy. Combination anti-retroviral therapy—two nucleoside analogues plus a protease inhibitor—is recommended for HIV-infected patients with symptomatic HIV disease, patients with low or rapidly declining CD4 lymphocyte counts and patients with a 'viral load' in excess

Table 15.4. Specific anti-HIV treatment

Class	Drug name
Nucleoside analogue reverse transcriptase inhibitor	Zidovudine (AZT) Zalcitabine (ddC) Didanosine (ddI) Stavudine (D4T) Lamivudine (3TC)
HIV proteinase inhibitor or protease inhibitor	Saquinavir Ritonavir Indinavir Nelfinavir
Non-nucleoside reverse transcriptase inhibitor	Nevirapine

Table 15.5. Treatment of opportunistic infections

PCP*	High-dose co-trimoxazole, i.v. corticosteroids
Tuberculosis	Rifampicin ± isoniazid ± pyrazinamide ± ethambutol
MAI	Ethambutol + clarithromycin + rifabutin
Cat scratch disease (bacillary epithelioid angiomatosis)	Erythromycin
Syphilis	Penicillin
Cytomegalovirus*	i.v. ganciclovir, i.v. foscarnet
Fungi—disseminated*	i.v. amphotericin ± flucytosine, itraconazole
Salmonellosis*	Ciprofloxacin
Giardiasis	Metronidazole
Isosporiasis*	Co-trimoxazole
Cryptosporidiosis	Nothing effective, ?spiramycin
Toxoplasmosis*	Sulphadiazine + pyrimethamine

*Many opportunistic infections require long-term therapy to prevent relapse.

of 5 000–10 000 HIV RNA copies/ml. Ideal management remains to be defined by clinical trial.

Prophylaxis against opportunistic infection. PCP is prevented with inhaled pentamidine, monthly, and oral co-trimoxazole, daily. Acyclovir will prevent HSV and HVZ infections.

Candidiasis is controlled with topical nystatin/amphotericin or oral fluconazole.

Other clinical manifestations of HIV infection (see Tables 15.6–15.10).

Treatment of HIV-related Kaposi's sarcoma

Local therapy comprises radiation (800 cGy single dose), cryotherapy (liquid nitrogen) and intralesional chemotherapy (vinblastine).

Systemic therapy is with vincristine, vinblastine, etoposide (VP16), adriamycin, bleomycin and liposomal daunorubicin or alpha-interferon.

Table 15.6. HIV infection and the lower respiratory tract

Disease	Clinical manifestation	Chest X-ray
Pneumocystis carinii pneumonia (PCP)	Chronic pneumonia cough, dyspnoea, fever, cyanosis	Normal, focal infiltrate, interstitial infiltrate
Mycobacterium tuberculosis		
Early	Cough, fever	Upper lobe (alveolar infiltrate)
Late	Cough, fever	Hilar and mediastinal lymphadenopathy

Table 15.6 cont. HIV infection and the lower respiratory tract

Disease	Clinical manifestation	Chest X-ray
Atypical mycobacteria	Cough, fever, weight loss	Diffuse interstitial infiltrate or normal
Viral, e.g. CMV	Cough, fever	Interstitial infiltrate
Fungi (*Aspergillus*, *Cryptococcus*, *Histoplasma*)	Fever	Diffuse, nodular infiltrate Single nodules
Pyogenic bacteria (*Strep. pyogenes*, *Staph. aureus*, *Haemophilus*, *Moraxella*, *Legionella*)	Cough, fever, pleuritic pain	Consolidation Pleural effusion
Kaposi's sarcoma		Nodular infiltrate Pleural effusion Lymphadenopathy
Lymphoma	Fever, weight loss	Pleural effusion
Chronic lymphoid interstitial pneumonitis	Cough, dyspnoea	Interstitial infiltrate

Table 15.7. Dermatological manifestations of HIV infection

Infectious disorders	
Bacterial	*Staph. aureus*—bullous impetigo, ecthyma, folliculitis, hidradenitis, abscess, cellulitis Primary and secondary syphilis Bacillary angiomatosis (cat scratch bacillus *Rochalimaea bartonella*)
Viral	Chronic persistent HSV, I and II Recurrent polydermatomal VZV (shingles) Molluscum contagiosum—pox virus Warts—human papilloma virus
Mycobacteria (atypical)	Ulceration Pustules, nodules—MAI
Fungi (yeasts)	Intertrigo—*Tinea* Chronic fungal paronychia Nodules, pustules of systemic fungal infection Seborrhoeic dermatitis Ectoparasites—scabies
Non-infective disorders	Drug eruptions Kaposi's sarcoma

Table 15.8. Gastrointestinal disease and HIV infection

Mouth	Oropharyngeal candidiasis Herpes simplex, herpes varicella zoster, hairy leukoplakia Papilloma virus, periodontitis, gingivitis, recurrent aphthous ulcers, Kaposi's sarcoma, non-Hodgkin's lymphoma
Oesophagus (dysphagia, pain on swallowing)	Candidiasis, herpes simplex, CMV, aphthous ulcers
Stomach	Kaposi's sarcoma, non-Hodgkin's lymphoma
Hepatobiliary disease	Acalculous cholecystitis, gangrenous cholecystitis, granulomatous hepatitis, TB, chronic hepatitis B, sclerosing cholangitis (*Cryptosporidium*), hepatitis C

Table 15.9. Bowel disease and HIV infection

Malabsorption, diarrhoea, abdominal pain ± fever	*Salmonella, Shigella, Campylobacter* *Giardia intestinalis, Isopora belli,* *Cryptosporidium* Microsporidiosis, Encephalitozoon CMV *Mycobacterium avium* *Strongyloides* AIDS enteropathy
Proctocolitis, diarrhoea ± blood and slime, fever	CMV colitis, herpes simplex, *Chlamydia,* *Cryptosporidium*, MAI, *Entamoeba* histolytica, rectal gonorrhoea, *Treponema* *pallidum*

Table 15.10. CNS manifestations of HIV infection

Brain	Primary HIV infection—meningoencephalitis
	AIDS dementia complex
	Opportunistic CNS infection:
	Toxoplasma gondii encephalitis
	Cryptococcal meningitis
	Progressive multifocal leucoencephalopathy (polyoma JC virus)
	Herpes simplex encephalitis
	Fungal abscess
	Neurosyphilis
	Mycobacterium tuberculosis tuberculoma
	CMV ventriculitis
	Neoplasms
	Primary CNS lymphoma
	Metastatic lymphoma
	Kaposi's sarcoma
	Stroke disease
	Embolic—marantic endocarditis
	Thrombotic—vasculitis, lupus anticoagulant
	Haemorrhagic—thrombocytopenia
Spinal cord	Vacuolar myelopathy—sensory disturbance, gait instability, hyperreflexia
	Acute myelopathy—lymphomatous compression, TB spinal abscess, herpes zoster myelitis
Peripheral nerves	Distal symmetrical polyneuropathy—sensory glove/stocking numbness, paraesthesiae, dysaesthesiae (late onset)
	Inflammatory neuropathies—early onset, patchy motor and sensory
	Lumbosacral polyradiculopathy—CMV
Muscle	Polymyositis—proximal muscles, wasting, marked fatigue, pain
	Zidovudine-related—rare

16

GENITOURINARY MEDICINE

A. Jane Scott, Patrick K. Taylor

Sexually transmitted diseases (STD) are conditions transmitted during sexual intercourse or close sexual contact. The scope of genitourinary medicine (GUM) has expanded to include several other conditions not necessarily sexually transmitted. Despite worldwide increases in many of these diseases, the position in the UK remains fairly satisfactory, mainly because of the service established in 1917 as a result of the Venereal Diseases Regulations Act. Unlike most other hospital departments, patients may attend without a referral letter and confidentiality is still legally enforced under the updated 1974 Act.

The spectrum of disease has shifted in the last few years from bacterial to viral infections and Fig. 16.1 indicates current proportions of disease seen. Changing disease patterns are regularly monitored by the Department of Health. Current figures, between 1994 and 1995, show major concern regarding chlamydial infection, which increased by 7%, and wart virus

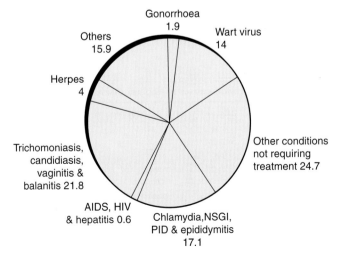

Fig. 16.1 Approximate proportions of disease seen in genitourinary clinics, 1995.

infection, first attacks of which rose by 5%. After an average annual fall of 17% over the last 3 years, cases of gonorrhoea have risen again by 5%. However, new cases of first attack genital herpes fell by 2%, the first annual fall since 1989. Partner notification (contact tracing) remains an important control aspect of asymptomatic carriers within the sexually active population. This must be coupled with health education and the urging of groups at increased risk, e.g. prostitutes, to attend for regular examination. Control of all these diseases depends upon good medical management, including accurate diagnosis, effective treatment and follow-up, contact tracing and a period of sexual abstinence during treatment.

VAGINAL DISCHARGE

Vaginal discharge is the most frequent presenting complaint in women. Investigation of STD in women is by taking swabs for culture, Gram-stained smears and a wet preparation in saline. A high vaginal specimen alone will readily identify the common causes of vaginitis (Table 16.1) but an endo-cervical specimen is necessary to detect both gonorrhoea and Chlamydia. The organisms responsible for these two infections also colonise the urethra and specimens from this site significantly increase pick-up rates. The three most common causes of vaginal discharge are summarised in Table 16.2. Where the history is unclear or urinary pathology suspected, a midstream specimen of urine (MSU) is of additional help. Women with STD have an increased risk of developing cervical intraepithelial neoplasia (CIN) and regular cervical cytological screening should be ensured.

Both male and female patients presenting with genital ulceration should have exudate from the lesion examined by darkfield microscopy for *Treponema pallidum* and a viral culture sent for herpes simplex. It is a wise precaution to take blood for syphilis serology not only in these patients but in all clinic attenders, especially if prescribing antitreponemal antibiotics.

Having performed the above investigations it is justifiable to prescribe antibiotics without awaiting the results of the laboratory tests, should the clinical picture indicate necessity for immediate treatment.

Table 16.1. Common causes of vaginal discharge

Physiological	Sexual stimulation, ectropion
Traumatic	
Physical	Self inflicted
Chemical	Douching
Infective	*Candida, Trichomonas, Gardnerella,* gonorrhoea, non-specific, puerperal, atrophic vaginitis, retained tampon
Candida often secondary to pregnancy, diabetes, antibiotics	
Neoplastic	
Benign	Polyp
Malignant	Carcinoma of cervix or corpus uteri

Table 16.2. The three most common causes of vaginal discharge

	Candida albicans	Gardnerella vaginalis (Bacterial vaginosis)	Trichomonas vaginalis
Cause	Fungus	Bacterium	Protozoon
Incubation	12–24 hours	24–48 hours	7–28 days
Symptoms			
Dysuria	Often	Occasional	Often
Discharge	White, thick, 'cheesy' odourless	Yellow, thin, frothy, malodorous	Yellow, thin profuse, malodorous
Irritation	Present	Absent	Often
Signs			
Vulvitis	Often	Absent	Often
Cervicitis	Often	Often	Usually
Investigations	Gram-smear, culture, check for glycosuria	Gram-smear, culture	Wet smear, culture
Treatment	Local cream and pessaries, e.g. clotrimazole, oral antifungals, e.g. fluconazole	Metronidazole Clindamycin cream	Metronidazole
Male contacts	Dysuria, balanitis, phimosis Treat	Asymptomatic, balanitis No treatment	Asymptomatic carrier Treat

URETHRAL DISCHARGE

Gonorrhoea, an infection with *Neisseria gonorrhoeae*, and non-gonococcal urethritis comprise most cases of sexually transmitted urethral discharge in men (Table 16.3); 50% of non-gonococcal cases are caused by *Chlamydia trachomatis*. Microscopy of a Gram-stained smear can differentiate gonococcal from non-gonococcal urethritis with 90% accuracy. A urethral swab for gonorrhoea and a specimen for Chlamydia should also be sent for microbiological examination. First-voided urine samples provide a very effective method of diagnosis for chlamydial urethritis. A sub-prepucial smear may demonstrate *Candida* or anaerobes.

Symptoms and signs

Incubation is 1–10 days in gonorrhoea and 7–14 days in Chlamydia. Only 5% of infected men are asymptomatic. Most men develop dysuria and mucoid or purulent urethral discharge. Proctitis is common in homosexuals. Pharyngitis may occur where oral intercourse is involved.

Gonorrhoea is asymptomatic in 70% of women and Chlamydia in 90%.

Table 16.3. Common causes of urethral discharge

Physiological	Prostatorrhoea
Traumatic	
Physical	Masturbation
Chemical	Alcohol
Infective	
Gonococcal	
Non-gonococcal (NGU)	
NSU	Chlamydial or non-chlamydial
Other	*Trichomonas, Candida, Gardnerella,* viral, e.g. herpes, secondary to urinary tract infection (UTI), urethral stricture
Neoplastic (uncommon)	Urethral lesions

There may be dysuria or vaginal discharge. Diagnosis should always be confirmed bacteriologically.

Complications

These are comparatively rare and can be prevented by effective early treatment. Local complications include prostatitis, acute epididymitis, periurethral abscess, urethral stricture and urethrophobia (constant fear of infection) in men.

Ascending infection gives rise to pelvic inflammatory disease (PID), which is the most serious complication for women, and 10% will present evidence of involvement of one or both fallopian tubes, usually subacutely. Lower abdominal pain and tenderness is present with thickening and tenderness of the affected tube. Infertility can follow bilateral PID due to fibrosis, leading to tubal blockage. Differential diagnosis is ectopic pregnancy, and torsion of an ovarian cyst.

Ophthalmia neonatorum is a complication in neonates. Both gonorrhoea and Chlamydia are transmitted during birth, and the infected baby will develop conjunctivitis 2–10 days later.

Systemic complications of gonorrhoea include arthritis, septicaemia and endocarditis. Those of chlamydial infection are perihepatitis (Fitz Hugh–Curtis syndrome) and cervical dysplasia. NGU can lead to Reiter's disease (Ch. 12).

Investigations

Men should not micturate for 3 hours prior to urethral tests.

1. Gram-stained smears and cultures for gonorrhoea from the urethra in men, and the cervix and urethra in women.
2. Enzyme-linked immunosorbent assay (ELISA) for Chlamydia.
3. Wet vaginal smear and culture for *Trichomonas vaginalis* in women.
4. Smears and cultures from other sites if indicated, e.g. rectum, pharynx.

Treatment

Penicillin is the drug of choice in gonorrhoea giving over 90% cure rates. A suggested schedule is amoxycillin 3 g stat orally with 1 g probenecid (to delay excretion). If there is penicillin allergy or non-treponemicidal therapy is required, ciprofloxacin 500 mg orally stat or spectinomycin 2 g i.m. stat is suitable.

Beta-lactamase-producing *N. gonorrhoeae* strains appear from abroad occasionally. These produce the enzyme beta-lactamase which destroys penicillin. Drugs of choice for these strains are ciprofloxacin 500 mg orally stat, spectinomycin 2 g i.m. stat or cefuroxime 1.5 g i.m. stat. *All* patients are then treated with oxytetracycline 500 mg 6-hourly for 1 week.

Fifty per cent of all patients with gonorrhoea develop post-gonococcal urethritis (PGU), which is NGU occurring concomitantly with gonorrhoea. Most chlamydial and non-specific urethritis (NSU) infections respond to tetracyclines. The suggested schedule is oxytetracycline tablets 250 mg 6-hourly for 10 days. Erythromycin 500 mg 6-hourly for 14 days should be used in pregnancy or tetracycline allergy. Ofloxacin 200 mg 12-hourly for 10 days may be used as an alternative. Consorts of patients with non-specific infection should be treated routinely after exclusion of other infection.

PID should be treated with doxycycline 100 mg b.d. for a minimum of 2 weeks and metronidazole 400 mg b.d. for 5 days following treatment for gonorrhoea if necessary.

Prognosis

Reinfection with *N. gonorrhoeae* and *C. trachomatis* after successful treatment occurs as many contacts are not traced. Relapses of NSU often occur for no apparent reason.

GENITAL WARTS (CONDYLOMATA ACUMINATA)

Genital warts are usually caused by sexual transmission of the human papilloma virus (HPV). There are over 50 types of HPV, four of these (types 6, 11, 16 and 18) showing preferential tropism for the genitoanal area. Types 6 and 11 occur mainly in benign lesions, and only rarely in cervical carcinoma, while with types 16 and 18 the reverse is true. Warts fall into three clinical types (acuminate, papular and flat) although there is often transition between them. The mean incubation is about 3 months.

The argument continues as to whether genital warts cause cancer. The evidence to date is only suggestive of a role in CIN and little else. It is possible that HPV and smoking acting as co-factors may have some role.

Symptoms and signs

Initially small lesions are often encouraged by discharge, and increase in size becoming filiform or hyperplastic.

Investigations

Routine cervical cytology and colposcopy if the cytology is abnormal.

Differential diagnosis

Condylomata lata, molluscum contagiosum, anal skin tags and haemorrhoids.

Basis of treatment

The predisposing causes, e.g. discharge, should be removed. Trichloracetic acid or podophyllotoxin can be applied locally.

Cryotherapy, using a metal probe or liquid nitrogen spray, or electro-cautery may be used for severe cases.

Sexual contacts should also be examined.

Prognosis

Treatment may be prolonged and recurrences occur.

HERPES GENITALIS

Genital herpes is usually sexually transmitted. Most infections are caused by herpes simplex virus type 2 but type 1 infections, usually associated with oral cold sores, are not uncommon.

In common with other herpes viruses, herpes simplex exhibits a degree of latency when, following the initial attack, the virus quickly reaches the dorsal root ganglion, where it lies dormant. Recurrent episodes may occur by reactivation of the virus from this site.

Symptoms and signs

Following 4–5 days' incubation, prodromal itching or burning may occur at any genital site, preceding groups of vesicles which form painful ulcers. These become larger erosions which crust over before healing after 2–3 weeks. Painful regional lymphadenopathy occurs in 20% of cases.

Complications

These include urethritis, cervicitis, proctitis, urinary retention and dissemi-nated infections (more severe in immunocompromised subjects). Most patients suffer recurrent episodes (less severe than the initial attack) due to reactivation of the virus. Known trigger mechanisms for this are stress, illness (especially viral), trauma, photosensitivity (avoid sun beds or solariums). Many recurrences have no obvious precipitating factor. Frequency and duration of attacks vary, decreasing over several years and eventually ceasing completely.

Neonatal infection may occur if maternal lesions are present at birth. Transmission is during birth resulting in dermatitis, meningitis or encepha-litis, which can lead to brain damage. This is very rare in the UK and, with careful monitoring around term, a decision to perform caesarean section is sometimes taken to exclude fetal risk.

Investigations

Viral culture, darkfield examination and cervical cytology.

Differential diagnosis

Table 16.4 shows the common causes of genital ulceration.

Table 16.4. Common causes of genital ulceration

Herpes	Erosive balanitis	Tropical STD (chancroid, donovaniasis, lymphogranuloma venereum)
Syphilis (primary, secondary, tertiary)	Behçet's syndrome (orogenital ulceration)	
Trauma	Lipschutz ulcer	Carcinoma
Candida	Drug eruptions	

Basis of treatment

In primary attacks, the treatment of choice (if started within 5 days of onset) is aciclovir 200 mg five times daily for 5 days. Two further antiviral drugs have recently been introduced, famciclovir and valaciclovir (metabolised to aciclovir), which have a less frequent dosage regimen. Attention to hygiene using normal saline bathing to prevent secondary infection and analgesia with paracetamol or anaesthetic creams is usually also necessary.

In recurrent cases many patients require no treatment; others do well using only anaesthetic cream and saline bathing. For patients with a prodrome, episodic aciclovir tablet therapy may be used for each attack but in patients suffering severe attacks every 4–6 weeks, continuous prophylaxis is available with aciclovir tablets, the dosage titrated to levels just preventing attacks. The newer antivirals (famciclovir and valaciclovir) may prove more effective and acceptable to patients due to longer intervals between doses.

Most patients have little trouble from recurrent episodes but some become bitter, angry or obsessed with the disease, resulting in severe psychological problems which require counselling.

SYPHILIS

Syphilis is a sexually transmitted infection caused by the spirochaete *T. pallidum* acquired on direct contact with an early lesion. The incubation period is 9–90 days. Since treponemes are present in the surface lesions of early (but not late) syphilis, it is infectious only in the primary, secondary (following initial dissemination of treponemes to all body tissues) and early latent stages (Table 16.5).

The essential process is that of an endarteritis obliterans leading to erosion of the surface of the lesion.

Latent syphilis

This follows the untreated secondary stage lasting between 2 years and a lifetime (average 10–15 years). There are no clinical signs, the diagnosis being made on serological grounds. Ultimately, routine serological tests may only be weakly positive or even negative.

Table 16.5. Stages of syphilis and their main symptoms

Stage	Symptoms
Acquired	
Early infectious (first 2 years of infection)	
Primary	Chancre (painless, indurated, ulcer), lymphadenopathy (local, painless, rubbery), rectal or vaginal chancres may not be noticed
Secondary (6–8 weeks after primary)	Malaise, mild pyrexia, lymphadenitis, rash (dull red/coppery maculopapular, non-itchy, often on palms and soles; can mimic any other rash), condylomata lata (fleshy warty lesions), mucous patches (oro-genital ulcers), moth-eaten alopecia
Early latent	No clinical signs, serology +ve, mucocutaneous relapses can occur
Late non-infectious (3–40 years after initial infection)	
Late latent	No clinical signs, serology +ve
Tertiary	Gumma
Cardiovascular syphilis	Aortic incompetence, aortic aneurysm, coronary ostial stenosis
Neurosyphilis	Tabes dorsalis, general paralysis of the insane, meningovascular
Congenital	
Early infectious (first 2 years of life, there is no primary stage)	
Symptomatic	Rash, mucous patches, condylomata lata, snuffles (nasal discharge, obstruction), failure to thrive, hepatosplenomegaly, periostitis, lymphadenopathy, meningitis
Latent	No clinical signs, serology +ve
Latent non-infectious (aged 2 years onwards)	
Latent	With or without stigmata
Symptomatic	(as for acquired infection)
	Gummatous (especially palate), cardiovascular, CNS
Stigmata (residual abnormalities due to early or late congential infections presenting in later life)	
	Interstitial keratitis, Hutchinson's teeth, eighth nerve deafness, facial bone deformities

Differential diagnosis

Dermatoses, in secondary syphilis, and other causes of genital ulcers (see Table 16.4).

Investigations

Darkfield microscopy is used to identify *T. pallidum* in serous exudate. Later stages need confirmation using serological tests (Table 16.6): VDRL

Table 16.6. Current serological tests for syphilis

VDRL	TPHA	FTA-Abs	Probable diagnosis
+	–	–	Biological false positive (BFP) Repeat to exclude primary syphilis
+	–	+	Primary syphilis (? positive darkfield)
+	+	+	Secondary syphilis or beyond (usually untreated) VDRL titres often high in secondary syphilis
–	+	+	Treated, partially treated or past history of treated syphilis

Similar patterns occur in yaws, bejel and pinta

VDRL = venereal disease research laboratory test; TPHA = *T. pallidum* haemagglutination assay; FTA-Abs = fluorescent treponemal antibody absorption test.

for non-specific anti-treponemal antibodies, and TPHA and FTA-Abs for specific antibodies to pathogenic treponemes.

In latent and late syphilis, CSF examination (to exclude neurosyphilis) and X-ray of the chest (to exclude cardiovascular changes) and long bones are often advised.

Late syphilis

This is now relatively rare as effective early treatment halts progression of the disease. In 35% of untreated patients clinical signs of late syphilis will develop between 3 and 40 years after the initial infection. Fifteen per cent will develop tertiary syphilitic ulcers (gummata), 10% neurosyphilis, 10% cardiovascular syphilis and the remainder will continue as non-infectious latent cases.

Congenital syphilis

Routine antenatal blood tests and treatment of women during pregnancy has made congenital syphilis rare in the UK. It is most commonly seen in early maternal infections and placental transmission to the fetus takes place after the fourth month of pregnancy. If the mother is treated soon enough this usually treats the fetus at the same time.

Stages are similar to acquired syphilis but there is no primary stage. Investigations are as for acquired syphilis.

Treatment

The treatment of choice is procaine penicillin 1.2 megaunits i.m. daily for 14 days in early syphilis increasing to 21 days in late syphilis. Doxycycline or erythromycin may be used but for a longer duration in cases of penicillin allergy.

Fifty per cent of patients with early syphilis develop the Jarisch–Herxheimer reaction, of uncertain origin, about 6 hours after the first injection only, consisting of fever, malaise, headache and often rigors, lasting only a few hours. Patients should be warned of this. It is less frequent but may be more serious in late syphilis, therefore small doses of prednisone are given for 24 hours preceding and 2 days after the first injection to prevent this occurring.

In congenital syphilis babies should be given 200 000 units penicillin per 450 g bodyweight divided over a period of 10 days. Adults are treated as for late acquired syphilis.

Clinical and serological follow-up should be continued for at least 2 years.

Prognosis
In early syphilis the cure rate approaches 100% in patients who become serologically negative and remain so for 2 years.

HEPATITIS B VIRUS INFECTION (see Ch. 9)

HIV INFECTION AND AIDS (see Ch. 14)

17

ADVERSE DRUG REACTIONS AND ACUTE POISONING

Clive J. C. Roberts

ADVERSE DRUG REACTIONS

An adverse drug reaction is any unwanted effect resulting from a drug's use in treatment. This definition excludes deliberate and accidental overdose.

Common examples of drug reactions include nausea with digoxin therapy, bronchospasm with beta-adrenoceptor blockers, ataxia and drowsiness with phenytoin, bleeding with warfarin, dry cough with angiotensin-converting enzyme (ACE) inhibitors, cholestatic jaundice with chlorpromazine, gastric ulcer with non-steroidal anti-inflammatory drugs (NSAIDs) and morbilliform rash with ampicillin. *Most drug reactions mimic naturally occurring conditions and are consequently difficult to detect early in drug development.* Occasionally drugs cause specific conditions not previously recorded, e.g. the eosinophilic myalgic syndrome caused by tryptophan and the oculomucocutaneous syndrome caused by practolol. These also often go undetected because they are of low incidence and totally unexpected.

Epidemiology

Adverse drug reactions account for 4% of hospital admissions, 1 in 1000 deaths in medical wards and occur in 10–20% of in-patients. In general practice it is estimated that adverse reactions may occur in up to 5% of patients. They are more frequent in patients aged over 65 years because:

1. functional impairment leads to erratic drug taking
2. multiple pathology attracts polypharmacy
3. decreased hepatic and renal capacity leads to relative drug accumulation
4. impaired CNS and CVS function leads to increased sensitivity to drug effects.

The drugs most commonly implicated are oral anticoagulants, NSAIDs, corticosteroids, anti-hypertensives, antibiotics, diuretics and insulin.

Drug reactions result from specific sets of circumstances relating to the drug's pharmacology, to predisposing features in the patient and to the care taken in choosing the right drug at the right dose.

CLASSIFICATION

Predictable reactions (type A):

1. can be predicted from the known pharmacology of the drug
2. may be common within pharmacological groups
3. are due either to excessive action at the target receptor or to action at a non-target receptor (Table 17.1)
4. are related closely to the amount of drug in the body
5. are determined by dose and by pharmacokinetic and pharmacodynamic factors (e.g. greatly reduced dose of warfarin needed in liver disease)
6. are common, accounting for 75% or more of all adverse effects
7. are largely avoidable with care.

In unpredictable (type B) reactions:

1. the effect is unrelated to established pharmacological effects
2. the effect may not be shared within pharmacological groups
3. the effect may be serious organ damage (e.g. pulmonary fibrosis with sulphasalazine)
4. there is a poor relationship to dose
5. they are uncommon and difficult to detect in drug development
6. they cannot be avoided if the drug is used (Table 17.2)
7. patient idiosyncrasy is a major factor.

Type A and B reactions account for the major commonly encountered adverse effects. However, some reactions depend on dose but are not obviously related to their pharmacological effects (Table 17.3), e.g. ototoxicity with streptomycin and nausea with digoxin. Some therefore prefer

---

Table 17.1. Some examples of predictable drug reactions

Excessive therapeutic effect	
Bone marrow depression	Azathioprine
Syncope	ACE inhibitors
Heart block	Digoxin
Hypoglycaemia	Chlorpropamide
Poor wound healing	Corticosteroids
Cardiac arrhythmias	Thyroxine
Effect at non-target receptor	
Micturition difficulty	Amitriptyline
Tremor	Salbutamol
Renal impairment	ACE inhibitors
Diabetes	Corticosteroids
Asthma	Beta-blockers
Constipation	Verapamil
Diarrhoea	Misoprostol

Table 17.2. Some examples of unpredictable drug reactions (with incidences where known)

Retroperitoneal fibrosis (1/250)	Methysergide
Pseudomembranous colitis (1/1000–1/10 000)	Clindamycin
Aplastic anaemia (1/6000)	Chloramphenicol
Jaundice (1/10 000)	Halothane
Deep venous thrombosis (1/10 000) ⎫	Combined oral
Myocardial infarction (1/10 000) ⎬	contraceptive
Pulmonary embolism (1/20 000) ⎭	
Aplastic anaemia (1/10 000–1/20 000)	Phenylbutazone
Cholestatic hepatitis (2/100)	Chlorpromazine
Myositis	Simvastatin
Visual impairment (1/200)	Ethambutol
Hepatic damage	Amiodarone
Marrow suppression	Mianserin

Table 17.3. Some examples of drug reactions that are difficult to classify

Gastric erosions	Aspirin and NSAIDs
Azoospermia	Sulphasalazine
Oral candida infection	Inhaled corticosteroids
Hyponatraemia	Carbamazepine
Dystonia and dyskinesia	Metoclopramide
Unproductive cough	ACE inhibitors

to consider reactions as simply dose-dependent or dose-independent. Even this classification fails. For example the blood abnormalities and proteinuria that occurred in a small percentage of patients given captopril have now virtually disappeared following use of lower doses. Lupus syndrome caused by hydralazine, although rare, occurs when high doses are used in poor metabolisers of the drug.

Fetal abnormality

Teratogenic drugs cause abnormalities of structural development of the fetus if given during the first 3 months of pregnancy e.g. amelia and phocomelia (absent or deformed limbs) as caused by thalidomide. Teratogenic effects are difficult to detect and extreme caution must be exercised in using drugs during pregnancy.

Many drugs cross the placenta and exert an effect in the fetus that may be harmful (Table 17.4). Easily predicted effects are from warfarin, sul-

---

Table 17.4. Examples of drugs thought to be harmful in pregnancy

Known or suspected teratogens

Phenytoin, oral anticoagulants, griseofulvin	Various congenital malformations
Sodium valproate	Neural tube defects
Heparin	Osteoporosis
Tetracycline	Dental discoloration
Alkylating agents, methotrexate	High risk of congenital abnormalities
Penicillamine	Fetal abnormalities reported
Etretinate	Congenital abnormalities

Drugs causing adverse effects on the fetus

ACE inhibitors	Oligohydramnios, impaired renal function and hypotension
Streptokinase	Placental separation
Chlorpropamide	Neonatal hypoglycaemia
Benzodiazepines	Depressed neonatal respiration, drowsiness and hypotonia, withdrawal syndrome
Beta-blockers	Neonatal bradycardia
NSAIDs	Closure of ductus arteriosus in utero, possibly pulmonary hypertension, prolonged labour

---

phonylureas, carbimazole, corticosteroids, barbiturates and benzodiazepines. ACE inhibitors cause fetal death in some animal species and have caused oligohydramnios in human pregnancies as well as neonatal hypotension and renal failure.

Allergy and 'pseudoallergy'

Acute hypersensitivity reactions occur when release of histamine and other mediators follows the interaction of drug antigen and IgE antibody (B lymphocyte produced) on the surface of mast cells or circulating basophils. Rashes, oedema, bronchospasm and cardiovascular collapse may follow. Such reactions require previous exposure to the drug which, acting as a hapten, becomes antigenic after combining with a protein.

Serum sickness syndrome is a less acute form of reaction which results from the damaging effects of circulating immune complexes. IgG or IgM antibody combines with antigenic drug and, if present in excessive amounts, may lodge in blood vessels giving rise to systemic and local inflammation. Interstitial nephritis is a common manifestation.

Delayed hypersensitivity is T lymphocyte mediated, e.g. contact dermatitis.

Some drugs can produce a reaction that mimics allergy on first encounter. Aspirin and other NSAIDs, for example, are capable of causing release of histamine and other mediators in susceptible individuals without immuno-logical mechanisms being involved. The syndrome of flushing, urticaria, angio-oedema, rhinitis, asthma and hypotension can resemble anaphylaxis. This 'pseudoallergy' may follow the administration of morphine, barbiturates, radiographic contrast media and other agents.

Dependence and withdrawal reactions

Psychoactive agents such as the benzodiazepines and barbiturates cause tachyphylaxis, psychological and physical dependence and when stopped can cause a withdrawal syndrome ranging from anxiety and insomnia to delirium and convulsions.

Other drugs may cause problems when discontinued. For example myocardial ischaemia may occur if beta-adrenoceptor agents are stopped suddenly.

FACTORS PREDISPOSING TO DOSE-DEPENDENT REACTIONS

Pharmacokinetic variation leads to reduced blood concentrations and therapeutic failure, or elevated concentrations and adverse effects. Pharmacodynamic variation (sensitivity of the receptor to a given concentration of drug) will have a similar effect. Genetic factors, disease processes, drug interaction and ageing are the main sources of variation (Tables 17.5–17.8).

Increased bioavailability

This term describes the fraction of orally administered drug that arrives in the systemic circulation. It depends on pharmaceutical formulation, the fraction absorbed from the gastrointestinal tract and the proportion metabolised as it passes through the liver from the portal circulation (presystemic metabolism or 'first pass' effect). Drugs that are extensively and rapidly metabolised by the liver normally have reduced bioavailability. However, if that metabolism is impaired by enzyme inhibition (e.g. by cimetidine), liver disease or in the elderly or if blood is shunted around the liver, as in chronic liver disease, excessively high drug concentrations occur after oral administration (Table 17.6). This applies to certain beta-blockers, calcium-channel blockers, opioids, anti-depressants and sedatives.

Reduced hepatic clearance

The steady-state blood concentration of any drug is determined by the rate of clearance by its organ of elimination (usually the liver or kidney) irrespective of the distribution volume. Most liver injuries cause impairment of drug metabolism but inter-individual variation is so wide that changes may be minor. When synthetic function is impaired, as indicated by a fall in serum albumin or prolongation of clotting, serious drug accumulation of highly lipid-soluble agents may occur, e.g. CNS depressant drugs. Some drugs impair the clearance by the liver of others, e.g. cimetidine and azapropazone are both inhibitors of the metabolism of warfarin and phenytoin.

Table 17.5. Examples of adverse drug interactions with mechanisms

Reduced absorption
    of phenytoin   by sucralfate
    of digoxin   by cholestyramine

Increased bioavailability
    of levodopa   by metoclopramide
    of labetalol, propranolol, nifedipine and   by cimetidine
    nortriptyline

Decreased hepatic clearance
    of phenytoin, warfarin and tolbutamide   by azapropazone
    of theophylline, pethidine, chlormethiazole,   by cimetidine
    phenytoin, warfarin

Increased hepatic clearance
    of corticosteroids, warfarin, tolbutamide   by barbiturates, phenytoin,
    and the oral contraceptive   carbamazepine, rifampicin
                 and griseofulvin

Competition for renal excretion
    of chlorpropamide   by phenylbutazone
    of methotrexate   by probenecid and NSAIDs
    of digoxin   by quinidine

pH-dependent increase in renal excretion
    of aspirin   by antacids

Increased effects through electrolyte changes
    of digoxin   by diuretics
    of diuretics   by corticosteroids
    of spironolactone   by captopril

Increased effect by mutual potentiation at the target organ
    of beta-blockers   by verapamil
    of warfarin   by aspirin
    of anti-hypertensives   by nitrates
    of phenothiazines   by benzodiazepines

Decreased effect by mutual antagonism at the target organ
    of insulin and tolbutamide   by thiazide diuretics and
                 corticosteroids
    of levodopa   by phenothiazines
    of diuretics   by indomethacin
    of valproate   by phenothiazines
    of adrenergic neurone blockers   by tricyclic anti-depressants

Hypertensive crisis
    with MAOIs   and ephedrine etc. and
                 tyramine-containing foods
    with adrenaline   and beta-blockers

Table 17.6. Mechanisms of adverse drug effects in chronic liver disease with examples

Increased CNS sensitivity leading to risk of encephalopathy
  Morphine, benzodiazepines, phenothiazines
Impaired hepatic function leading to increased drug sensitivity
  Warfarin, chlorpropamide, aspirin
Exacerbation of fluid and electrolyte abnormalities
  Diuretics, NSAIDs, magnesium trisilicate mixture, carbenoxolone
Constipating agents leading to increased risk of encephalopathy
  Amitriptyline, codeine
Increased bioavailability due to reduced metabolic capacity and porto-systemic shunting
  Chlormethiazole, opioids, propranolol, labetalol, nifedipine, verapamil
Decreased elimination
  Phenytoin, theophylline, methotrexate
Possibly decreased protein binding
  Corticosteroids
Risk of hepatotoxicity leading to worsening of condition or diagnostic confusion
  Paracetamol, chlorpromazine, methyldopa, fusidic acid, simvastatin, monoamine oxidase inhibitors, etc.

A disproportionate rise in drug concentration of phenytoin can result from a small change in dose or minor inhibition of enzymes. Some metabolic pathways are under genetic control, e.g. acetylation of drugs such as hydralazine and isoniazid can be classified as slow and fast. Slow acetylators tend to experience adverse effects (lupus syndrome and peripheral neuropathy respectively) whilst fast acetylators may suffer therapeutic failure. There is also evidence for genetic polymorphism in determining some hepatic drug oxidising enzymes.

Increased hepatic clearance

Induction of enzymes by barbiturates, rifampicin, carbamazepine, phenytoin and others results in reduced levels of warfarin, sulphonylurea and other drugs. The result is decreased efficacy in the first place but if the dose has been titrated to the patient's requirement and the inducer is then stopped, overdosage may occur and cause bleeding or hypoglycaemia.

Impaired renal excretion

The clearance of many drugs is proportional to renal function. Dose adjustment in renal failure takes account of the therapeutic margin of the drug, the degree of renal failure, the need for a loading dose and the distribution volume together with any risks particular to the condition (Table 17.7). Renal function tails off with ageing and drug interaction may occur in the kidney.

Table 17.7. Mechanisms of adverse drug effects in chronic renal failure with examples

Impaired elimination leading to predictable drug toxicity	Amiodarone, atenolol, benzylpenicillin, digoxin, metformin, glibenclamide
Increased sensitivity	Anti-psychotics, opioids
Exacerbation of renal impairment	ACE inhibitors, acyclovir, aspirin, cisplatin, gentamicin, tetracycline, clofibrate
Exacerbation of metabolic derangement	Acetazolamide, carbenoxolone, loop diuretics, magnesium trisilicate mixture, NSAIDs, spironolactone
Increased incidence of rashes	Ampicillin, amoxycillin, pivampicillin, allopurinol, sulphonamides, sulphasalazine, nalidixic acid

Table 17.8. Some genetically determined drug reactions

Condition	Precipitating drugs	Adverse effect
Glucose-6-phosphate deficiency	Quinine, sulphonamides, nitrofurantoin, dapsone	Haemolysis
Porphyria (hepatic)	Barbiturates, griseofulvin	Attack precipitated
Malignant hyperpyrexia	Halothane, suxamethonium	Hyperthermia, muscle rigidity, acidosis
Trisomy 21	Atropine	Increased response

Increased drug sensitivity

The elderly may become confused by normal doses of sedative drugs or hypotensive in response to vasodilators. They bleed more frequently with aspirin and suffer bone marrow depression more readily with mianserin and co-trimoxazole. Diuretics cause more electrolyte abnormalities in the aged. Organ failure—cardiac, respiratory, renal and hepatic—creates conditions in which specific reactions to drugs may occur, e.g. sedating drugs should not be given to patients with ventilatory failure, calcium channel blockers may exacerbate cardiac failure, constipating drugs may be harmful in liver failure and potassium-retaining diuretics can be lethal in renal failure. Adverse drug interactions may also result in excessive drug sensitivity and some reactions are genetically determined (Table 17.8).

PREVENTING DRUG ADVERSE EFFECTS

The following principles of prescribing should reduce the risks:

1. assess the risk-to-benefit ratio when about to prescribe
2. identify pharmacokinetic and pharmacodynamic risk factors in the patient, e.g. liver disease, concurrent drugs, etc.
3. always ask about allergy
4. avoid drugs if possible in pregnant women or those seeking pregnancy
5. avoid polypharmacy in the elderly by establishing priorities
6. use new drugs only when the evidence for advantage is convincing
7. keep up to date with information in publications
8. explain to patients the objectives and possible consequences of treatment
9. stop drugs that have become unnecessary.

DETECTING DRUG ADVERSE EFFECTS

Adverse effect monitoring during early development and clinical trials of drugs cannot identify all risks. Post-marketing surveillance is mandatory. Detailed investigations should be made when a suspicious number of reports is received.

ACUTE POISONING

In 1994, 2378 people died in England and Wales from acute poisoning; of these, 1704 were confirmed suicides. Most of the remainder are likely to have been acts of self-harm although successful suicide may not have been intended. Amongst the drug overdoses, tricyclic antidepressants, paracetamol with or without dextropropoxyphene, and benzodiazepines are frequently recorded. Chlormethiazole, phenothiazines, morphine, diamorphine and methadone account for a significant number but salicylates are less commonly involved than previously. About 85% of the deaths occur outside hospital. Approximately 35% more women than men are admitted to hospital after poisoning but twice as many men than women die after poisoning. Suicidal and parasuicidal behaviour is common in teenagers and the incidence in the over 60-year-olds is twice that in the younger age groups. The peak incidence of death from poisoning is between the ages of 25 and 35 years.

As many as 20% of poisoned patients seen in A & E departments are not admitted. Acute poisoning has been called the 'modern epidemic' and most doctors will see numerous cases, virtually all of whom will be acts of self-harm.

Management of poisoning

Some poisonings (e.g. with chlormethiazole) are best treated by supportive measures. Others (e.g. with paracetamol) require administration of specific antidotes. In the UK, information on common poisonings is available in the *British National Formulary*, in specific texts and from the National Poisons Information Centres.

Principles

1. prevent further absorption of ingested poisons
2. sustain bodily functions and treat complications as they arise
3. administer antidotes or take measures to increase the elimination of the poison if appropriate
4. provide psychiatric or social assistance.

The order in which these principles are applied depends on the clinical state of the patient and the nature of the poison ingested.

Methods for reducing drug absorption

Gastric lavage and the administration of emetics retrieves a substantial amount of drug in only a small number of patients and then only when performed within 2 hours for most poisonings. These procedures are not without hazard. They should be employed only when a seriously toxic dose has been ingested within 2 hours or within 4 hours for salicylates, tricyclics or opiates, which delay gastric emptying. They are contraindicated in corrosive or petroleum distillate ingestion or in known oesophageal or gastric disease. Gastric lavage should not be performed in uncooperative patients because of the risk of oesophageal perforation. The only acceptable emetic is syrup of ipecacuanha and this must not be given to patients whose consciousness is impaired. Salt must not be used as fatal hypernatraemia is well documented.

Administration of chelating agents (e.g. desferrioxamine for iron poisoning) or adsorbents (e.g. Fuller's earth for paraquat ingestion) have major importance in preventing absorption. Recently the use of activated charcoal has increased because it dramatically reduces the absorption of many drugs if given within 1 hour and significantly reduces it if given later. It also has a place in increasing drug elimination (see below). Activated charcoal does not adsorb alcohols, inorganic acids or alkalis, iron or lithium.

Intensive supportive treatment

Specific therapies do not exist for many poisonings, particularly CNS depressants. Lives can be saved by careful monitoring of vital functions and provision of support and treatment of complications (Fig. 17.1). Level of consciousness, heart rate, blood pressure, respiration and state of peripheral perfusion should be recorded regularly. Good nursing care is essential. Hypothermia should be identified by rectal temperature measurement with a low reading thermometer. If minute respiratory volume falls below 4 litres and blood gas levels change, artificial ventilation should be undertaken. Hypotension should be dealt with by first ensuring ventilation and hydration are adequate. The foot of the bed should be raised and only if these measures fail should infusion of inotropic agents be considered. Cardiac arrhythmias, dystonias and convulsions should be managed conventionally.

Methods for increasing drug elimination

Forced diuresis is of no value and can be hazardous but urinary alkalinisa-

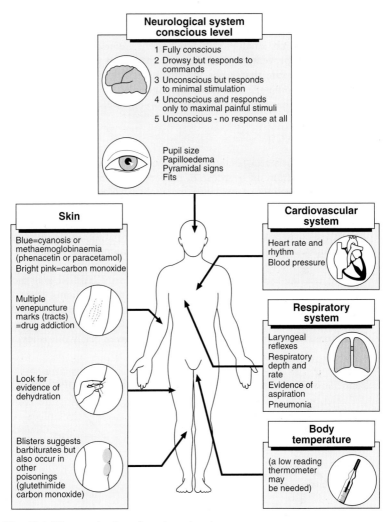

Fig. 17.1 The examination of a poisoned patient.

tion increases the elimination of aspirin and is a useful part of therapy (see below).

Dialysis and haemoperfusion may increase the clearance of the drug from the blood but this is meaningless for drugs with wide distribution as the actual amount of drugs removed is small. These techniques are therefore rarely used. Dialysis effectively removes salicylates, lithium, methanol and ethylene glycol. Haemoperfusion involves the passage of blood through an adsorbent material such as activated charcoal or a polystyrene resin. This technique removes barbiturates, carbamazepine, disopyramide and theophylline.

Repeat-dose activated charcoal enhances the non-renal elimination of many drugs. Not only drug which is secreted into bile, but also large amounts which diffuse into small intestinal secretions are held within the gut and their reabsorption prevented. Therefore for maximum efficacy, charcoal should be given at a rate that keeps the small intestine filled. The technique has been shown to be effective for poisonings with aspirin, theophylline, phenobarbitone, carbamazepine, digoxin, meprobamate, phenytoin and others.

PARACETAMOL

Hepatic necrosis and acute hepatic failure sometimes associated with renal failure result from an overdose of paracetamol, which is safe in therapeutic doses. The product of oxidative metabolism (N-acetyl benzoquinonimine) binds to hepatocyte proteins and damages the cell (Fig. 17.2). In normal doses this product is conjugated with glutathione and does no harm. In overdose the alternative metabolic pathways for paracetamol—sulphation and glucuronidation—become saturated and glutathione becomes depleted. Thus excessive amounts are produced and reduced amounts removed. Patients taking enzyme-inducing drugs, alcohol, the malnourished and those with pre-existing liver disease are at greater risk from paracetamol overdose. The two antidotes commonly used act as precursors to glutathione. N-acetyl cysteine must be given intravenously and causes occasional hypersensitivity reactions. Methionine is cheaper and can be given orally but is less reliable.

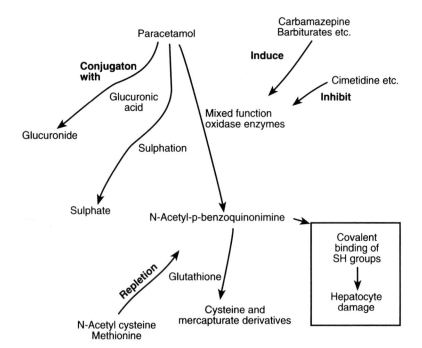

Fig. 17.2 Metabolism and mechanism of paracetamol toxicity.

Paracetamol poisoning has several important distinctive characteristics:

1. It is common, perhaps the most common poisoning encountered in the UK.
2. It is dangerous—hepatic necrosis is recorded with as little as 10 g.
3. Symptoms develop late.
4. Measurement of blood concentration of drug accurately predicts toxicity.
5. Early administration of antidote saves lives.

All doctors should be familiar with the procedure for dealing with this emergency as shown in Fig. 17.3—and consider even liver transplantation.

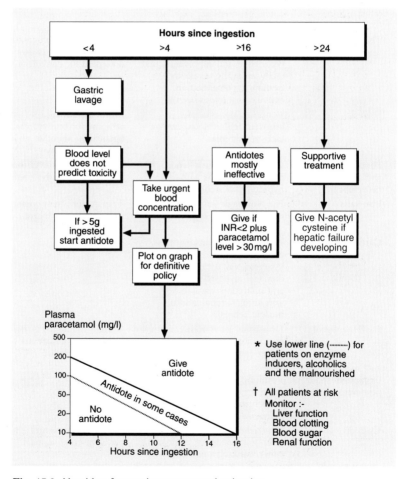

Fig. 17.3 Algorithm for treating paracetamol poisoning.

Table 17.9. Characteristic features and main points in management of certain poisonings

Poison	Main effects	Supportive treatment
Amitriptyline and other tricyclic antidepressants	Tachycardia, hypotension, conduction defects, arrhythmias, excitation, hyperreflexia, coma, respiratory depression, pupillary dilatation, micturition problems	Avoid anti-arrhythmics unless CVS embarrassment; treat convulsions with diazepam, hydrate and maintain oxygenation
Benzodiazepines	Coma without respiratory failure	General measures Beware pneumonia in elderly
Morphine and other opioids	Profound respiratory depression, coma, hypotension, pupillary constriction, pulmonary oedema	Maintain airway, oxygenation
Theophylline	Vomiting, abdominal pain, diarrhoea, tachycardia, ventricular and supraventricular tachycardia, hyperreflexia, tremor, hyperventilation, convulsions, hypokalaemia	Potassium supplementation, beta-blockers for tachyarrhythmias, diazepam for convulsions
Digoxin	Vomiting, drowsiness, atrioventricular block, cardiac tachyarrhythmias	Monitor plasma potassium; atropine for bradycardia; lignocaine, amiodarone or atenolol for tachyarrhythmia
Phenothiazines and other neuroleptics	Coma, convulsions, acute dystonic reactions with hyperreflexia, oculogyric crises	Diazepam for convulsions benztropine for dystonia
Iron salts	Haemorrhagic gastritis, encephalopathy, hepatic necrosis	Transfusion, treat convulsions and circulatory failure
Carbon monoxide	Impairment of consciousness, coma, hypertonia and hyperreflexia, focal neurological damage, myocardial ischaemia and infarction, cardiac arrhythmias, renal failure, muscle necrosis	
Ethylene glycol	Drunkenness, vomiting, coma, convulsions, cardiac failure, pulmonary oedema, acute renal failure	Correct metabolic acidosis Correct hypocalcaemia with i.v. calcium gluconate
Organophosphorous pesticides	Vomiting, sweating, salivation, pupillary constriction, bronchospasm, muscle twitching, diarrhoea, convulsions	
Cyanide	Headache, anxiety, dyspnoea, pulmonary oedema, confusion, coma, cardiovascular collapse	Maximum concentration oxygen, cardiovascular support

See text for aspirin, other salicylates and paracetamol.

Methods for increasing elimination	Antidote
None	Physostigmine, best avoided
None	Avoid flumazenil (antidote) in mixed overdoses (when deaths due to sudden unmasking of effects of tricyclics reported)
None	Naloxone in repeated doses
Repeated activated charcoal Resin haemoperfusion	
Repeated activated charcoal	Digoxin-specific Fab antibody fragments
None	
Intragastric and intravenous desferrioxamine according to serum iron	
100% oxygen with artificial ventilation Hyperbaric oxygen in severe cases	
Consider dialysis	Infuse ethanol to inhibit breakdown to toxic products
Remove contaminated clothes Wash skin	Atropine, pralidoxime
	Amyl nitrite and sodium thiosulphate Consider dicobalt edetate followed by dextrose i.v.

SALICYLATES

Poisoning with aspirin and other salicylates is common and dangerous. Symptoms and signs may be misleading and active treatment is indicated. Measurement of the drug level has a predictive value and can be used as a guide to the need for active treatment. The lethal acute dose in an adult is 20–25 g.

The toxic effects of salicylates are complex and include acid–base disturbances, uncoupling of oxidative phosphorylation with inhibition of the production of high energy phosphates and disordered glucose metabolism. Initial respiratory alkalosis from increased rate and depth of respiration causes loss of bicarbonate and accompanying loss of sodium, potassium and water. This results in failure to buffer the subsequent metabolic acidosis caused by the interference with normal cell metabolism.

The symptoms and signs may not be apparent until the poisoning is well advanced. Nausea, vomiting and tinnitus progressing to deafness are common. Fever, flushed skin and sweating and hyperventilation may give way to excitability and agitation. The patient is usually dehydrated and blood tests may reveal hypokalaemia, hyponatraemia, alkalosis or acidosis, hyperglycaemia or hypoglycaemia and sometimes hypoprothrombinaemia. Pulmonary oedema and CNS depression are late and sinister signs.

Salicylate preparations tend to clump in the stomach. Gastric lavage up to 12 hours after ingestion is therefore worthwhile. The rate of elimination of aspirin can be greatly increased by repeated administration of activated charcoal and by urinary alkalinisation. The latter relies on ionisation of salicylate within the nephron tubule, which renders it non-lipid-soluble and non-diffusible. Maintenance of hydration is also important but large volume diuresis is unnecessary and can be hazardous.

Plasma salicylate concentration should be determined. If less than 50 mg/100 ml, oral rehydration is all that is required. However, a repeat estimation is advisable if the first was taken less than 6 hours from ingestion. If greater than 90 mg/100 ml or if there are CNS signs or pulmonary oedema, then haemodialysis is performed. Between these values 50 g of activated charcoal should be given every 4 hours. In young or middle-aged people, in the absence of hypotension, heart failure or renal impairment, urinary alkalinisation is carried out by infusing 500 ml 1.4% sodium bicarbonate over 1 hour, followed by 500 ml 5% glucose with 20 mmol potassium chloride over 1 hour. Both are repeated until the plasma salicylate is below 40 mg/100 ml. Urinary output and pH must be monitored and the rate of infusion adjusted. If the procedure is prolonged, regular measurement of plasma electrolytes is required so that adjustments in the rate of potassium infusion can be made.

OTHER POISONINGS

Brief details of examples of other poisonings with drugs and some non-ingestants are given in Table 17.9.

18

INBORN ERRORS OF METABOLISM

Richard Harvey

The inborn errors of metabolism are a group of genetic disorders in which there is abnormal accumulation or deficiencies of particular substances in the body, usually as a result of malfunction of an individual enzyme or transport protein.

Most of the more serious of these disorders are carried as autosomal or X-linked recessive traits, because potentially lethal dominant genes tend to disappear through natural selection. The incidence of the clinical disorder reflects the prevalence of the causative abnormal gene, which often shows considerable variation, with markedly increased incidences of various disorders in isolated communities or in those which tend to intermarry. Thus there is a high incidence of lipid storage disorders (e.g. Tay–Sachs disease) in Ashkenazi Jews, of glucose-6-phosphate dehydrogenase deficiency in Greeks and Italians and of variegate porphyria and hypercholesterolaemia in Afrikaaners.

Table 18.1. Factors that should suggest the possibility of inborn metabolic disease

---

Persistent vomiting (may suggest pyloric stenosis, but with acidosis rather than alkalosis)

Poor feeding, failure to thrive

Severe illness in neonatal period, suggestive of septicaemia

Unexplained drowsiness, fits, coma

Jaundice or hepatomegaly

Metabolic acidosis

Odd smell

Unexplained hypoglycaemia, hyponatraemia or neutropenia

Delayed development or mental retardation

Family history of death in early life

Consanguinity

Symptoms worse after feeds or improved on glucose/saline

Table 18.2. Abnormalities of miscellaneous plasma proteins/enzymes

Protein	Normal function	Deficiency state
Tissue non-specific alkaline phosphatase (TNSAP)	Bone mineralisation	Hypophosphatasia
Pseudocholinesterase	Participates in destruction of some synthetic choline esters	Succinylcholine sensitivity
C1 esterase inhibitor	Inhibits activity of the complement component C1	Hereditary angio-oedema
Alpha-1-antitrypsin	Inhibits damaging effect of trypsin on lungs	PiZ allele produces abnormal antitrypsin which cannot be secreted and accumulates in hepatocytes
Factor VIII	Blood clotting	Haemophilia A (classical haemophilia)
Factor IX	Blood clotting	Haemophilia B
Von Willebrand factor	Transport of factor VIII and platelet activation	Von Willebrand's disease
Immunoglobulins	Agammaglobulinaemia	All Ig classes very low Plasma cells absent
Selective IgA deficiency	—	Both plasma and secretory IgA deficient, other Ig classes normal
Thyroxine-binding globulin (TBG)	Transport of thyroxine	TBG deficiency

Clinical features	Inheritance
Abnormal bone mineralisation, often rather like rickets. Premature loss of deciduous teeth. Variable severity	Variable: several alleles interact
Succinylcholine is a popular muscle relaxant used in anaesthesia	Autosomal recessive
Normal persons given usual dose develop apnoea for 3–4 min In homozygous pseudocholinesterase deficiency apnoea often lasts over 30 min, necessitating artificial ventilation	Heterozygotes are mildly affected
Attacks of angio-oedema and/or atypical abdominal pains May be fatal if laryngeal oedema occurs Fresh plasma has been used to interrupt a severe attack Stanazolol (an anabolic steroid), in small oral doses, effectively prevents attacks	Dominant, varying penetrance
Liver cirrhosis and early-onset emphysema	Autosomal recessive Heterozygotes are mildly affected
Easy bruising and bleeding, haemarthrosis etc	X-linked recessive
Easy bruising and bleeding, haemarthrosis etc.	Autosomal: dominant and recessive forms occur
Recurrent pyogenic infections	X-linked recessive
Enteropathy with malabsorption, like coeliac disease, bacterial respiratory tract infections	Autosomal recessive
Thyroid function normal but total serum thyroxine low, so may lead to incorrect diagnosis of hypothyroidism TSH level is normal	Dominant

Diagnosis and screening

Most of the more serious inborn errors of metabolism present in early life and should be diagnosed as early as possible, partly because in some cases early treatment may be life-saving or may prevent permanent brain damage, and partly because, even if no treatment is available, the risk in future pregnancies can be assessed and the parents counselled appropriately. Clinical features which suggest the possibility of an inborn error of metabolism are listed in Table 18.1.

Unfortunately, it is impractical to screen all babies for all disorders. It is only worth finding an inborn error if it is potentially serious yet has an effective treatment available, and it is probably not worth looking in a newborn baby for disorders seen in fewer than 1 in 50 000 live births. Screening can obviously be more intensive in an ill baby (Table 18.1), and in families with an affected member, in children of consanguineous marriages or in mentally retarded individuals. In one screening programme in New England, 19 000 infants were screened, yielding 38 cases of hypothyroidism, 3 cases of phenylketonuria, 2 cases of homocystinuria and 1 each of galactosaemia and maple syrup urine disease. Screening costs were $0.80 for hypothyroidism and $1.20 for amino acid disorders.

Problems of carrier detection, prenatal diagnosis, counselling and the possibility of future genetic therapy are discussed in Chapter 19. Because of the relatively large number of inborn errors of metabolism, they have been grouped in this chapter in a series of tables which are self-explanatory (Tables 18.2–18.6). The rarest disorders have been excluded, and in some cases a single example has been included of a group of related disorders which are described more fully elsewhere in this book (e.g. haemophilia A).

Table 18.3. Inborn errors of amino acid metabolism

Condition	Defective enzyme	Biochemical and clinical consequences
Phenylketonuria	Phenylalanine 4-hydroxylase	Phenylalanine (PA) accumulates in the body fluids, phenylpyruvate and derivatives are excreted in urine Severe mental deficiency, epilepsy, eczema Normal development possible if given low PA diet within first few months of life, continued long-term
Alkaptonuria	Homogentisic acid oxidase	Homogentisic acid accumulates in body fluids, and is excreted in urine Urine goes dark brown or black on standing, e.g. staining nappies Cartilage and sclerae may darken (ochronosis) and osteoarthritis appears from second or third decade Prognosis good without treatment
Homocystinuria	Cystathionine β-synthetase	Homocystine accumulates and is excreted in urine Mental retardation, dislocation of lenses, tendency to arterial and venous thromboses Treatment: methionine restriction, high-dose pyridoxine
Albinism	o-diphenol-oxidase	Lack of melanin in skin, hair and eyes, resulting in nystagmus, photophobia, skin carcinomas Treatment is symptomatic (avoid sun, wear dark glasses)
Tyrosinosis	p-hydroxy-phenylpyruvic acid oxidase	Tyrosine accumulates Rapid liver enlargement, cirrhosis and, usually, death in infancy due to hepatic failure Chronic types known—these develop renal tubular lesion with acidosis and vitamin-D-resistant rickets Prognosis poor, however treated
Maple syrup urine disease	Branched chain ketoacid decarboxylase	Accumulation of valine, leucine and isoleucine with urinary excretion of their derivatives (characteristic smell) Severe cerebral degeneration with early death Milder form occurs which may be helped by diet low in the 3 amino acids
Goitrous Cretinism (several types)	Tyrosine iodinase, Coupling enzyme, Iodotyrosine deiodinase	All types develop goitre and mental retardation of variable severity Replacement therapy with L-thyroxine is completely effective

Table 18.4. Some inborn defects of transport mechanisms

Disorder	Site of defect	Biochemical abnormality
Cystinuria and small intestine	Proximal renal tubule and jejunal absorption of	Defective tubular reabsorption dibasic amino acids (cystine, ornithine, arginine, lysine)
Hartnup disease	Proximal renal tubule and small intestine	Defective tubular reabsorption and jejunal absorption of most monoaminomonocarboxylic and acidic amino acids Deficiency of nicotinamide (derived from tryptophan) results in pellagra
Juvenile Fanconi syndrome	Proximal renal tubule	Fanconi syndrome = defective tubular reabsorption of most amino acids, glucose, phosphate and bicarbonate
Cystinosis	Lysosomal membrane	Fanconi syndrome
Distal renal tubular acidosis	Distal renal tubule	Defective acidification of urine
Proximal renal tubular acidosis	Proximal renal tubule	Defective bicarbonate reabsorption (may be associated with Fanconi syndrome)
Hypophosphataemia	Proximal tubule	Renal phosphate wasting
Liddle's syndrome	Distal renal tubule	Increased Na^+/K^+ exchange
Pseudohypo-parathyroidism	Proximal renal tubule, bone	Resistance to action of PTH, causing hypocalcaemia and hyperphosphataemia
Nephrogenic diabetes insipidus	Renal collecting duct: abnormal vasopressin receptor or mutation in aquaporin-2 water channel	Failure to reabsorb water in response to vasopressin
Renal glycosuria	Proximal renal tubule	Reduced tubular reabsorption of glucose
Iodine trapping defect	Thyroid	Inability to take up iodine from plasma
Wilson's disease (hepatolenticular degeneration)	Liver	Defective copper transporter protein in liver, with failure to secrete copper into bile

Inheritance	Clinical effects	Treatment
Recessive Heterozygotes often asymptomatic	Formation of cystine calculi	High fluid intake, reduced sodium intake, alkalinisation of urine, D-penicillamine
Recessive	Pellagrous rash of face and extremities, (photosensitive) and cerebellar ataxia with falling attacks	Nicotinamide
Variable (may also be secondary to other genetic disease, or acquired)	Failure to thrive, vomiting, thirst, acidosis, hypovolaemia, rickets	Alkalis, vitamin D
Recessive	As for Fanconi syndrome plus eye damage. Variable severity	Alkalis, vitamin D
Various (and may be acquired)	Failure to thrive, hypokalaemia (causing muscle weakness), nephrocalcinosis and urolithiasis	Potassium citrate
	Rickets, osteomalacia, growth retardation	High dose alkali
X-linked recessive	Vitamin-D resistant rickets/ osteomalacia	Phosphate supplementation
Autosomal dominant	Hypertension, hypokalaemia	Amiloride
Dominant, varying penetrance	Onset in first or second decade: tetany, fits, cramps, mental retardation. Basal ganglia and extra-articular calcification. Short metacarpals	Vitamin D and calcium supplements
X-linked recessive (V_2 receptor); autosomal recessive (aquaporin-2)	Recurrent dehydration and hypernatraemia causing mental retardation if untreated	High intake of water. Thiazide diuretics
Dominant	None. May result in mistaken diagnosis of diabetes mellitus. Glucose tolerance test will distinguish the two	None required
Various	Goitrous cretinism	L-thyroxine
Recessive	Copper accumulates and is deposited in tissues. Initially liver, then brain, cornea and later kidneys are affected. Very variable clinical picture, with cirrhosis, hepatitis, haemolysis, tremor, slurred speech and Fanconi-like renal disease	D-Penicillamine

Table 18.4 *cont.* **Some inborn defects of transport mechanisms**

Disorder	Site of defect	Biochemical abnormality
Congenital lactase deficiency	Small intestine	Inability to hydrolyse lactose This type much less common than acquired lactase deficiency
Congenital sucrase–isomaltase deficiency	Small intestine	Inability to hydrolyse sucrose and isomaltose

Table 18.5. Genetic disorders of collagen synthesis

Disorder	Defect
Marfan's syndrome (arachnodactyly)	Abnormal fibrillin formation
Ehlers–Danlos syndrome	Several different types, some with known defective enzyme (e.g. type VI, lysyl hydroxylase)
Osteogenesis imperfecta (fragilitas ossium, brittle bone disease)	Impaired synthesis of type I procollagen Several types, of varying severity
Pseudoxanthoma elasticum	Uncertain—probably a defect in transcription Several types
Cutis laxa	Uncertain, possibly lysyl oxidase deficiency

Inheritance	Clinical effects	Treatment
Recessive	Symptoms develop soon after first milk feed. Misery, abdominal colic and acid diarrhoea (lactic acid formed from unabsorbed lactose)	Lactose-free diet
Recessive	Most present in infancy, with diarrhoea at weaning, some later Acute diarrhoea after sucrose and sometimes after starch	Sucrose-free, starch-reduced diet

Clinical features

Long thin limbs and fingers, high arched palate, dislocated lens, lax joints
Weak arteries, leading to aneurysmal dilatation of aortic arch with resulting rupture, aortic valve incompetence
Dominant, varying penetrance

Various combinations of fragility and hyperelasticity of skin, easy bruising, 'cigarette paper' scars, hyperextensible joints with dislocations, poor tensile strength of aorta, gut and eye, leading sometimes to spontaneous rupture of any of these
Various different types of inheritance

Dwarfism, weak brittle bones, many deformities from fractures
Sclerae may be blue
May be severe type (fractures in utero, early death) or relatively mild

Small soft flat yellowish papules parallel to skin folds, especially sides of neck, axillae
Linear 'angioid' streaks in retina
Tendency to bleed spontaneously into gastrointestinal tract
Prone to hypertension, atheroma

Loose inelastic skin, hanging in folds
Hypermobility of joints
X-linked recessive or dominant

Table 18.6. Miscellaneous inborn errors of metabolism

Condition	Nature of disorder	Clinical features
Galactosaemia	Galactose-1-phosphate uridyl transferase deficiency	Normal at birth, but with milk (lactose) ingestion progressive accumulation of galactose causes hepatosplenomegaly and mental deficiency Cured by galactose-free diet if started early enough
Leucine-induced hypoglycaemia	Mechanism uncertain	Protein (leucine) ingestion causes hypoglycaemia, with fits and brain damage Prevented by adequate carbohydrate intake with proteins
Von Gierke's disease	Glycogen storage disorder (one of several types) due to glucose-6-phosphatase deficiency	Retarded growth, accumulation of glycogen in the liver and kidneys Frequent carbohydrate feeds, ? liver transplant
McArdle's syndrome	Deficiency of muscle glycogen phosphorylase	Muscle pain on exercise, relieved by oral glucose
Hurler's syndrome	Mucopolysaccharidosis (one of several types). A lysosomal storage disease	Dermatan sulphate and heparin sulphate progressively accumulate, with coarse facial features, hepatosplenomegaly, skeletal changes and mental retardation
Tay-Sachs disease Gaucher's disease and Niemann-Pick disease	Lipidoses (three of several types)	Accumulation of various lipids (specific for each type) in brain, liver, spleen, etc. Usually recessive disorders occurring in Jews Most get dementia, epilepsy and blindness (cherry-red spot at macula) with early death, but in Gaucher's disease there is a chronic adult form consistent with a normal lifespan

19

GENETICS AND MOLECULAR MEDICINE

Peter Lunt, Charles R. V. Tomson

Why does a particular person develop a particular disease at a particular time? There are few diseases, whether rare or common, where genetic factors do not play some part. This is most obvious in conditions that follow Mendelian inheritance patterns, which, although individually often quite rare, together account for a certain proportion of chronic medical problems. Some cases of more common conditions also occur in families due to inheritance of a single faulty gene, and such families are important to recognise because of the high risk conferred. Features that may suggest a significant genetic component in disease presentation are:

1. positive family history
2. unusually early onset
3. separate bilateral presentation in paired organs
4. abnormal function of several organs
5. congenital abnormality
6. learning problems.

For many other people with a common disease, genetic factors contribute to susceptibility, and advances in medical genetics over the past decade are now beginning to identify some of the particular genetic polymorphic variants involved. The Human Genome Project, which aims to have sequenced all 10^4–10^5 transcribed genes in the human genome by 2002, raises hopes of rapid advance in the possibilities for targeted disease prevention and treatment.

However, the most immediate genetic advances have been in the identification of the genes and mutation mechanisms involved in the rarer conditions due to single faulty genes. In many of these, a molecular genetic test can now provide the definitive diagnosis and replace more invasive clinical investigations. Although most 'Mendelian' mutations remain constant within a family, we know now that others do not, which can help explain the variation in severity of presentation seen within some families. Other conditions may arise from a faulty gene being present in only some cells in the body, or from cryptic chromosome aberration, or mutation in mitochondrial DNA. Molecular genetics is therefore now in routine diagnostic use for single gene conditions, or for identification of specific viruses or bacteria. Genetic testing, particularly if prior to the onset of clinical symptoms, or used antenatally, carries unique ethical considerations, and protocols being established for single gene conditions must also apply to any proposed future molecular genetic test for disease susceptibility.

DISEASES CAUSED BY CHROMOSOMAL ABNORMALITIES

The 46 chromosomes constituting a normal human karyotype each have a short arm ('p') and a long arm ('q') joined at the centromere. The karyotype is studied by light microscopy following staining, allowing recognition of characteristic light- and dark-stained bands, which are numbered to allow accurate designation of missing, duplicated or translocated chromosome segments. The nomenclature also provides a framework for describing the location of disease genes, e.g. Marfan's syndrome (at 15q21) is caused by mutation in the fibrillin gene located in band 21 of the long arm of chromosome 15. Increasingly, light microscopy may be combined with the use of fluorescently tagged DNA probes (for fluorescent in-situ hybridisation or 'FISH') to detect microdeletion or duplication of DNA in a particular chromosome band (e.g. microdeletion at 22q11 is an important cause of some forms of congenital heart defect).

Chromosome abnormalities may be unbalanced (with gain or loss of genetic material) or balanced (with rearrangement but no net gain or loss of genes), and can involve the 22 autosomes or the sex chromosomes. Autosomal abnormalities occur in 1/150 live births, and excepting balanced re-arrangements, invariably cause learning difficulty, dysmorphism and often multiple congenital abnormality, and may have increased susceptibility to other medical conditions. Sex chromosome abnormalities occur in around 1/500 adults, but usually without congenital malformation, and only a mild, if any, learning problem. Many first-trimester miscarriages are due to non-viable chromosomally abnormal conceptuses. Recurrent miscarriage or a live birth with an unbalanced rearrangement can be due to one parent having a balanced translocation. This may often be inherited, but only affect the carrier if the chromosome breakpoints disrupt an important gene. Such cases have been pivotal for mapping and cloning certain disease genes (e.g. a 1/17 translocation helped to clone the neurofibromatosis (NF1) gene at 17q11).

Some chromosome abnormalities occur as mosaics, where, as a result of nondisjunction during mitosis in the developing embryo, only some cells have an abnormal karyotype. These may require skin fibroblast culture for recognition, since the abnormal cells may not be present in blood. Other conditions with an apparently normal chromosome complement may be due to both copies of one chromosome being inherited from the same parent (uniparental disomy). This affects genes whose copies differ in expression according to the parent of origin (through genomic imprinting by parent-specific methylation of DNA).

AUTOSOMAL TRISOMIES

These disorders have a whole extra chromosome.

Trisomy 21 (Down syndrome) is the most common and occurs in 1/700 births, but is more frequent in older mothers (e.g. 1/100 at 40 years). Affected children or adults have moderate to severe mental retardation (IQ 25–50), a typical facies, short stature and other dysmorphic features. Associated problems often include hypotonia, congenital heart disease (ventricular septal defect (VSD), AV canal, Fallot's tetralogy), duodenal atresia, Hirschsprung's disease, cataract, and an increased incidence of leukaemia or Alzheimer's disease, with lifespan limited to 35–50 years. Mosaic trisomy 21 tends to have milder problems. The age-dependent risk for a mother for having a trisomy-21 baby can be estimated according to the alphafetoprotein level measured in her blood at 17 weeks' gestation, to facilitate a couple's decision of whether or not to have fetal chromosome analysis by amniocentesis.

Trisomy 13 (Patau's syndrome) and **trisomy 18** (Edward's syndrome) result in multiple malformations and neonatal or infant death.

Trisomy 8, occurring as a mosaic, has only mild to moderate retardation, and is compatible with a normal lifespan. Characteristically there are small patellae, deep plantar creases, finger flexion contractures and often hydronephrosis.

SEX CHROMOSOME ABNORMALITIES

These disorders occur in 1 in 500 live births. A chromosome test for diagnosis may be predicting infertility, and must be preceded by careful counselling, particularly for adolescents.

Turner's syndrome (45,XO) has an incidence in liveborn females of 1/2500. It is probably the most common chromosome abnormality at conception, but > 95% of 45, XO embryos abort spontaneously. Clinical features, in addition to gonadal dysgenesis, usually include short stature, neck webbing, pigmented naevi, absent pubertal development and infertility; aortic coarctation and horseshoe kidney are also often present. In infants the only abnormality may be lymphoedema. Growth hormone and oestrogen treatment improve growth and sexual development; pregnancies have been sustained following egg donation.

Klinefelter's syndrome (47,XXY) affects 1 in 550 males, and causes tall stature, small male genitalia, hypogonadism and infertility, often with gynaecomastia and a female body hair distribution. IQ is 85–90% of expected, but shyness and behavioural difficulties are common.

Triple X syndrome (47,XXX) occurs in 1 in 800 females, often as a chance finding or causing mild mental retardation. Premature ovarian failure may occur.

XUY syndrome is present in 1 in 1000 men, typically with tall stature, but normal sexual development and fertility. IQ is 85–90% of expected. The prevalence is increased five-fold amongst prison inmates, possibly reflecting impulsive, immature behaviour.

XX males, or XY females. There are men and women (respectively) where the chromosomal sex is opposite to the phenotypic sex. Infertility is inevitable. Testicular feminisation in 46,XY women is an X-linked recessive condition due to mutation in the androgen receptor gene. Pubertal growth and development is normal, but the uterus is absent.

MICRODELETION SYNDROMES

Deletion of a small section of chromosomal material, too small to be detected by conventional microscopy of chromosome preparations, is responsible for several dysmorphic syndromes associated with mental retardation, e.g. Shprintzen syndrome or Williams syndrome.

Microdeletions are detected by FISH, in which a DNA probe for the deleted region binds to only one of the particular chromosome pair. Owing to genomic imprinting (p. 464), the clinical presentation may differ according to which parent's copy of the chromosome region is lost, either from deletion or from a trisomic conception reducing to uniparental disomy. At 15q11 loss of the paternal copy causes Prader–Willi syndrome (hypotonia, obesity, hypogenitalism, retardation); loss of the maternal copy gives Angelman syndrome (retardation, ataxia, characteristic EEG and facies).

Shprintzen (Di George) syndrome is caused by a microdeletion at 22q11 and typically includes submucous cleft palate, congenital heart defects (truncus arteriosus, Fallot's tetralogy, VSD, right aortic arch), hypoparathyroidism, small or absent thymus, mild to moderate learning problems, long fingers and characteristic facies.

ACQUIRED CHROMOSOMAL ABNORMALITIES

Many leukaemias are associated with acquired chromosomal abnormalities; the most common is the Philadelphia chromosome, a balanced translocation between chromosomes 9 and 22 which causes expression of a chimaeric oncogene, resulting in chronic myeloid leukaemia. Monosomy 7 is often seen in myeloid leukaemia in childhood, presumably indicating myeloid cells that have acquired mutation in one copy of a tumour suppressor gene on chromosome 7, and proliferated following loss of the second copy. Increasingly, detection of these specific somatic chromosome abnormalities is by molecular or FISH techniques.

DYSMORPHIC SYNDROMES

A 'dysmorphic or malformation syndrome' is a recognised combination of morphological defects, usually of genetic origin. They are usually defined by the presence of major features (e.g. polydactyly, cleft palate or cardiac defects) with other minor features (e.g. transverse palmar crease), but rarely with all features in any one case. Minor dysmorphic features occur in 10% of the population but the presence of three or more increases the likelihood of an associated major malformation.

DISEASE CAUSED BY SINGLE GENE MUTATIONS

The coding part of each gene which is transcribed and spliced into mRNA is arranged in several different sections termed 'exons' separated by non-translated 'intron' sequences. Gene expression is subject to regulation according to age, body site and physiological conditions, and for large genes can include alternative ways of splicing exons in different tissues (e.g. the dystrophin gene transcript differs in brain and muscle).

Genetic mutations can disrupt gene function in several ways, including:

1. Point mutation, causing an amino acid substitution ('mis-sense') or a stop codon ('nonsense').
2. Deletion of all or part of the DNA sequence, leading to absence, truncation or other shortening of the protein product. Deletion of an exact multiple of three bases from exons within a gene may leave a partially functional protein product (e.g. in Becker muscular dystrophy).
3. Insertion of extra bases, causing a reading error in all subsequent nucleotide triplets ('frameshift') unless three or a multiple of three bases are inserted.
4. Trinucleotide repeats: expansion of a normal tandemly repeated triplet sequence of nucleotides, either within or outside the transcribed region of a gene, affecting expression of the gene.
5. Mutation in an intron, affecting splicing of transcribed RNA from exons.
6. Alteration of gene regulation, either through mutation in transcription promotor sequenes, or through 'position effects' due to alteration in local chromosome structure (e.g. in facioscapulohumeral muscular dystrophy).
7. Mutation in DNA replication error repair (RER) genes, allowing somatic mutations to build up during normal mitotic cell divisions (e.g. in dominantly inherited colon cancer).
8. Mitochondrial DNA replication or electron transport chain component synthesis can be affected by mutation in certain nuclear genes or mutation in mitochondrial-specific t-RNA, resulting in a mitochondrial disorder.

At cellular level, mutations usually cause a reduction in the amount of functional protein product (e.g. in most inborn errors of metabolism), but may increase the amount (e.g. in paraproteinaemias) or confer a novel function (e.g. in activation of certain cancer-causing oncogenes).

PATTERNS OF INHERITANCE (Fig. 19.1)

Autosomal dominant

This occurs when one faulty copy of a gene is sufficient to cause the condition, for example by an altered protein introducing a gain of function, or

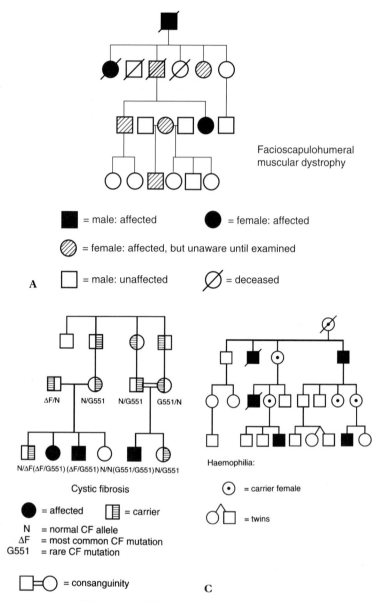

Facioscapulohumeral
muscular dystrophy

■ = male: affected   ● = female: affected

⊘ = female: affected, but unaware until examined

A   □ = male: unaffected   ∅ = deceased

ΔF/N   N/G551   N/G551   G551/N

N/ΔF(ΔF/G551) (ΔF/G551) N/N(G551/G551)N/G551

Cystic fibrosis

Haemophilia:

● = affected   ▥ = carrier

⊙ = carrier female

N   = normal CF allele
ΔF   = most common CF mutation
G551 = rare CF mutation

= twins

B   □—○ = consanguinity   C

Fig. 19.1 Patterns of inheritance. (**A**) Autosomal dominant inheritance;
(**B**) autosomal recessive inheritance; (**C**) X-linked recessive inheritance.

disrupting the integrity of a membrane or protein complex. Patients inheriting
the faulty gene will not all show the disease to the same extent, and may
sometimes remain asymptomatic. Both sexes are affected equally, and offspring are each at 50% risk. Isolated cases can be due to new mutation,

non-penetrance in a parent, germ-line mosaicism for the mutation in a parent, or incorrectly assumed paternity.

Autosomal recessive

A person is affected only if both copies of the gene are faulty, although not necessarily with the same mutation. The mutations usually cause loss of function, but with 50% of the gene product being sufficient for normal cell function. Both parents must be heterozygous 'carriers', and further children will be at 1 in 4 risk. Usually the condition is only seen in a single full sibship in a family, since the risk to offspring of an affected person, or in other branches of a family, is low. The exception is where the disease gene is prevalent in the population (e.g. in a particular ethnic group) or where a couple come from the same extended family ('consanguinity'). New mutation is rare.

X-linked recessive

Faulty genes on the X-chromosome usually cause loss of function. The disease affects males who inherit the faulty gene in the mother's egg. New mutation (or maternal germ-line mosaicism) will account for one-third of isolated cases where the condition is lethal; in at least two-thirds of cases the mother is a carrier and further sons will be at 50% risk. An affected male cannot pass the disease to male offspring, but all his daughters will be carriers. Females can be affected if they have Turner's syndrome (45,XO), if the father is affected and the mother is a carrier, if a chromosome translocation cuts through the disease gene, or if a carrier has disproportionate inactivation of the normal X-chromosome.

Maternal inheritance

This is seen in some diseases caused by mutations in mitochondrial DNA (mtDNA). Each mitochondrion contains 2–10 copies of a circular DNA molecule, which through intra-mitochondrial synthesis encodes some of the subunits of proteins in the mitochondrial respiratory chain, as well as the DNA sequence for mitochondrial-specific tRNA molecules. This information is transmitted exclusively by mothers, as spermatozoa pass only their nucleus into the egg at fertilization. Defects of mitochondrial DNA can be inherited, arise by new mutation, or accumulate with age, causing a spectrum of diseases characterised by lactic acidosis, muscle weakness (including ophthalmoplegia) and several central nervous system disorders. Mitochondrial dysfunction may also present with common disease symptoms such as diabetes, cardiomyopathy, neutropenia, epilepsy and possibly Parkinson's or Alzheimer's disease.

Multifactorial/polygenic inheritance

Most common conditions are associated with a slight increase above population risk for other family members. This is usually due to genetic polymorphic variation in the population, where certain combinations of normal variant alleles confer increased genetic susceptibility to the disease, onset of which may be triggered by environmental factors. The same alleles may well have other beneficial effects, accounting for their frequency in the population. Typically the genetic risk increases with: proximity to the index case, increased number of cases in the family, increased severity or earlier onset in the index case, or the index case being of the less commonly affected sex. Increasingly, some of the polymorphic alleles that contribute to multifactorial susceptibility to disease are being characterised, including in diabetes, venous thrombosis, coronary thrombosis, Alzheimer's disease and inflammatory disease. Potential application of this knowledge will require careful evaluation before its use should be contemplated in influencing routine clinical practice.

A small proportion of common disease (e.g. breast or colon cancer) occurs in families where a single faulty gene confers a very high risk, usually following dominant inheritance. At-risk relatives in these families are often at close to 50% risk and often now wish to explore genetic predictive testing. Clues to a high-risk single gene family may be: unusually early age at onset, bilateral presentation and strong family history.

USE OF MOLECULAR GENETICS IN MEDICINE

Molecular genetics can be used in clinical medicine in several ways:

1. establishing a diagnosis in a symptomatic patient
2. prediction for a family member at known high risk of a single gene disorder
3. testing for genetic susceptibility in multifactorial disease
4. screening for genetic disease in a population at low-risk
5. screening for disease susceptibility in the general population
6. treatment of genetic disease
7. research into disease mechanisms and inheritance
8. research into normal cellular processes.

ESTABLISHING A DIAGNOSIS IN A SYMPTOMATIC PATIENT

DNA testing can be either direct or indirect. A direct DNA test detects mutation within a gene and can be used diagnostically. An indirect test, which recognises genetic polymorphic variation in or adjacent on a chromosome to a disease gene, can only be used to track the disease gene through a family. The availability of a direct DNA test with high specificity for a single gene condition can enable diagnosis from a blood sample alone. This is becoming possible for an increasing number of conditions as the genes for them are cloned. Already this can replace otherwise invasive or expensive clinical diagnostic investigation, particularly in certain neurological and neuromuscular diseases. To exclude a diagnosis requires that the test also be highly sensitive. How easily a given genetic disease can be tested for depends on whether it is always caused by exactly the same mutation; has a uniform or prevalent type of mutation mechanism; or whether numerous different types of mutation (or even mutations on different genes) can cause the same phenotype. Diseases always caused by a uniform mutation mechanism, such as trinucleotide repeats, can be diagnosed or excluded with certainty. Diseases such as cystic fibrosis (CF), which can be caused by several different mutations on the same gene (p. 77), can be diagnosed in most cases, but the diagnosis cannot currently be excluded by genetic testing. Conditions in which large numbers of mutations in a large gene can cause disease, such as Marfan's syndrome (p. 474), or are genetically heterogeneous with mutation possible in one of two or more genes, such as autosomal dominant polycystic kidney disease, cannot currently be tested for by direct DNA tests in a routine service setting. Table 19.1 lists some of the more important examples of single gene conditions, according to their mutation mechanisms, and sensitivity of specific diagnosis. These are discussed in more detail below.

EXACTLY THE SAME MUTATION(S) IN EVERY CASE

Achondroplasia and Apert syndrome
These are two skeletal dysplasias that follow autosomal dominant inheritance, but are usually seen as a new mutation occurring in fibroblast growth factor genes, respectively FGFR3 at 4p16 and FGFR2 at 10q25. In each case the mutation always occurs at the same site in the gene, and interestingly always in sperm, never in the egg. Specific DNA diagnosis is therefore made very easy.

UNIFORM MUTATION MECHANISM: TRINUCLEOTIDE REPEATS

Several neurological disorders always arise from expansion of normal runs of a tandemly repeated trinucleotide sequence. Invariably the repeated triplet is a glutamine codon; translation would produce an extended polyglutamine tract. The length of the DNA repeat can be readily detected by DNA techniques, enabling a specific diagnostic test for the disorder. Correlation exists between the severity of clinical presentation (or earliness of age at onset) and expansion size, allowing some prediction of prognosis. The expansion is often unstable at meiosis, tending to become larger in the offspring than the parent, and hence leading to a younger age at onset with each generation (a phenomenon termed 'anticipation'), particularly if each parent passing on the faulty gene is of the same sex. Paternal transmission gives younger onset in Huntington's disease and spino-cerebellar ataxias; maternal transmission gives younger onset in myotonic dystrophy and more severe learning problems in fragile X syndrome.

Facioscapulohumeral muscular dystrophy
This dominant neuromuscular disorder has a so far unique mutation

Table 19.1. Mutation mechanism and sensitivity of routine diagnostic DNA test in some single gene conditions

Condition	Gene	Gene locus
Autosomal dominant		
Myotonic dystrophy	Myotonin	19q13
Huntington's disease	Huntingtin	4p16
Spino-cerebellar ataxias	SCA 1,2,3	3 sites
Charcot–Marie–Tooth disease	PMP22	17p11
Facioscapulohumeral muscular dystrophy	(D4F104S1)	4q35
Achondroplasia	FGFR3	4p16
Apert syndrome	FGFR2	10q25
Tuberous sclerosis	TSC1 or 2	16p or 9q
Neurofibromatosis	NF1	17q11
Marfan syndrome	Fibrillin 15	15q21
Adult polycystic kidney disease	APKD1 or 2	16p or 4q
Autosomal recessive		
Friedreich's ataxia	Frataxin	9q13
Juvenile Batten disease	CLN3	16
Spinal muscular atrophy	SMN	5q21
Cystic fibrosis	CF	7q32
Sickle cell anaemia	β-globin	11p
Haemochromatosis	HLA-H	6
α-$_1$antitrypsin deficiency	Pi	14q32
Congenital adrenal hyperplasia	CYP21	6p21
Phenylketonuria	PKU	12q
X-linked recessive		
Fragile X syndrome	FRAXA	Xq28
Bulbo-spinal muscular atrophy	Androgen receptor	Xq21
Duchenne/Becker muscular dystrophy	Dystrophin	Xp21
Mitochondrial		
Leber's hereditary optic neuropathy	(complex I) ND4/ND1/ND6 mitochondrial	

mechanism involving deletion of integral numbers of copies of a very large (3.3 kb) repeat. This is located at the tip of chromosome 4q, and may well act through affecting chromosome structure locally.

PREVALENT MUTATION MECHANISM

Homozygosity for deletion of exon 7 in the survival motor neuron gene at 5q21 accounts for over 95% of cases of **spinal muscular atrophy**. Deletion of exons from the dystrophin gene (Xp21) causes 70% of cases of X-linked **Duchenne** or **Becker muscular dystrophy**, the severity of muscle weakness depending on whether the number of deleted bases is a multiple of 3 or not. In **familial adenomatous polyposis coli**, mutations in the APC gene (5q12) tend to be nonsense mutations leading to a truncated protein product.

Mutation type	Inheritance	Sensitivity of DNA test
Trinucleotide repeat	Aut.dom.	100%
Trinucleotide repeat	Aut.dom.	100%
Trinucleotide repeat	Aut.dom.	100%
Gene duplication	Aut.dom	>50%
3.3 kb repeat deletion	Aut.dom	>90%
Mis-sense point mutation	Aut.dom	>95%
Mis-sense point mutation	Aut.dom	>95%
Various	Aut.dom	No DNA test
Various	Aut.dom	No DNA test
Various	Aut.dom	No DNA test
Various	Aut.dom	No DNA test
Trinucleotide repeat	Aut.rec.	>90%
1 kb deletion	Aut.rec.	73%
Deletion of exon 7	Aut.rec.	>95%
3-base deletion/other	Aut.rec.	65%
Mis-sense point mutation	Aut.rec.	100%
Mis-sense point mutation	Aut.rec.	87%
Mis-sense point mutation	Aut.rec.	High
Aberrant splicing/recombinant pseudogene	Aut.rec.	50%
Various	Aut.rec	<50%
Trinucleotide repeat	X-rec.	>95%
Trinucleotide repeat	X-rec.	100%
Deletion of exons	X-rec.	70%
One of three mis-sense point mutations	Mitochondrial	>70%

MULTIPLE DIFFERENT MUTATIONS POSSIBLE—SOME MORE PREVALENT

In CF (p. 77) a common 3-base pair deletion results in deletion of phenyl-alanine at the 508th amino acid position along the peptide chain. This mutation (dF508) accounts for 70% of carriers in northern Europe; a further 10–15% carry other relatively common mutations which can readily be tested for. Over 300 rarer CF mutations can also occur.

MULTIPLE DIFFERENT MUTATIONS POSSIBLE—EACH FAMILY SPECIFIC

Confirmation of diagnosis by DNA testing is not yet practicable in the many conditions where each family may have a different mutation.

Neurofibromatosis type 1
This is caused by autosomal dominant mutation in the neurofibromin gene at 17q11, and presents with multiple light brown ('café-au-lait') skin patches and neurofibromas on peripheral nerves. Tumours of tissues derived from neural crest, including phaeochromocytomas, may occur. A large head circumference and learning problems may be present.

Marfan's syndrome
This is caused by a dominant mutation in the fibrillin gene at 15q21, and can cause tall stature, long digits, scoliosis, chest deformity, lax ligaments, high-arched palate, myopia, lens dislocation, mitral valve prolapse and aortic aneurysms and dissection. It is important to examine all first-degree relatives of an index case and to offer regular echocardiographic screening to enable prophylactic replacement of the ascending aorta if it is widening. The multiplicity of possible mutations usually precludes direct DNA testing, and diagnosis must rely on imperfect clinical criteria.

GENETIC HETEROGENEITY

The possibility that mutation in different genes may be responsible for the same clinical condition in different families complicates molecular diagnostic testing.

Tuberous sclerosis
This can be caused by autosomal dominant mutations in either of two genes at 16p13 or 9q34. Clinical presentation is the same, with hamartomas in the brain, resulting in epilepsy and/or mental retardation; in the heart causing rhabdomyomas; and in the kidneys, causing cysts and angiomyolipomas. Skin signs include facial adenoma sebaceum, depigmented ('ash-leaf') patches and nailbed fibromas.

Adult polycystic kidney disease and hereditary non-polyposis colon cancer
These are two other conditions exhibiting genetic heterogeneity.

DIAGNOSTIC DNA TESTS

The methods used for recognition of known mutations in diagnostic testing depend on the properties of the specific mutation. Broadly these divide into:

1. Hybridisation of denatured single strand test DNA with DNA probes complementary to either the mutant sequence or the normal sequence.
2. Failure of a DNA probe complementary to the exon sequence to bind to single strand DNA deleted for that sequence.
3. Detection of altered length of a DNA fragment following cutting by a restriction enzyme, where the particular DNA sequence required for cleavage by that enzyme is introduced or removed by the mutation.

4. Measurement of the size of a DNA fragment containing a tandem trinucleotide repeat.
5. Detection of an altered DNA fragment size due to deletion or insertion of a DNA sequence within it.

To detect the test DNA, each of these methods can either use a DNA sample extracted from the whole genome, or first amplify DNA from the particular exon of the gene to be studied. If using whole genome DNA, a radioactively labelled DNA probe is hybridised with the test DNA after first incubating this with the restriction enzyme, running the DNA fragments along an electrophoretic gel, and then soaking them up onto a membrane by Southern blotting. Amplification of DNA can be achieved by the polymerase chain reaction technique (PCR).

The PCR technique

This uses two synthetic oligonucleotide 'primers' chosen to be complementary in sequence to the two DNA strands at sites closely flanking the site under test. The primers and test DNA are incubated *in vitro* with DNA polymerase and nucleic acids to allow replication of the DNA between the primer sites. Since the primers are present in excess compared with the test DNA, the process is self-perpetuating and leads to a doubling of the number of copies of the DNA sequence between the primers with each round of replication. The process is controlled by alternate heating and cooling of the reaction mixture.

PCR not only often avoids the need for radioisotopes, but is far quicker than Southern blotting, and has now superseded this in many test procedures as it is usually superior for detecting specific point mutations. Direct sequencing of DNA would always now only be done on pre-amplified DNA, but is not usually required in tests for uniform or prevalent mutation. On its own, however, PCR cannot reliably test for mutation across stretches of DNA of greater than 250 bases. It is also exquisitely sensitive to any similar contaminating DNA sequence, and therefore for diagnostic and predictive use, especially for detection of trinucleotide repeats above 60 copies, or in any prenatal test, PCR would usually be backed up by a Southern blotting technique on genomic DNA.

For conditions without a uniform mutation mechanism, screening for mutation in a gene is only feasible as a routine diagnostic service test if a few known mutations are relatively frequent and together account for a majority of carriers or of patients with the condition (e.g. mutations at nucleotides mt11778, mt3460, mt14484 in the mitochondrial genome account for 70–90% of patients with Leber's hereditary optic neuropathy). Otherwise the complete testing of a gene to identify or exclude a possible unique mutation would in most cases currently be impracticable. Current mutation detection techniques are detailed below, but wider service application for diagnostic testing must await development of more efficient and financially robust methods.

Alternatives to direct testing for genetic mutations include using a nucleic acid probe to test for abnormal mRNA ('Northern blotting') or using immunostaining against the encoded protein product ('Western blotting'). These can be done either from electrophoresis of tissue homogenates (e.g. staining for peroxisomal alanine; glyoxylate aminotransferase in liver biopsies in suspected primary hyperoxaluria) or increasingly by immunofluorescent staining on tissue biopsy sections (e.g. for dystrophin in muscle biopsy in suspected Becker or Duchenne muscular dystrophy). The disadvantage compared with DNA testing is that both techniques require access to the tissue in which the gene is normally expressed.

GENETIC TESTING IN FAMILIES

Genetic testing for family members at risk of inheriting a gene mutation is now potentially possible for most single gene disorders. Common reasons for requesting genetic prediction are:

1. For someone without symptoms to find out if they have inherited a serious late-onset disorder such as Huntington's disease, where:
   (i) surveillance screening can be targeted to those at certain risk (e.g. annual colonoscopy in adolescents at risk of familial polyposis coli), and/or preventative treatment may be possible (e.g. prophylactic removal of the ovaries in familial ovarian cancer); or
   (ii) they have adult offspring whose risk depends on their result, or seek informed reproductive choice, including the option of prenatal testing, or the freedom and confidence to have a family; or
   (iii) other 'life' choices can be made more easily through removal of uncertainty. While a 'good' result will bring relief from anxiety, for some this can be tempered by 'survivor guilt' if a sib has a 'bad' result.
2. To clarify whether uncertain clinical symptoms may be due to the disease.
3. To find out if someone is a carrier of a recessive or X-linked gene mutation, where they wish to know the risk of passing the genetic disease to their offspring, and whether prenatal testing is possible.
4. To predict the severity of a disease, its prognosis, or determine the most appropriate treatment according to the mutation involved.

Predictive genetic testing within families can be either by direct or indirect DNA methods.

Direct testing

As a test for the exact mutation in the gene known to be involved in a particular family, direct tests are accurate and, with increasing availability as genes become cloned, are the preferred choice in almost all cases. However, a fully sensitive direct test requires either that the family-specific mutation has already been characterised in that family, or will inevitably be of a uniform mutation type. Tests of high specificity but lesser sensitivity may be considered for conditions where a few mutations are prevalent, but DNA is not available from other family members. For example, in cystic fibrosis (CF), the most common mutation is a 3-base pair deletion (ΔF508) which can be readily detected. Some rarer CF mutations can also be detected routinely, enabling ready identification of 80–85% of CF carriers.

Family-specific mutation detection in a known affected family member or gene carrier can be difficult labour-intensive work, and currently limits the conditions for which direct genetic testing can be offered on a service (as opposed to research) basis, to those where the efficiency of detection (sensitivity vs. effort) is likely to be highest. For conditions such as CF in which a few mutations are relatively common, these will be tested for first. In juvenile Batten disease, homozygosity for a 1 kb deletion in the CLN3 gene accounts for over 70% of cases; in Xp21 muscular dystrophy it is relatively easy to screen an affected male for deletion of exons from the dystrophin gene, observed in over 70% of cases.

A similar 'best guess' approach can be used to choose the technique for mutation detection if no common mutation is found. The 'gold standard' would be DNA sequencing of a series of PCR products covering the whole gene. Although this can be automated, it would be slow and technically demanding. Therefore one of several techniques is used to first identify the approximate position of the mutation along the gene, followed by PCR amplification and sequencing of only the relevant exon. These different techniques may:

1. Compare the folding pattern of single-stranded DNA from the patient with the normal pattern ('single strand conformation polymorphism, 'SSCP').
2. Allow the DNA from the patient to reanneal with normal DNA and test either for reduced stability of the resulting 'heteroduplex' DNA (by denaturing gradient gel electrophoresis, 'DGGE') or for sensitivity to chemical cleavage at the mismatch site.
3. Use in vitro protein synthesis to test for a premature chain termination codon (nonsense mutation) in the mRNA from the patient ('protein truncation test', 'PTT').

A variant DNA sequence is further checked for its predicted effect on the encoded peptide, and its frequency in the normal population, to ensure that it would be pathogenic rather than a normal polymorphic variant.

Indirect testing

In diseases in which the exact mutation is not known, or in which numerous mutations in a gene can cause the disease, it is usually impractical to test for the causative mutation. However, through relying on genetic linkage, if it is possible to identify a 'marker allele' which is on the same chromosome and in the near vicinity of the mutated gene, it may be possible to determine how that allele 'tracks with' the disease in question in the subject's family. For instance, in a particular family, if all affected family members inherit marker allele 'a' together with the disease gene from their relevant parent, and their unaffected sibs inherit the parent's other copy of the marker, it makes it highly likely that the disease gene in the family is 'tracking' with marker allele 'a'. A test subject inheriting 'a' from their disease gene-carrying parent is highly likely also to have inherited the faulty gene, provided that the parent's other marker allele can be distinguished from allele 'a'.

Since the marker locus is polymorphic in the normal population, the particular allele tracking with the mutated copy of the disease gene will differ in different families. In any one family the high-risk marker allele will also be found to occur by chance on normal chromosomes. The best markers to use are therefore ones where the number of different possible alleles is maximal. These tend to be sites of tandemly repeated dinucleotide sequences (e.g. CACACACACA ...), which have a very variable copy number, producing different lengths of PCR product.

Indirect testing is only possible with the availability of DNA samples from multiple family members, and therefore relies on their cooperation, whether affected or unaffected. It may also prove inaccurate for several reasons, including recombination between the marker allele and the gene causing the disease, the possibility of genetic heterogeneity resulting in the wrong gene being tracked in the family, or incorrectly assigning paternity. It is inappropriate in cases of new mutation.

Even with characterisation of disease genes there may always remain a particular use of indirect testing. This is in prenatal exclusion testing, where a parent at 50% risk for a late-onset dominant disorder wishes to have a prenatal test to ensure there will be no risk to their child, but does not wish to know if they will develop the disease themselves.

ETHICAL ASPECTS OF GENETIC TESTING

A genetic test for diagnosis or prediction of risk for one person inevitably also affects others, including through possible discovery of non-paternity. Genetic testing should therefore always be voluntary with informed consent, and supported by counselling. Children aged under 18 years should not be tested, particularly for a late-onset disorder, unless treatment could be offered. Invasive prenatal diagnosis is only acceptable for a serious disorder and where the result would alter the management of the pregnancy, individual patient views being respected, including in antenatal screening programmes. Testing for susceptibility genes to multifactorial disease remains problematic at any age until such tests have a high predictive value. The potential for genetic discrimination in insurance risk assessment is of concern, and in the UK is currently under governmental surveillance.

Genetic counselling

This is the assessment and discussion of information pertaining to genetic risk with a person or couple who may be at risk of having inherited or of passing on a genetic disorder, often so that they can take informed decisions relating to personal prediction or to reproductive options. Assessment of risk depends on age and pedigree structure, combined with results of clinical examination and investigation, increasingly involving molecular genetic testing. Correct genetic advice relies on accuracy of diagnosis, which should be confirmed by direct molecular testing where applicable. For the wider family, a patient should in general be helped to inform unknowing relatives about potential genetic risk, with counselling support, particularly if disease could be prevented or treated.

GENETICALLY DETERMINED SUSCEPTIBILITY TO DISEASE

There are few if any diseases in which there is no genetic variation in susceptibility. It has long been known that the human lymphocyte antigen HLA-B27, present in 5% of the normal population, is found in 90% of men with ankylosing spondylitis (AS), conferring a relative risk of AS of 170 × in men with HLA-B27. Increasingly, in studying common diseases, it is being found that particular polymorphic alleles show alterations in frequency in patients with the disease compared with their frequency in an unaffected control population. The assumption tends to be made that the alleles found to be increased in frequency in the disease confer an increase in susceptibility to the disease, particularly where the polymorphism occurs in a gene whose protein product seems likely to be involved in the disease process. A few illustrative examples are listed here.

Autoimmune disease

Most autoimmune diseases demonstrate association with antigens of the HLA system, including type 1 diabetes and rheumatoid arthritis. The particular antigen associated varies between different populations, suggesting that a gene closely linked to the HLA locus, rather than the HLA antigen itself, is conferring susceptibility. Genetic abnormalities in the complement system are associated with systemic lupus erythematosus.

Infection

Inherited differences in the control of cytokine production appear to influence susceptibility to, and severity of, and infectious disease. For instance, a polymorphism causing increased production of tumour necrosis factor alpha is associated with increased risk of death from cerebral malaria. Recently, a mutation in the interferon-γ gene was found to be associated with increased susceptibility to mycobacterial infection. Susceptibility to the 'new variant Creutzfeldt-Jakob disease', a prion disease thought to be associated with bovine spongiform encephalopathy, appears to be higher in patients homozygous for methionine at position 129 of the PrP gene.

Thrombosis

Deficiency in anticoagulant proteins (protein C, protein S, antithrombin III), inherited in each case as a dominant condition, can cause an increased tendency to arterial and venous thrombosis. A particular polymorphic allele in the factor V gene (factor V Leiden, FVL), which causes resistance to activated protein C, occurs heterozygously in 4% of the UK population, but in 15–20% of cases of deep venous thrombosis (DVT) (p. 351) conferring a relative risk of 4–6 for DVT in persons heterozygous for FVL. FVL should therefore be suspected in patients who develop DVT without obvious predisposing cause. Screening the general population for FVL would not, however, yet be appropriate, since if only 10% of people with FVL develop DVT, it would be a poor predictor of this.

Dementia

Early-onset Alzheimer's disease can be inherited as a dominant condition, due to mutation in one of at least three genes. In late-onset Alzheimer's disease the ε4 allele of the apolipoprotein E gene is more frequent in patients (40%) than in age-matched controls (12%), conferring a 5 × relative risk.

Atherosclerosis

Familial hypercholesterolaemia, which follows dominant inheritance, is due to mutations in the low density lipoprotein (LDL) receptor, which cause impaired catabolism of LDL. Other more common lipid disturbances, including familial combined hyperlipidaemia and familial hypertriglyceridaemia with low HDL-cholesterol, appear to be polygenic. Genetic factors affecting thrombosis may also be important, e.g. a polymorphism in the platelet membrane glycoprotein IIIa present in 39% of patients with coronary artery disease compared with 19% of controls is associated with a 2.8 × increased risk of coronary thrombosis (or 6 × increased risk if aged under 60 years).

MOLECULAR ASPECTS OF CANCER

Although there will undoubtedly be many genetic polymorphisms conferring an increased cancer risk, most cancer genetic research has concentrated either on the events in somatic cells that initiate benign or malignant transformation, or on identifying single genes in which inherited mutation confers a very high cancer risk, often following dominant inheritance in families. Development of cancer is a multi-step process, and usually requires mutation to develop in both copies of a gene (Knudson's 'two-hit hypothesis') or in two different genes. Mutations may be inherited at parental meiosis ('constitutional') or be acquired during normal mitotic cell division ('somatic'). Acquired 'somatic' mutations can include:

1. activation of proto-oncogenes (genes that promote cell division) (e.g. *ras*)
2. decreased expression of tumour suppressor genes, which control programmed cell death ('apoptosis')
3. altered function of DNA repair genes, allowing the accumulation of somatic mutations. For instance, mutation in the p53 gene on 17p13.1 is found in 50–80% of human cancers. The normal product from this

gene arrests cell division or causes apoptosis in cells that have acquired DNA mutations, and also acts as a transcription factor, controlling gene expression.

INHERITED CANCERS

There are rare families where a mutation in p53 follows dominant inheritance, leading to a variety of types of cancer presenting at a young age in affected family members (Li Fraumeni syndrome). Around 1 in 20 cases of breast cancer are due to inheritance of a dominant gene mutation, typically in the genes BRCA1 (on 17q21) or BRCA2 (on 13q12). Such cases tend to have a relatively young onset (< 45 years), are often bilateral, and usually have a positive family history. Numerous distinct family-specific mutations have now been identified in BRCA1 or BRCA2; those in BRCA1 usually also confer an increased risk of ovarian cancer. Dominantly inherited colon cancer may occur in familial adenomatous polyposis coli (APC), or in hereditary non-polyposis colon cancer (HNPCC). A mutation in the APC gene, which controls apoptosis, allows somatic mutations in other key genes controlling cell proliferation to result in cancer. The normal APC gene would ensure apoptosis of cells carrying these mutations. HNPCC is caused by mutations in several mismatch repair genes. Somatic mutations in APC are commonly seen in HNPCC patients.

Clinically it is important to offer physical screening tests (particularly of the bowel in APC or HNPCC) to family members known to be at 50% risk of inheriting a dominant cancer-gene. The availability of predictive genetic testing in these cases can enable 50% of those at risk to have relief from anxiety and release from further screening, while the 50% found to have inherited the faulty gene will know that screening can be preventative.

OTHER APPLICATIONS OF MOLECULAR GENETICS

Diagnosis of infectious disease

The PCR is now used routinely in the diagnosis and quantification of HIV infection (p. 421) and hepatitis C (p. 287) in blood samples. Other applications include the rapid diagnosis of viral encephalitis and meningitis using CSF, and the diagnosis or confirmation of tuberculosis.

Monitoring response to cancer treatment and bone marrow transplantation

Molecular polymorphisms can be used to differentiate between donor and host cells after bone marrow transplantation in the treatment of leukaemias or certain metabolic disorders. Detection of somatic mutations characteristic of an individual tumour cell line, such as the Philadelphia chromosome translocation, can be used to show the spread of malignant cells in a biopsy, or monitor blood for relapse of leukaemia.

Medical research

Molecular genetic techniques have been fundamental to many of the advances made in medicine over the past 10–15 years, and will certainly continue to be so for the forseeable future. For many rarer single gene conditions, methods used to identify the gene continue to include:

1. study of large families by genetic linkage analysis using polymorphic markers known to map very close to possible candidate genes
2. finding a patient with the disease who also has a unique chromosome rearrangement
3. study of possible candidate genes for mutations
4. identifying diseases to fit with peptides predicted from the genome sequence.

Advance has come not only in the mapping and cloning of single genes, and in our understanding of mutation mechanisms, but in study of the expression of genes involved in the whole range of disease processes. For instance, study of the control of inflammation has been transformed by the ability to study expression of genes controlling adhesion of inflammatory cells, the expression of cytokines, and the control of programmed cell death. Completion of the Human Genome Mapping Project (by the year 2002) will enable sequencing of all human genes, and lead to a vastly improved understanding of genome organisation, gene control and genetic susceptibility. This will not only revolutionise diagnostic investigation, but lead to a much clearer understanding of normal cellular processes and morphogenesis. Improved treatments based on altering control of gene expression or replacing faulty genes can be anticipated.

Forensic medicine and anthropology

Detection in human biological material of polymorphic DNA alleles at multiple sites recognised by a single DNA probe provides a genetic profile (DNA fingerprint) that can be used to estimate the likelihood that a specimen is from a particular individual. On a population level, the 'relatedness' of different human populations can be estimated by comparing the allele frequencies of polymorphic markers.

COMMUNITY AND POPULATION GENETICS

PREVALENCE OF GENETIC DISEASE

Up to 30% of the population may have raised genetic susceptibility to develop multifactorial disease. In a few people this susceptibility will be due to a single faulty gene, conferring high risk to other members of those families. Although individual genetic diseases are rare, there are many of them, and up to 5% of the population has a genetic mutation causing disease. Two of the most common examples are familial hypercholesterolaemia (1 in 500) and early-onset breast cancer due to BRCA1 mutation (1 in 600), both of which are autosomal dominant. For autosomal recessive conditions the incidence of carriers approximates to $2 \times \sqrt{(\text{disease incidence})}$. Thus, for CF with a UK birth incidence of 1/2000, carriers are found to be very common in the general population (1 in 22). For rarer recessive conditions, carriers are less frequent (1/160 for a typical incidence of 1/100 000).

The prevalence of a genetic disease is increased by a high rate of new mutation (e.g. neurofibromatosis) or by a selective advantage conferred to carriers of the mutation (e.g. decreased susceptibility to malaria in haemoglobinopathy carriers, or possibly, protection against cholera in CF carriers). This is balanced by selection against the disease due to reduced reproductive fitness of the affected person. In small or closed communities a mutation may be prevalent because of the community's isolation. For many other mutations, competing selective factors may operate, but are as yet poorly understood. Although there might be concern that advances in medical treatment of diseases that previously would have prevented reproduction could increase the prevalence of the causative mutations, the effect at population level for recessive conditions in particular will be negligible.

POPULATION SCREENING FOR GENETIC DISEASE

Screening apparently healthy individuals for genetic disease is only justified if:

1. early detection allows earlier and more effective treatment
2. the mutation is sufficiently common to justify the costs and anxieties generated by screening
3. the disease can be detected reliably, either because it is caused by a single mutation or because the phenotype is characteristic. In particular the likelihood of a false positive result, with the consequent inevitable anxiety, must be very low, i.e. the test must have very high specificity.

Screening should always be voluntary, except in statutory screening of babies or children for a handicapping condition where prophylactic treatment is preventative. Examples where screening is justified include neonatal biochemical screening for phenylketonuria (in which early institution of a phenylalanine-restricted diet prevents brain damage), congenital hypothyroidism and voluntary haemoglobinopathy carrier screening in susceptible racial groups. Neonatal screening for CF may be justified, as there is evidence that early diagnosis and treatment improve prognosis, as well as alerting couples to the risk of having another affected child. In other recessive conditions, owing to their low birth incidence, even with a uniform or prevalent mutation, screening for carrier status is unlikely to become available except within extended families. Any proposed wider screening programme for common disease risk (e.g. diabetes, cancer or neural tube defect) would need to be justifiable ethically, as well as scientifically and financially.

MANAGEMENT OF GENETIC DISEASE

Information, both for patients and for the society in which they live, is crucial for the optimal management of genetic disease. Support groups now exist for most genetic conditions, and provide information and support for patients and their families, as well as acting as pressure groups and supporting research into the condition.

Reproductive choice

The options available to a couple at risk of having a child with a serious genetic disease are:

1. avoidance of pregnancy by contraception or sterilisation (and consideration of adoption)
2. prenatal testing (by genetic techniques and/or detailed ultrasound scanning) and selective termination of pregnancy
3. preimplantation testing of a single cell from the embryo by PCR technique following in vitro fertilisation (IVF)
4. artificial insemination by donor (AID), if the father carries the abnormal gene
5. using donor eggs (if the mother is the carrier of the abnormal gene) for IVF or gamete intrafallopian transfer (GIFT)
6. accepting the risk, receiving counselling, and proceeding with the pregnancy.

Treatment of genetic disease

In addition to general supportive treatment, specific therapies to correct or ameliorate the genetic defect are available in some diseases, e.g., low phenylalanine diet in phenylketonuria, liver or bone marrow transplantation for a variety of metabolic diseases, heart–lung transplantation in CF. It may be possible to alter or induce the expression of abnormal genes or to induce expression of genes that may compensate for the faulty gene (e.g. eutrophin in muscular dystrophy). In diseases that predominantly affect one organ, an alternative to organ transplantation which may become practicable in the future is the insertion of normal genetic material into the cells of the affected organ ('gene therapy'). This has been achieved in one patient with familial hypercholesterolaemia where a faulty gene for the LDL receptor has been replaced in some liver cells. Such treatment will require detailed knowledge of the affected gene, the control of its expression and the ability to monitor this expression. The difficulties of delivering the gene to the target organ and of avoiding immuno-rejection of the gene product will need to be overcome. Although viral vectors are currently under study as the most promising way of inserting new genetic material into somatic cells, it is the search for appropriate vectors able to deliver the modified gene to a target organ in vivo which presents the greatest challenge for 'gene therapy'.

20

CARE OF THE ELDERLY
Gordon K. Wilcock

Many of the disorders that afflict our elders will be covered elsewhere. Common symptoms in the elderly, rather than specific diseases, and one or two other important areas will therefore form the substance of this chapter.

CONFUSION AND DEMENTIA

Confusion is common in the elderly. It is important to differentiate between a confusional state induced by another illness, e.g. a urinary tract or respiratory infection or a drug toxicity, and the more chronic conditions that cause dementia. The two can of course co-exist as both are common.

ACUTE CONFUSIONAL STATES

These tend to occur suddenly, presenting over a relatively short period, e.g. days rather than weeks or months. The patient is often ill or has been recently prescribed different drugs or an increased dose of his or her usual medication.

The most common infections are those of the respiratory and urinary tracts but infection anywhere could be responsible. Endocrine disorders, a raised blood urea level, electrolyte abnormalities and an elevated calcium level may also cause confusion. If a metabolic cause is discovered, the underlying reason should be sought.

Medication is a potent cause of confusion in the elderly. Particularly important in this respect are antidepressants, anticonvulsants, anti-Parkinsonian treatment, beta-blockers and hypnotics.

Several other conditions may present with confusion, although less commonly. These include anaemia of any cause, especially if it has arisen relatively suddenly, neurological abnormalities such as a subdural haematoma, space-occupying lesions, cerebrovascular events, and cardiac failure. Some of these usually present with a more chronic deterioration and are more likely to cause dementia than an acute confusional state.

A careful history, taken from a reliable third party if possible, physical examination and basic screening investigations will often establish the diagnosis. Treatment depends upon the underlying cause.

DEMENTIA

Dementia is diagnosed when the patient has global intellectual dysfunction. This of course means more than memory loss and can include difficulty in using language, difficulty with simple tasks such as subtracting serial sevens, disorientation in time and space, apraxias for day to day activities, and so on. The prevalence is around 2% of those aged 65–70 rising 10-fold to 20% by the age of 80 and over. It is usually insidious and progressive.

In a small proportion of people there is a treatable component to the aetiology, e.g. hypothyroidism, vitamin B_{12} and folate deficiency, neuro-syphilis, etc. More usually it is caused by an irreversible condition such as Alzheimer's disease, multiple small strokes or Lewy body disease. Even if the underlying cause is untreatable, much can be done to help support the patient and his or her carers, e.g. by referral to the local branch of the Alzheimer's Disease Society.

General principles of management of the agitated confused patient

It is helpful to nurse the subject in a light and simple environment, and to relate to him or her with a kindly approach, carefully explaining what is about to happen, even if one feels the patient may not understand this.

If treatment is required for disturbance or wandering at night, chlorme-thiazole or triclofos sodium are often useful. Benzodiazepines should be avoided if possible, resorting to the short-acting preparations only if essential. Agitation or restlessness during the day may respond to small doses of thioridazine or promazine. These can also be used at night if necessary. Side-effects of phenothiazines include Parkinsonism, postural hypotension, photosensitivity, jaundice and the development of tardive dyskinesia.

CONSTIPATION

Many old people are very conscious of their bowel habit, or lack of it, and become anxious if they do not have a daily evacuation. Reassurance that this is not always necessary may help, but rarely does. However, alteration in bowel habit, especially if accompanied by other symptoms, particularly weight loss, may indicate the presence of serious bowel pathology.

Causes of constipation

Many elderly people, especially women, have taken purgatives for most of their lives. It is this group that are often difficult to treat. Like so many other problems in older people, however, constipation is often multifactorial in origin. Amongst the important contributory factors are impairment of mobility; drugs, especially those with an anticholinergic action, those which contain codeine or other opiate derivatives and some iron preparations; hypothyroidism, depression and some lesions of the gastrointestinal (GI) tract. A diet lacking in fibre may also play a part.

DEAFNESS

Although there are many age-associated degenerative changes in the auditory mechanism and pathways, it is surprising how frequently there are simple contributory factors that are remediable. In general, older people lose the ability to hear the higher frequencies first, may suffer hypersensitivity to loud noises, and develop impairment of the ability to discriminate between different noises.

Assessment and management

Routine examination of cranial nerve function will ascertain whether there is likely to be a remedial cause, e.g. wax in the external auditory meatus. Wherever there is any doubt, hearing is best assessed by an audiometrician.

A hearing aid can make an important contribution to the quality of life of the wearer. Modern technology allows improved performance in relation to the telephone, radio and television. Most modern aids are also able to make use of the induction loops that are installed in many public places, allowing the wearer to participate fully in public meetings, etc.

It is important to face people with impaired hearing during conversation, as they become increasingly reliant upon non-verbal cues to communicate.

FALLS

Falls are a common medical problem of the elderly, responsible for many admissions to hospital, and frequently result in fractures of the hip and wrist in osteoporotic females. There are many causes (Table 20.1), and not infrequently the aetiology is multifactorial.

Table 20.1. Specific causes of falls

Cardiovascular system	Dysrhythmia, postural hypotension, myocardial infarction
Central nervous system	Cervical spondylosis, peripheral neuropathy, posterior column impairment, extrapyramidal disorders, cerebellar ataxia, epilepsy, visual impairment, TIA/stroke
Musculoskeletal system	Any form of arthritis, proximal myopathy

Enquiries should be made specifically about the following four points in the history: vertigo/giddiness, accident hazards, loss of consciousness, relation to posture. These are obvious pointers to specific aetiological factors. Postural hypotension most commonly results from the use of drugs, especially antidepressants, anti-Parkinsonian agents, diuretics and hypotensive agents. Other causes include hypocalcaemia, autonomic dysfunction secondary to diabetes mellitus, Parkinson's disease, etc. Treatment involves attention to the underlying cause, the use of compression stockings and if necessary fludrocortisone.

Treatment

This will depend upon the underlying cause. Where it is not possible to remedy the problem, instruction from a physiotherapist coupled with careful attention to the day to day environment is essential. In some cases an alarm system will help those who have fallen, to summon assistance.

IMMOBILITY

As is the case for falls, this is often multifactorial in aetiology.

Specific causes of immobility

A patient complaining of generalised weakness may well have a myopathy, especially that accompanying osteomalacia, electrolyte imbalances and malignancy. Frequently encountered neurological lesions include Parkinsonism, peripheral neuropathy and undetected cerebrovascular damage. Postural hypotension may also lead to an elderly person refusing to walk, as may other cardiovascular and also respiratory problems which reduce exercise tolerance. Minor foot problems are often overlooked and it is important not to forget that dementia and depression may also lead to immobility. Many old people who have a history of falling will take to their bed or chair and refuse to move because they are frightened of further accidents.

Treatment

As is the case with so many problems in older people, diagnosis and treatment of the underlying cause is the most important factor. In addition, inpatient rehabilitation is usually necessary as even a few days in bed will make it very much more difficult for an elderly person to get back on his or her feet. This will allow the patient access to daily physiotherapy, occupational therapy and medical and social assessment.

An important part of the treatment of an immobile patient is to prevent pressure sores, venous thromboses, hypostatic pneumonia, constipation, contractures and other consequences of being bed- or chair-bound.

INCONTINENCE OF URINE

Incontinence of urine is a frequent problem. Unless there is an obvious cause it is very helpful to chart the pattern of the incontinence, relating it to time of day, meals, drinks, etc. It is also important to ensure that it really is incontinence and not pseudoincontinence. The latter occurs when a person cannot get to the toilet in time, e.g. after a potent diuretic or with urgency of micturition from a urinary tract infection. This also arises when a patient has difficulty finding the toilet, e.g. in the middle of the night.

Treatment

This depends upon the underlying cause. From a practical point of view these are best divided up in the elderly as follows:

1. Retention with overflow: commonest causes are prostatic hypertrophy in men, faecal impaction and drugs, especially those with an anticholinergic action such as antidepressants and anti-Parkinsonian treatment.
2. Stress incontinence and senile vaginitis. Stress incontinence in the elderly usually requires a gynaecological referral as pelvic floor exercises are rarely successful in women over 80. A pessary may be helpful. Senile vaginitis is treated with a local oestrogen preparation although some patients respond better to an intermittent course of oral oestrogens.
3. Mental impairment: incontinence occurs commonly in people who are confused, whatever the cause. Sedative drugs taken at night may also impair the level of consciousness such that the patient sleeps through the need to void urine.
4. The uninhibited neurogenic bladder: this is a common cause resulting in the patient being unable to control spontaneous bladder contractions. It is best diagnosed with a cystometrogram. The incontinence is often accompanied by frequency and urgency. It may respond to flavoxate, but often environmental modification, e.g. a bedside commode, will prove more useful.

Many patients have incontinence for which the cause is not immediately apparent. Wherever treatment has failed it is important to consider whether or not referral to a specialist urodynamic unit would be helpful. Assistance from the incontinence advisory nurse will often help.

VISUAL IMPAIRMENT

Normal ageing changes affect the eye, for example the increasing difficulty with accommodation and the reduction in visual acuity that many people notice. Spectacles help the former; the latter rarely interferes with normal day to day vision significantly and is helped by adequate lighting.

Causes of visual impairment

Three conditions are particularly important as they occur commonly. Cataracts rarely cause total blindness and progress slowly. Once day to day life is significantly impaired on their account, the patient should be referred for surgery.

Acute glaucoma, often heralded by severe pain as well as blurring of vision, is an emergency requiring immediate referral for specialist treatment.

Retinal degeneration may be caused or aggravated by diabetes or hypertension, as in younger patients, and should be treated similarly. It is more usually the result of senile macular degeneration which can be helped by visual aids, e.g. a magnifying glass, strong reading spectacles and good lighting.

Any sudden deterioration in visual ability should lead to specialist referral unless this is inappropriate, e.g. the field deficit resulting from a stroke.

RHEUMATIC DISEASES IN THE ELDERLY

The elderly suffer from a different spectrum of diseases (Table 20.2). The clinical presentation is often atypical, minor rheumatic disease on top of other disorders cause a major disability, there are more problems with drug side-effects and polypharmacy, and the social consequences are worse.

Normal ageing changes may be mistaken for disease, e.g. the elderly hand resembles that in rheumatoid arthritis.

'Abnormal' investigations are not always significant in the elderly: e.g. radiographic osteoarthritis, chondrocalcinosis, hyperuricaemia, rheumatoid factor, antinuclear antibodies and mild elevation of the ESR.

Not all symptoms should be attributed to old age, and a careful diagnosis should be made. The priority is to maintain independence and avoid side-effects of treatment.

Table 20.2. Causes of rheumatic diseases in the elderly

Soft-tissue rheumatism, chiefly adhesive capsulitis

Osteoarthritis

Polymyalgia rheumatica

Crystal arthropathies: diuretic-induced gout, pseudogout

Trauma: unsteadiness, poor eyesight

Osteoporosis

Rheumatoid arthritis: tends to be more severe, may have a polymyalgic onset or present with diffuse swelling of the hands and forearms

Iatrogenic, e.g. haemarthrosis from anticoagulation, drug-induced systemic lupus erythematosus

Others: hypothyroid arthropathy, pain from Parkinson's disease, post-hemiparesis pain, septic arthritis

---

21

PSYCHIATRY

David Nutt, Caroline Bell

Psychiatric illnesses are prevalent both in the community at large and throughout medicine in general. Patients who are psychiatrically unwell complain of a wide variety of symptoms and present not only to psychiatrists but also to family doctors, casualty and other medical or surgical departments. This means that all doctors, whatever their specialty, will inevitably see patients with a psychiatric illness. This may be a psychiatric disorder mimicking a medical one, e.g. panic attacks with chest pain and palpitations presenting as cardiovascular disease, or a psychiatric problem in response to a physical illness, e.g. depression after a myocardial infarction. Effective diagnosis and management is crucial in both situations and is the aim of this chapter. We first describe the key features of the most common psychiatric disorders and then give practical guidelines for their differential diagnosis and management.

It should be remembered that psychiatric illness does not usually occur in isolation but as a consequence of the interaction of a variety of factors (biological, psychological and social) (Fig. 21.1), all of which may need to be addressed over the course of treatment.

ORGANIC STATES

ACUTE ORGANIC DISORDERS (ACUTE CONFUSIONAL STATES, DELIRIUM)

Acute organic disorders are quite common occurrences on medical and surgical wards and are particularly prevalent in the elderly. The cardinal sign is clouding of consciousness, which is shown clinically by disorientation and poor attention. Other common features are listed in Table 21.1. The symptoms all tend to develop acutely over hours/days and fluctuate over the course of the day, typically being worse at night.

Acute organic disorders are caused by a variety of factors which have in common the fact that they all result in a metabolic disturbance in the areas of the brain responsible for consciousness. Some of the causes are listed in

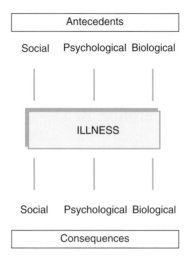

Fig. 21.1 The biopsychosocial model.

Table 21.1. Features of acute organic states

- Disorientation in time, person and place, e.g. do not know what time it is, where they are or who you are
- Inability to maintain attention, e.g. questions have to be repeated to be understood
- Disorganised thinking, e.g. rambling, incoherent speech
- Perceptual disturbances, e.g. misinterpretations, particularly visual
- Psychomotor activity disturbed, e.g. can be restless and irritable or have difficulty keeping awake

---

Table 21.2. It is worth remembering that although infections used to be the most common cause, drug intoxication and alcohol withdrawal now head the list.

Investigations
These are aimed at finding the underlying cause: full blood count (FBC), urea and electrolytes (U&E), liver function tests (LFTs), blood glucose, appropriate blood cultures, blood gases, ECG and chest X-ray. Also consider lumbar puncture, skull X-ray, computed tomography (CT) and magnetic resonance imaging, as indicated.

Treatment
This consists of good, consistent nursing care in a well-lit room to reduce disorientation and perceptual disturbance and treatment of the underlying cause, e.g. infection, fluid imbalance, thiamine deficiency (with i.m. injec-

Table 21.2. Causes of acute organic disorders

Toxins
Alcohol/alcohol withdrawal (delirium tremens)
Opiates, amphetamines, cocaine, ecstasy, LSD, solvents
Prescribed drugs—steroids, digoxin, L-dopa, anticholinergics, diuretics, psychotropics
Lead, manganese, mercury

Infections
General—pneumonia, urinary tract, septicaemia
Cerebral—meningitis, encephalitis

Hypoxia
Heart failure, myocardial infarction (MI)
Respiratory disorders

Metabolic disorder
Electrolyte disturbance
Uraemia
Hepatic failure
Hypoglycaemia
Porphyria

Endocrine
Hypothyroid
Hypercalcaemia

Vitamin deficiency
Thiamine (Wernicke-Korsakoff syndrome)

Trauma
Head injury

Epilepsy
Psychomotor seizure
Postictal state

Vascular disease
Transient ischaemic attack (TIA), cerebrovascular accident (CVA)
Hypertensive encephalopathy

tions). Sedate as necessary using diazepam or chlordiazepoxide, and if fits occur, treat with i.v. diazepam. Marked psychotic symptoms are treated with neuroleptics, e.g. haloperidol 1.5–5 mg t.d.s.

CHRONIC ORGANIC DISORDERS (DEMENTIA)

Dementia is very common with a prevalence of 5% in the population aged over 65 increasing to 20% in the 85 and over age group. The diagnosis is made on the basis of the history from the patient (as far as is possible) and relatives and a careful examination of their mental and physical state. Patients with dementia have a global deterioration of all mental functions with the essential feature of impairment of short- and long-term memory occurring in clear consciousness. Other associated features are listed in Table 21.3.

In practice the cause is most often Alzheimer's disease or multi-infarct dementia. A list of causes with their characteristic features is given in Table 21.4.

Table 21.3. Features of dementia

- Impairment in short-term memory—inability to remember a name and address after 5 minutes
- Impairment in long-term memory—inability to remember past personal information, e.g. what they did yesterday, or facts of general knowledge, e.g. name of the queen, well-known dates
- Thinking muddled—difficulty in defining words and thinking abstractly, e.g. explaining meaning of a metaphor
- Disturbances of other higher cortical functions, e.g. dysphasia—difficulty finding or understanding words, apraxia, e.g. difficulty dressing
- Affective lability
- Personality change, e.g. alteration or accentuation of premorbid traits
- Impaired judgement, social or sexual disinhibition

Especially in the elderly, depression can present with a very similar picture with poor concentration and memory (pseudodementia) and can be difficult to differentiate. They may perform better on tests of cognitive function if they are given more time—patients with dementia do not improve however long they have. If the diagnosis is still in doubt, a trial of antidepressant medication (without anticholinergic effects) should be used.

Investigations
These are aimed at identifying treatable causes: FBC, B_{12} and folate, erythrocyte sedimentation rate (ESR), U&E, LFT, calcium, TFT (thyroid function tests), syphilis serology, HIV (at risk), chest X-ray, CT/MRI.

Treatment
Treat any underlying treatable causes.

Pharmacological. Anticholinesterases, e.g. Donepezil, may improve cognitive function in carefully selected patients. Antipsychotics can help wandering and night disturbance. Use carbamazepine for seizures.

Psychological. Memory aids and lists.

Social. Careful explanation to relatives; physical aids in the home; day care; respite admissions; Alzheimer's Disease Society.

The prognosis is bad with a relentless deterioration and death in 2–5 years.

PSYCHOSIS

The concept of psychosis implies lack of insight and being out of touch with reality, e.g. having delusions or hallucinations. The acutely psychotic patient may also be acutely disturbed and difficult to manage and may require compulsory admission.

Table 21.4. Causes of dementia

Degenerative

Alzheimer's disease	More common in women, memory impairment early and prominent, relentless progress, intellectual and personality deterioration, parietal lobe dysfunction, e.g. apraxias and extrapyramidal signs occur later
Creutzfeldt-Jakob disease	Personality change with depression and fatigue, memory loss, parietal signs, seizures, neurological signs prominent
Pick's disease	Frontal and temporal lobes—personality deterioration, disinhibition and dysphasia common, memory and neurological deterioration later
Huntington's chorea	Autosomal dominant gene on chromosome 4, chorea and mental changes (paranoid psychosis, personality change, global dementia) often develop independently, 50% present with psychiatric not physical symptoms
Normal pressure hydrocephalus	Memory impairment, slowness and apathy, unsteady gait, incontinence
Subcortical dementia	Seen in e.g. Parkinson's disease (Lewy body dementia), Wilson's disease; affects frontal lobes—personality change, depression, apathy, forgetfulness, ataxia, fluctuating levels of consciousness, visual hallucinations, marked deficits in attention and visuospatial performance

Vascular

Multi-infarct dementia	Slightly more common in males, acute onset with stepwise deterioration, fluctuating impairment worse at night, insight often retained and depression common, evidence of vascular disease elsewhere

Toxins
Alcohol

Infections
Late syphilis
Chronic or subacute encephalitis
AIDS

Metabolic
Liver and kidney failure
Metastatic or non-metastatic cancer, lymphomas

Vitamin deficiency
Thiamine
B_{12} or folate

Endocrine
Hypothyroidism
Hypo- and hyperparathyroidism

Trauma

Punch drunk syndrome	Repeated mild head injuries, e.g. horse riding; intellectual and personality deterioration with cerebellar, pyramidal and extrapyramidal signs

MANIA/HYPOMANIA

The manic/hypomanic description may be used to indicate degree of severity, or presence of delusions or hallucinations, manic being the more severe form. Both usually occur as part of a bipolar illness, i.e. alternating with episodes of depression, and there is often a positive family history. The features of a manic or hypomanic episode are listed in Table 21.5.

Investigations
These are aimed at finding any organic cause (Table 21.6): urine drug screen, FBC, U&E and CT/MRI as indicated.

Treatment
Pharmacological. If the patient is very disturbed, recommendations for management of the violent patient (see p. 511) are followed.

Acute: antipsychotics, e.g. droperidol; lithium: aim for a level of 0.8—it takes 3 or 4 days for therapeutic effect.

Table 21.5. Features of mania

- Persistently elevated or irritable mood
- Decreased need for sleep, e.g. feels rested after only 3 hours sleep—often the earliest sign
- Racing thoughts
- More talkative with 'pressure of speech'
- 'Flight of ideas'—jumps from one theme to the next but a link can be seen
- Distractible
- Inflated self-esteem or grandiosity
- Increased activity—rushing around and not feeling a need to rest or eat
- Excessive involvement in pleasurable or risk-taking activities, e.g. spending sprees, sexual overactivity or disinhibition, foolish business ventures
- Psychotic features, if they occur, are mood congruent—delusions and hallucinations are grandiose, e.g. they believe they are more gifted than others, hear voices saying 'You are the son of God'

Table 21.6. Some organic causes of mania

Toxins and drugs
Steroids
Amphetamines, cocaine

Neurological
Frontal tumour
Multiple sclerosis
Temporal lobe epilepsy

Infections

Maintenance: lithium at a level of 0.5–0.8 reduces the likelihood of recurrences. Regular, i.e. 3-monthly, blood checks for lithium level, renal and thyroid function are carried out.

Other. Regular contact is needed to assess the mental state. The patient may need rehabilitation as described below if illness is severe and recurrent.

SCHIZOPHRENIA

The prevalence of schizophrenia is about 1%. The median age of onset is 28 years for males and 32 years for females and it has a marked genetic component. The symptoms of schizophrenia are divided into positive and negative types (Table 21.7).

Positive symptoms present acutely and often result in intervention because they are so abnormal. They typically respond to antipsychotics. The negative symptoms, although in some ways less obvious, are usually chronic and probably even more damaging, affecting all aspects of the patient's life. Negative symptoms respond less well to antipsychotics and may be augmented by extrapyramidal side-effects.

Acute psychotic states can be caused by other organic conditions listed above as causes of mania, and need to be excluded by appropriate investigations.

Treatment
Pharmacological. If violent, the patient is managed as described in a later section (p. 511).

Acute: antipsychotics, e.g. haloperidol, trifluoperazine, risperidone, olanzapine zuclopenthixol acetate; anticholinergics, e.g. procyclidine, may be required to counteract extrapyramidal side-effects.

Table 21.7. Features of schizophrenia

Positive symptoms
Delusions—often paranoid or bizarre, e.g. being controlled by another force, thought broadcasting
Hallucinations, e.g. voices conversing with each other, running commentary
Incoherence—thoughts have no obvious connections
Catatonic behaviour—take up odd postures
Physically disturbed and violent
Negative symptoms
Social isolation or withdrawal
Marked lack of initiative, interests or energy
Impairment of personal hygiene
Blunted or inappropriate affect—unconcerned about things that should provoke emotion, or the emotion provoked is inappropriate, e.g. laughing at distressing news
Vague digressive speech

Maintenance: antipsychotics orally or as depot to improve compliance.

Resistant cases: atypical antipsychotic, clozapine (requires blood monitoring because of risk of agranulocytosis).

Other. The aim is to avoid over- or understimulation. Regular contact is required to assess mental state and rehabilitation using day hospitals and sheltered workshops should be provided. The family will need help to understand the illness and reduce their expressed emotion.

Prognosis

Fifty-five per cent have a chronic course and 45% have an acute, improving course.

DEPRESSION

Depression is a very common clinical problem affecting 1 in 10 people during their lifetime. It is very important with such a serious and prevalent condition to recognise the symptoms and to treat it effectively. The longer depression exists, the more damage and suffering it does to the patient, their family and society and the more resistant to treatment it becomes. The fact that depression is often precipitated by a life event and is thus understandable leads many doctors to believe that it does not warrant treatment. This is not the case—all episodes of clinical depression should be treated. Various other factors, in addition to the immediate precipitant, also contribute to the onset of depression (biological sensitivity, genetic predisposition, personal vulnerability and psychodynamic issues) and must also be addressed.

The essential feature of depression is either depressed, low mood or a loss of interest or pleasure (anhedonia) in almost all usual activities. It is often accompanied by other features, listed in Table 21.8.

Some patients have an 'atypical depression' with reversed diurnal mood

---

Table 21.8. Features of depression

- Depressed mood—often worse in morning
- Anhedonia—inability to enjoy themselves or feel pleasure
- Poor appetite with weight loss
- Sleep disturbance with onset insomnia, disrupted sleep and early morning waking
- Fatigue or loss of energy
- Decreased libido
- Difficulty concentrating
- Psychomotor retardation (slowing thoughts and actions) or agitation
- Feelings of worthlessness or guilt
- Recurrent ideas of death and suicide

variation, i.e. feeling worse in the evening, increased appetite and hypersomnia, 'leaden paralysis' and hypersensitivity to criticism.

Investigations

These are aimed at excluding organic causes, listed in Table 21.9: FBC, U&E, calcium, TFT, iron, B_{12}/folate, and CT/MRI, as indicated.

Treatment

Antidepressants are increased to the maximum does tolerated and continued at this dose for 6–8 months. An explanation is given of any likely side-effects and the delay of 2–3 weeks in therapeutic response. The choice of antidepressant is important and is based on likely side-effects and consequent tolerability, any coexisting medical problems and suicide risk (safety in overdose) (see Table 21.10).

Electroconvulsive therapy (ECT). Despite its bad publicity, ECT remains a very effective treatment for depression, particularly where rapid results are required, e.g. the patient is not eating or drinking, in post-partum illness, in the elderly and where delusions or hallucinations are prominent.

Psychological treatments. Cognitive therapy aims to change the patient's negative thoughts about themselves and the world using techniques where thoughts are identified, recorded in a diary and then challenged with alternatives. It is the most effective of the psychological approaches but even so is only effective in mild to moderate cases. There is no evidence that other forms of unstructured counselling are beneficial in depression.

Table 21.9. Organic causes of depression

Toxins and drugs
Methyldopa, clonidine, L-dopa, steroids, beta-blockers
Alcohol
Prolonged use of amphetamines, opiates

Infections
Post-influenza
Infectious mononucleosis

Endocrine
Hypothyroidism
Hyperparathyroidism
Cushing's syndrome
Addison's disease

Deficiency
Iron deficiency
B_{12} folate deficiency

Neurological
Multiple sclerosis
Parkinson's disease
Intracranial tumour

Table 21.10. Comparison of different antidepressant groups

	Side-effects	Coexisting medical conditions that contraindicate use	Safety in overdose
Tricyclics (TCAs)	Blurred vision, dry mouth, urinary retention, constipation, sedation, postural hypotension, tachycardia, arrhythmias, weight gain, tremor, sweating, sexual dysfunction, convulsions (rarely)	Glaucoma, prostatism, arrhythmia, recent MI	Not safe
Selective serotonin reuptake inhibitors (SSRIs)	Nausea, diarrhoea, headache, dizziness, anxiety exacerbation, sexual dysfunction		Safe in overdose
Monoamine oxidase inhibitors (MAOIs)	Postural hypotension dizziness, headache, weight gain, sexual dysfunction Interactions: tyramine-containing foods, sympathomimetics, pethidine, caution with other antidepressants	CVA, phaeochromocytoma	Not safe
RIMA, moclobemide	Headache, dizziness, nausea		Safer in overdose

ANXIETY DISORDERS

This is a group of conditions in which anxiety is experienced in response to different situations. They cause extreme distress and disability but are often seen as minor ailments not warranting treatment—this is not the case.

PANIC DISORDER

The essential feature of this condition is the occurrence of panic attacks, the symptoms of which are shown in Fig. 21.2. The symptoms are very somatic, which explains why patients so frequently present to casualty and other departments convinced they are dying or having an MI. The first panic attack is usually clearly remembered and often occurs out of the blue. The situation in which it first occurred is avoided as much as possible and whenever confronted again is associated with marked anticipatory anxiety. The patient typically avoids more and more situations, a condition known as agoraphobia. Patients often self-medicate with alcohol.

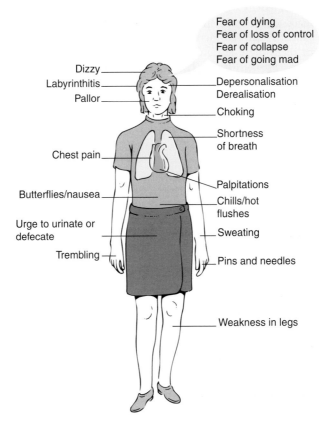

Fig. 21.2 Symptoms of panic.

Differential diagnosis
Excessive caffeine use, alcohol or benzodiazepine withdrawal, hyperthyroidism, phaeochromocytoma, cardiac arrythmias and temporary lobe epilepsy need to be considered.

Investigations
These are aimed at excluding the above conditions: FBC, macrocytosis with alcohol abuse, U&E, LFT, thyroid function tests (TFTs) and urine for metabolites of catecholamines.

Treatment
Education about the nature and symptoms of anxiety is helpful.

Pharmacological. SSRI or TCA starting with half the minimum dose (to prevent anxiety exacerbation) titrating up gradually according to response to as large a dose as tolerated. Cover for 2–3 weeks with benzodiazepine may be needed over this period. The effective dose is continued for 6–8 months and then the antidepressant tapered.

Psychological. Cognitive behavioural psychotherapy (CBT) is aimed at changing 'catastrophic misinterpretations' of bodily symptoms, e.g. when the patient's heart rate increases that they think they are having an MI, which makes them more anxious and causes the heart rate to increase further, setting up a vicious circle. The behavioural component involves drawing up a hierarchy of anxiety-provoking situations and then exposing the patient to them in a graded way, i.e. easiest first and repeating this until anxiety habituates.

SOCIAL PHOBIA

The essential feature of this disorder is the fear of social or performance situations when the patient feels they are under scrutiny and thinks they will do something humiliating or embarrassing. Typical situations are talking in groups, public speaking, eating or drinking in public, being watched while they work, talking to people in authority, e.g. their boss or doctors, and talking to someone of the opposite sex. The symptoms experienced are similar to those experienced in panic disorder but in particular they blush, sweat and shake—all very noticeable to other people, which makes things worse. It is a very disabling condition—patients are commonly depressed and often abuse alcohol (self-medication for anxiety). It interferes with all aspects of their lives, i.e. work (never going for promotion) and social life (half never marry).

Investigations
These are as for panic disorder.

Treatment
Education about the illness is helpful: patients often think they are unique.

Pharmacological. RIMA, moclobemide (first-line treatment as it is better tolerated), traditional MAOI or SSRI for 6–8 months.

Psychological. CBT, as described above. This is often done in groups which, at least initially, may be too anxiety-provoking. The best response probably occurs when medication and CBT are used in combination.

OBSESSIVE COMPULSIVE DISORDER (OCD)

The essential feature of this condition is the presence of obsessions and compulsions. Obsessions are unwanted, recurrent, persistent ideas, images or impulses that are repeatedly experienced. Compulsions are voluntary actions that are performed with a sense of compulsion—resistance results in a mounting feeling of tension. The content of obsessions and compulsions are often concerned with a fear of being contaminated, for example, leading to cleaning rituals, or harming others, e.g. parent having impulses to kill a loved child. The disorder is chronic with fluctuating exacerbations and is often complicated by depression.

Treatment

Pharmacological. A serotonergic antidepressant, e.g. SSRI or clomipramine is prescribed for at least 8 months at as high a dose as is tolerated.

Psychological. Behaviour therapy—graded exposure with response prevention.

POST-TRAUMATIC STRESS DISORDER (PTSD)

The essential feature of this disorder is the development of characteristic symptoms following exposure to an extreme traumatic stressor. The symptoms include persistent re-experiencing of the traumatic event, persistent avoidance of stimuli associated with the trauma and numbing of general responsiveness, and persistent symptoms of increased arousal. In taking a history the association with the event is usually obvious. PTSD is differentiated from acute stress disorder by its persistence: the symptoms of acute stress disorder resolve within a 4-week period. Depression quite commonly coexists with PTSD and should be enquired for in the history.

In the current climate of litigation it is likely that this condition will be cited frequently in the courts. If it is to retain its validity as a serious and disabling disorder, we need to ensure that the diagnosis is not in doubt and that clear criteria for its diagnosis are fulfilled.

The treatment of this condition is poorly researched; there have been no properly controlled trials and almost all open trials have been conducted on patients a long time after the causative incident; which may explain the poor outcome. A range of drugs have been reported to be helpful including benzodiazepines, TCAs, SSRIs and MAOIs. Long-term therapy appears to be indicated with doses in the same range as for other anxiety disorders. Treatment immediately following the incident should probably be a short course of a benzodiazepine to promote sleep and to help minimise mental rehearsal of the trauma that may lead to long-term problems.

Our practice is to use an SSRI or TCA as first-line treatment with the addition of a benzodiazepine for more enduring cases.

ACUTE STRESS DISORDER

This is anxiety in response to a recent extreme stress. Although in some respects it is a normal and understandable reaction to an event, the problems associated with it are not only the severe distress the anxiety causes but also the risk that it may evolve into a more persistent state.

The benzodiazepines work quickly and are particularly useful for the anxiety and sleep disturbance that are common in these states. It may well be that treating these symptoms when they are severe reduces the likelihood of their progression to a more persistent anxiety state. Drugs with a slow onset of action such as oxazepam causes less dependence and withdrawal than those with fast brain entry such as diazepam and lorazepam and so are probably the drugs of choice. There is the risk, however, that some patients once started on a benzodiazepine will find it hard to stop, so their use should be reserved for patients where extreme distress is disrupting their normal coping strategies.

SIMPLE OR SPECIFIC PHOBIA

This is fear of a circumscribed object or situation, e.g. spiders. Patients know the fear is irrational but panic whenever they are confronted with the feared object. The object is avoided at all costs with the consequence that their lives often become governed by the phobia, e.g. not going into rooms unless someone has checked that there are no spiders there.

Treatment
Psychological. Behaviour Therapy—graded exposure to the feared object.

GENERALISED ANXIETY DISORDER

The essential feature of this condition is chronic anxiety and worry associated with motor tension (restlessness, muscle tension), autonomic hyperactivity (palpitations, sweating, dry mouth, frequent urination), vigilance and scanning (exaggerated startle response, irritability, trouble falling or staying asleep). The anxiety is persistent, not the sudden, intense waves of panic experienced in panic disorder. It is often chronic with periods of exacerbation at times of stress.

Investigations
These are as for panic disorder.

Treatment

Pharmacological. Buspirone for 6–8 weeks is the first-line treatment. If there is no response, SSRI or TCA is prescribed. Benzodiazepines may be used for short-term exacerbations if all else fails.

Psychological. Teaching of anxiety management techniques may be helpful.

HYSTERICAL DISORDERS (CONVERSION AND DISSOCIATIVE)

The essential features of this group of disorders are symptoms and signs that suggest a physical disorder but for which there are no demonstrable organic findings. The symptoms of hysteria are often divided into conversion symptoms (mental energy converted into physical symptoms, e.g. blindness, paralysis, fits) and dissociative symptoms (dissociation between different mental activities, e.g. amnesia, multiple personality).

The symptoms are not produced deliberately but are created around the patient's ideas about illness, e.g. imitating symptoms of a relative who is ill, and there are often discrepancies between hysterical signs and symptoms and those of organic disease, e.g. the distribution of paralysis is not compatible with anatomical innervation. The symptoms usually confer some advantage on the patient (secondary gain), e.g. hysterical paralysis means not having to look after an elderly relative. It is also reported that patients with hysterical symptoms often show less distress than would be expected for their condition, which is described as 'belle indifference'.

The concept of hysteria gives rise to problems in clinical practice because it is often difficult to completely exclude physical pathology without extensive investigations and because hysterical symptoms can complicate true organic disease.

When the diagnosis is established, treatment is aimed at alleviating any underlying emotional disorder with explanation and reassurance that there is no serious organic disease. A team approach is often required, rewarding healthy behaviour without reinforcing the sick role.

SUBSTANCE ABUSE

ALCOHOL

The current guidelines for maximum alcohol intake per week are 21 units for men and 14 units for women (1 unit = 1 measure of spirit or 1/2 pint of beer). Drinking more than this is very common: of medical inpatients, 30% of men and 10% of women have a drinking problem with even higher rates on trauma wards where withdrawal is often missed. Occupations at particular risk include publicans, journalists, armed forces and doctors. Patients with anxiety disorders often self-medicate with alcohol, e.g. patients with social phobia drink several glasses before going into an anxiety-provoking situation.

It is vitally important to take an alcohol history from every patient. It should include the following—CAGE:

Criticism: has anyone criticised their drinking
Anger: have they ever felt angry when challenged that they have a drink problem
Guilt: have they felt bad about their behaviour
Eye opener: do they have a drink first thing in the morning to prevent withdrawal symptoms.

Alcohol dependence
The clinical features of the alcohol dependence syndrome are listed in Table 21.11.

Withdrawal symptoms
Withdrawal of alcohol in someone who is alcohol dependent causes a variety of symptoms: tremor, nausea, sweating, sleep disturbance, muscle cramps, mood disturbance (e.g. fear and depression), convulsions and perceptual distortions and hallucinations, which may progress to the syndrome of delirium tremens (DTs).

Delirium tremens typically occurs 2–4 days after stopping or reducing alcohol intake. Patients may have all the above symptoms and are very dis-

Table 21.11. Features of alcohol dependence syndrome

- Stereotyped pattern of drinking—drink to avoid symptoms of withdrawal
- Relief or avoidance of withdrawal symptoms by further drinking
- Prominence of drink-seeking behaviour—give priority to drinking over other considerations (social, financial, physical)
- Increased tolerance to alcohol—need more drink to give effect. At later stages tolerance may be suddenly lost as liver failure develops
- Repeated withdrawal symptoms
- Subjective awareness of compulsion to drink
- Reinstatement after abstinence—if start drinking again relapse is rapid and severe

turbed with vivid hallucinations, delusions, marked confusion, sleeplessness, agitation, fear and autonomic overactivity.

Alcohol-related disabilities

Physical disabilities include:
1. Liver damage: alcoholic hepatitis, cirrhosis
2. Gastrointestinal disorders: oesophageal varices, pancreatitis
3. Anaemia: iron deficiency, B_{12} and folate
4. Infection: TB, pneumonia
5. Neurological: Wernicke–Korsakoff syndrome (clouding of consciousness, ocular palsies and nystagmus, staggering gait, peripheral neuropathy) and Korsakoff syndrome (inability to form new memories, confabulation i.e. apparent recollection of imagined events, clear consciousness, peripheral neuropathy). Both are due to B1 (thiamine) deficiency
6. Dementia: global with frontal signs prominent.

Psychological. These include depression and suicide, anxiety (particularly in alcohol withdrawal) and violent behaviour.

Social. These include work difficulties, e.g. absenteeism on Monday mornings, marriage and family difficulties, social isolation, vagrancy and criminality.

Investigations
These are aimed at assessing damage: LFTs including gamma glutamyl transpeptidase (GGT), U&Es to detect electrolyte imbalance, FBC to show macrocytosis, increased carbohydrate deficient transferrin (CDT) and blood alcohol level.

Treatment

Detoxification. A withdrawal regimen is implemented with reducing doses of benzodiazepine, e.g. chlordiazepoxide or diazepam (DTs may require i.v.). Haloperidol is used if DTs are present, and anticonvulsants if there is a previous history of fits. Vitamins, particularly thiamine, and rehydration, are required and any infection should be treated.

Longer-term treatment is as follows:

Medication: Antabuse (disulfiram)—toxic acetaldehyde is produced when alcohol is ingested. New drugs such as acamprosate and naltrexone help reduce relapse once the patient has stopped drinking. Many alcoholics have an underlying anxiety disorder, e.g. social phobia, that responds to treatment.

Psychological: behavioural methods, group therapy, agencies, e.g. Alcoholics Anonymous (AA).

DRUGS

Dangers are secondary to i.v. use, e.g. AIDS and hepatitis B/C.

Opiates (morphine, heroin)

These are smoked, taken orally and injected i.v., i.m. or s.c.. They give an intensely pleasurable 'rush' followed after about an hour by drowsiness, relaxation, decreased libido and appetite. Tolerance and dependence occur rapidly. Unintentional overdoses can occur when the purity of the opiate is unknown. Withdrawal symptoms include craving, agitation, perspiration, rhinorrhoea, yawning, tachycardia, abdominal cramps and dilated pupils. They peak 24–48 hours after the last dose and subside after 7–10 days. Withdrawal symptoms may be controlled by using methadone given in decreasing doses. Benzodiazepines and lofexidine can also help. Some addicts do well on maintenance methadone.

Cocaine

This is sniffed (nasal ulceration may result), chewed and injected i.v. It produces euphoria, excitement and increased energy. It can also produce visual or tactile hallucinations of crawling insects (formication) and paranoid psychosis. Withdrawal can produce depression, insomnia and craving.

Crack is a purified form of cocaine smoked by releasing vapours when heated. It gives similar but intensified effects to cocaine, especially feelings of exhilaration and power. It is more addictive than cocaine with the user feeling compelled to continue to avoid feelings of depression.

Amphetamine

This is taken orally or injected i.v. It is a stimulant drug and used to be widely prescribed in the 1940s and 1950s for depression, fatigue and obesity. It causes increased arousal and excitement, reduced appetite, tachycardia, hyperreflexia and dilated pupils. Prolonged use can cause a psychosis with paranoid ideas and hallucinations. Withdrawal causes depression and fatigue.

Ecstasy is an amphetamine-like compound that increases energy and social interaction and, like amphetamine, can cause psychotic episodes. It impairs water balance and so can lead to terminal dehydration particularly when used in hot, sweaty conditions, e.g. night clubs.

Hallucinogens: lysergic acid diethylamide (LSD), mescaline

These are taken orally. Effects occur after about 30 minutes and last for several hours. They heighten perceptions of vision, colour, touch and sound and can cause hallucinations. They also cause pupils to dilate and peripheral blood vessels to constrict. A 'bad trip' causes frightening perceptual changes, despair and depression. Withdrawal symptoms do not occur although 'flashbacks' of hallucinations can be experienced for up to 1 year.

Cannabis

This is usually smoked but can also be taken orally with food or drink. Its effects occur after minutes and last for 6–12 hours. These include feelings of relaxation and well-being, increased appetite, lowered body temperature and perceptual changes with visual distortions. Cannabis may precipitate a psychotic episode and worsens schizophrenia but does not cause physical withdrawal symptoms.

Solvent sniffing

Solvents used include petrol, cleaning solvents, aerosols and glues, the base substances of which are commonly acetone and toluene. It mainly occurs in boys usually as a group activity. Inhalation causes initial euphoria followed by drowsiness and stupor if continued. It can cause perceptual disturbances, liver and CNS damage and death from cardiac arrhythmia or asphyxiation from the use of a plastic bag or vomiting.

EATING DISORDERS

ANOREXIA NERVOSA

This relatively common disorder has a prevalence of 1% in schoolgirls. It is more frequent in females with a female : male ratio of 15 : 1. The illness is probably a response to pressures for slimness plus family dynamic problems. The features of the disorder are:

1. refusal to maintain weight over the minimum for age and height, i.e. 15% below expected norm, by restriction of food intake, vomiting and use of laxatives
2. intense fear of gaining weight even though underweight
3. disturbance in body image—feels fat even though obviously not
4. amenorrhoea.

Weight loss is achieved by restricting intake, vomiting, laxative abuse or excessive exercise. There is often coexistent depression, anxiety and obsessional symptoms. Abnormalities on physical examination include bradycardia, cold extremities, peripheral cyanosis and fine lanugo hair on the trunk.

Investigations

These are to exclude, for example, thyrotoxicosis, malabsorption syndrome and neoplasm, and any consequence of weight loss, e.g. electrolyte imbalance.

Treatment

1. **Restoration of adequate nutrition**: admit to hospital if weight < 70% of normal expected. Carefully controlled calorie intake often with bedrest.
2. **Psychotherapy**: individual and family therapy is often required to resolve underlying issues.
3. **Medication**: newer antidepressants, e.g. SSRIs, may help reduce depression, anxiety and obsessive concerns.

Prognosis

Prognosis is poor—up to 5% die in 5 years and at least 50% have a chronic, relapsing illness often switching to bulimia.

BULIMIA NERVOSA

Again this is common, particularly in females. The age of onset is typically later adolescence or early adult life and is often preceded by a history of anorexia nervosa. The features of the syndrome are:

1. lack of control over food intake and binge eating (food of high calorie content) often associated with guilt afterwards
2. self-induced vomiting, laxative use or exercise to prevent weight gain
3. persistent over-concern with body weight and image.

Patients with bulimia are usually within the normal weight range (unlike those with anorexia). They also often have coexistent depression, anxiety and obsessional symptoms. Abnormalities on physical examination include calluses on the back of the hands from self-induced vomiting and erosion of dental enamel from frequent presence of gastric contents in mouth.

Investigations

Check for electrolyte imbalance as a consequence of frequent vomiting and laxative abuse.

Treatment

1. **Restoration of adequate nutrition**: reduction of frequency and severity of binges with the aim of achieving regular food intake.
2. **Psychotherapy**: cognitive behaviour therapy as an individual or group with the use of dietary diaries.
3. **Medication**: newer antidepressants, e.g. SSRIs, may help reduce depression, anxiety and obsessive concerns. The SSRIs, particularly fluoxetine, are also effective at reducing bingeing.

Prognosis

Prognosis is poor with frequent relapses and chronicity.

SLEEP DISORDERS

One third of our lives is spent asleep, but the reasons why we sleep are not yet fully understood. We have all experienced the effects of lack of sleep and can readily understand the distress caused by sleep disruption.

The diagnosis of the various sleep disorders is made from the history, asking the patient to keep a sleep diary of when they slept and what they felt about their sleep with the use of objective measures and sleep EEG recordings being made if necessary.

INSOMNIA

Complaints of insomnia are very common and include difficulty getting off to sleep, difficulty staying asleep and waking too early in the morning. Some causes of short-term insomnia are:

1. situational, e.g. going into hospital, before exams
2. stress, e.g. bereavement, stress at work
3. drugs, e.g. caffeine, beta-blockers, SSRI antidepressants at the start of treatment
4. drug withdrawal, e.g. benzodiazepines, alcohol
5. physical factors, e.g. pain, pregnancy, coughing, need to urinate (diuretics)
6. psychiatric disorders, e.g. depression (restless with early morning waking), hypomania (sleep less)
7. shift work.

Treatment
1. explanation and reassurance
2. identify and as far as possible remove/treat precipitating factors (see above)
3. educate re good sleep hygiene, i.e. regular bedtime and getting up, no caffeine just before or during the night, do not 'clock watch'
4. short-term hypnotic, e.g. zopiclone, or a short-acting benzodiazepine for 1–2 weeks.

The treatment of long-term insomnia can be very difficult because patients have often established a pattern of poor sleep hygiene and have become very anxious about their sleep and lack of it, spending large amounts of time and effort on 'trying' to sleep. Care should be taken to identify and treat any psychiatric disorders and any remediable precipitants removed. Further treatment often involves the use of a structured programme to change the patient's behaviour and thoughts about sleep. Taking this condition seriously may be important because chronic insomnia leads to a significant reduction in life expectancy.

OTHER IMPORTANT TOPICS

SUICIDE, DELIBERATE SELF-HARM AND ASSESSING SUICIDE RISK

Approximately 6000 deaths a year from suicide are recorded in the UK

Table 21.12. Risk factors for suicide

- Male
- Age over 40 years, recent increase in young men
- Single
- Unemployed
- Chronic, painful illness
- Previous suicide attempts
- Psychiatric conditions: depression
  - schizophrenia
  - alcohol abuse

although this is probably an underestimate of the true incidence. The risk factors for suicide are listed in Table 21.12 and need to be taken into account when assessing suicide risk.

Deliberate self-harm (DSH) describes the actions of patients who take or do something that mimics the act of suicide but does not have a fatal outcome. However, there is often real danger in these acts and a history of DSH is a predictor of successful suicide. Epidemiological studies have shown that the rates of DSH are highest in young women and the most common method used is self-poisoning under the influence of alcohol.

Assessment of suicide risk should be part of the clinical interview of all patients and is crucial in the assessment of anyone with depression (the disorder most commonly indicated) or after DSH. Key areas to cover are:

1. **Suicideal thoughts** should be asked about directly, e.g. 'Have you ever thought that life is not worth living, do you wish you could go to sleep and not wake up?'
2. **Suicide plans.** What method they intend to use—have they collected tablets, bought a rope to hang themselves, got a hosepipe to connect to the exhaust, etc.; have they left a note, put their affairs in order, told anyone of their plans or have they planned to do it in secret?
3. **Presence of risk factors for suicide.**

From the above the likelihood of suicide can be established and managed appropriately. The acutely suicidal patient needs to be kept safe and may need admission to hospital to achieve this. Treatable conditions, e.g. depression, need to be managed using medication and referral.

MANAGEMENT OF THE VIOLENT PATIENT

The differential diagnosis of the violent patient is difficult. Possible causes that need to be excluded include:

1. acute psychosis
2. drug/alcohol induced state
3. drug/alcohol withdrawal

4. other acute organic state
5. epilepsy.

However, it should also be remembered that violence does not necessarily indicate illness. The aim of management is to keep yourself and staff safe, prevent the patient harming him- or herself or others and to establish and treat the cause—a lot to achieve during a very stressful time.

Interview
1. Do not be alone with the patient.
2. Make sure there are sufficient trained staff to deal with the situation.
3. Make sure you and staff can exit the room.
4. Remain calm and avoid confrontation.
5. Talk and listen to the patient.

Restraint
1. Do not attempt restraint without an adequate number of staff.
2. Use staff trained in control and restraint techniques.
3. Use the minimum force necessary.
4. Never press on the neck, chest or abdomen.

Medication
The patient is sedated with benzodiazepine, e.g. lorazepam 2–4 mg i.v. ± neuroleptic, e.g. 20–40 mg droperidol i.m. and the underlying cause treated.

Very regular reviews are undertaken to assess the situation and physical state of the patient.

LIASION PSYCHIATRY

Liasion psychiatry is a subspecialty of psychiatry that deals with the interface between medicine and psychiatry. It reflects the reciprocal nature of this relationship: medical illnesses act as risk factors for the development of psychiatric disorders; psychiatric and medical problems commonly coexist, e.g. anxiety, depression and alcohol problems affect 12–18% of medical inpatients; the presence of a psychiatric disorder markedly affects the outcome of medical conditions, e.g. patients who are depressed after an MI have a much poorer recovery and an increased mortality than patients who do not get depressed; patients with psychiatric disorders have a higher incidence of medical illnesses, e.g. anxiety and depression increase the risk of cardiovascular disease; psychiatric disorders can mimic medical disorders and lead to wasted investigations and treatment, e.g. panic attacks presenting with chest pain and palpitations may lead to coronary angiograms!

The clinical component of liasion psychiatry is the assessment and management of psychological morbidity in all these situations and particularly:

1. patients presenting after deliberate self-harm
2. patients presenting to casualty departments with psychological problems

3. patients with psychological problems on medical, surgical, oncology and other wards.

The educational component is also very important to highlight the frequency and possible presentations of psychiatric illness within the medical setting.

Always be sensitive to a psychiatric explanation and diagnosis.

22

TROPICAL MEDICINE
Stuart Glover

MALARIA

Malaria is an acute and chronic disease caused by the obligate intracellular protozoan of the genus *Plasmodium*. There are four types of human malaria: *P. vivax*, *P. falciparum*, *P. ovale* and *P. malariae*. Malaria parasites are transmitted to humans by female anopheline mosquitoes, the definitive host for plasmodia.

Malaria is widespread in the tropics and subtropics causing an estimated two million deaths annually; 2000 cases are diagnosed each year in the UK. There were eight deaths in the UK from malaria during 1989 and 1990. *Falciparum* malaria accounts for 52% and *vivax* for 40% of the malaria diagnosed in Britain. It can on rare occasions be acquired at international European airports, during very brief stopovers in malarious airports (runway malaria), by blood transfusions and organ transplantation. Neonatal malaria is rare.

Pathology

Plasmodial trophozoites alter the deformability of red blood cells, which become sequestered in the microcirculation of the brain, myocardium, gut and kidneys with resultant ischaemia and organ dysfunction. With maturation of trophozoites to schizonts, red cells will rupture, contributing to anaemia. Tumour necrosis factor (TNF) levels rise with schizont release.

Symptoms and signs

The incubation period is 10–15 days for *falciparum* and as long as 24 months for *vivax*. The onset of symptoms is delayed by prior chemoprophylaxis, partial therapy and natural immunity.

Primary attacks in non-immune individuals are abrupt, causing:

1. cold stage (vasoconstriction): rigors, vomiting, rising temperature
2. hot stage (vasodilatation): dry and hot skin, severe throbbing headache, high fever > 40°C, restlessness and delirium
3. sweating stage: drenching sweat, rapid defervescence.

Fever is variable and irregular in *falciparum* and may even be absent. A tertian (every 48 hours) pattern occurs in established *vivax* and *ovale* malaria. Fever may cause delirium.

Other signs include splenomegaly, hepatomegaly with mild jaundice (caused mainly by haemolysis), anaemia and tachycardia with relative hypotension. Retinal haemorrhage is evidence of cerebral malaria, even in non-comatose subjects.

Investigations

Blood films, thick and thin, show intracellular trophozoites ('ring forms') and, in *falciparum*, crescent-shaped gametocytes. Full blood count reveals anaemia, thrombocytopenia and monocytosis. Eosinophilia does *not* occur in malaria.

Urinalysis for haemoglobinuria, urea and electrolytes for renal function, liver function tests (LFT) and blood sugar monitoring are also required.

Differential diagnosis

Irrespective of the clinical presentation or whether or not prophylactic anti-malarial drugs have been taken, a history of travel to an endemic area makes it mandatory to rule out malaria.

Malaria can and does mimic many other diseases such as typhoid fever, brucellosis, viral hepatitis, arboviral infections (dengue fever), viral haemor-rhagic fevers (Lassa fever), tick typhus and Q fever.

Treatment

P. vivax and *P. ovale* malarias are treated using the '10 tablet chloroquine course' (day 1: chloroquine base 600 mg stat; chloroquine base, 300 mg 8 hours later; days 2–3 chloroquine base 300 mg; then primaquine 15 mg daily for 14–21 days).

The treatment of *P. malariae* malaria is as for *P. vivax* but there is no need for primaquine.

Uncomplicated *P. falciparum* infections where the patient is able to swallow tablets are treated in chloroquine-resistant areas (now widespread) with quinine 10 mg salt/kg every 8 hours for 7 days, combined with tetra-cycline, 4 mg/kg q.d.s. or doxycycline 3 mg/kg daily for 7 days, or with mefloquine 15 mg base/kg followed by 10 mg base/kg 8–24 hours later.

Complicated *P. falciparum* infections where the patient is unable to swal-low are treated in chloroquine-resistant areas with quinine dihydrochloride 20 mg/kg loading dose i.v. infusion over 4 hours, followed by 10 mg/kg i.v. infusion over 4 hours every 8 hours until the patient is able to swallow and complete a 7-day course.

Other aspects of treatment include management in an intensive care unit with monitoring of the pulse, blood pressure (BP), central venous pressure (CVP), urine output, blood gases, blood sugar, renal and hepatic function, haemoglobin, platelet count, coagulation status, and conscious level (Glasgow Coma Scale), and prophylaxis and treatment of fits in cerebral malaria.

Prophylaxis

Recommendations are changed frequently as a result of changing patterns of drug resistance; the British National Formulary or a malaria reference laboratory should be consulted if in doubt.

1. Protection against mosquito bites is the key to prevention: this includes pyrethroid-impregnated mosquito nets, insect repellants (diethyltoluamide), use of long-sleeved clothing and trousers at night, and burning mosquito coils.
2. Countries where *P. falciparum* is sensitive to chloroquine: chloroquine (300 mg base weekly) plus proguanil (200 mg daily).
3. Countries where *P. falciparum* is resistant to chloroquine: either
   (a) mefloquine (250 mg weekly); or
   (b) proguanil (200 mg daily) plus chloroquine (300 mg base weekly); or
   (c) Maloprim (pyrimethamine 12.5 mg, dapsone 100 mg weekly) plus chloroquine (300 mg base weekly).

Prognosis

Vivax and *ovale* malaria are rarely fatal but relapses may occur unless treated with primaquine. Malaria *malariae* is associated with nephrotic syndrome. *Falciparum* malaria, if untreated, can be rapidly fatal in non-immune individuals.

Pregnant, primiparous women, children and asplenic patients are at increased risk of severe *falciparum* malaria. Sickle cell trait and thalassaemia appear to confer some protection.

Complications of *P. falciparum* malaria, many of which are associated with a poor prognosis, include cerebral malaria, which has a 20–50% mortality, acute renal failure (with or without oliguria and haemoglobinuria (blackwater fever)), hepatic failure, hypoglycaemia, hyperpyrexia, electrolyte abnormalities, pulmonary oedema, convulsions, retinal haemorrhages and superimposed Gram-negative septicaemia (algid malaria).

SCHISTOSOMIASIS (BILHARZIASIS)

Schistosomiasis is a very common parasitic infection caused by several species of intravascular trematodes or blood flukes. Three main species of schistosomes infect humans. *Schistosoma haematobium* is prevalent in Africa, the Middle East and Goa, and forms in the bladder venous plexus. *S. mansoni* is found in Africa, Arabia, Brazil, Surinam, Venezuela, the Caribbean, the Nile Delta and infects the inferior mesenteric veins. *S. japonicum* is restricted to China, the Philippines and Indonesia (Sulawesi) and infects the mesenteric veins.

Humans are the definitive host and main reservoir of *S. haematobium*, *S. mansoni* and *S. japonicum* but several mammals also host the latter. Various species of snail act as intermediate hosts.

Pathology

Adult worms remain in intravascular locations for years producing large numbers of ova. These ova penetrate the gut or bladder wall to be excreted to the environment, or become trapped within the organ walls where granulomata develop, or embolise to the liver, lungs or CNS where obstructive granulomata form.

Symptoms

Cercarial dermatitis or swimmers' itch may develop within a few hours of metacercariae penetrating the skin.

Acute schistosomiasis or Katayama fever occurs 3–8 weeks post-infection. It is immune complex mediated. Fever, prostration, diarrhoea, arthritis, lymphadenopathy, hepatosplenomegaly and massive eosinophilia can be fatal.

Established schistosomiasis (see Table 22.1)

Table 22.1. Schistosomiasis

	S. mansoni	*S. haematobium*	*S. japonicum*
Symptoms	*Gastrointestinal:* None or abdominal pain, diarrhoea, dysentery	*Bladder:* None or terminal haematuria, dysuria, nocturia, frequency, suprapubic pain	*Gastrointestinal:* Diarrhoea, dysentery, abdominal pain *CNS:* headaches, convulsions
Signs	Rectosigmoid polyps hepatosplenomegaly, ascites, oedema, cor pulmonale	Anaemia, chronic renal failure (obstructive uropathy) pulmonale	Hepato-splenomegaly, raised intracranial pressure, cor pulmonale
Investigation	Eosinophilia Stools: lateral spined ova Sigmoidoscopy: rectal 'snips' Barium enema Serology	Eosinophilia Urine and stools: terminal spined ova Rectal biopsy Cystoscopy: 'sandy patches' IVU Serology	Eosinophilia Stools: ova Rectal biopsy Serology CT scan: brain Intracranial granulomata which may be calcified
Treatment	Praziquantel 40 mg/kg in 2 divided doses	Praziquantel 40 mg/kg in 2 divided doses	Praziquantel 60 mg/kg in 3 divided doses
Prognosis	Colorectal cancer Pipe stem fibrosis of the liver Portal hypertension Oesophageal varices Cor pulmonale Spinal cord damage	Iron deficiency anaemia Hydronephrosis Hydroureter Fibrous/granulomatous ureteral strictures Bladder wall calcification Bladder papilloma/cancer *S. typhi* carriage in urine Urethral stricture	Oesophageal variceal haemorrhage Liver failure Appendicitis Space-occupying lesions in brain—convulsions

FILARIAL INFECTIONS

Lymphatic filariasis is caused by the nematode parasites *Wuchereria bancrofti*, *Brugia malayi* and *B. timori*. The adult macrofilariae live in lymph glands and vessels causing inflammation and subsequent obstruction. Adult females produce microfilariae which circulate in the blood and are transmitted by a variety of biting mosquitoes.

Loiasis is caused by infection with the filarial worm *Loa loa*, which is transmitted by deer flies of the genus *Chrysops*.

Onchocerciasis is a chronic filarial disease caused by *Onchocerca volvulus* and is transmitted by black flies of the genus *Simulium*. The disease affects the skin, eyes and lymph nodes.

Symptoms and signs (see Table 22.2)

Investigations

Blood films may show microfilariae and eosinophilia. A nucleopore membrane can be used to filter the blood to facilitate diagnosis. Serology will show

Table 22.2. Symptoms and signs of filarial infections ('filariasis')

Species of filarial parasite	Geography	Symptoms and signs
W. bancrofti (nocturnal periodicity)	Asia, Middle-East, Africa, South and Central America, the Caribbean	Acute filarial fever, funiculitis, epididymitis, orchitis, hydrocele, lymphadenitis, genital/limb oedema, elephantiasis, chyluria
W. bancrofti (diurnal subperiodicity)	Pacific islands, Polynesia	As above
B. malayi (nocturnal periodicity)	South-East Asia, Japan, China	Lymphadenitis (inguinal), retrograde lymphadenitis, distal elephantiasis, genitals spared
B. malayi (diurnal subperiodicity)	Malaysia	As for *B. malayi*
B. timori	Indonesia	Filarial abscess
Loa loa	West Africa	Calabar swellings, adult worms under skin and in conjunctivae
O. volvulus	Africa, Yemen, Central and South America	Dermatitis, nodules, keratitis and iritis, causing blindness

anti-filarial antibodies. Chest X-ray may show shadowing due to pulmonary eosinophilia (eosinophilic pneumonia).

Skin snips can be examined for onchocerciasis.

Prognosis

Onchocerciasis can cause blindness. Lymphatic filariasis causes elephantiasis, genital oedema and chylothorax.

Treatment

Diethylcarbamazine is given for 21 days increasing from 1 mg/kg to 6 mg/kg in divided doses over 3 days. Onchocerciasis is treated with ivermectin 150 µg/kg in a single dose. Re-treatment may be needed.

ENTERIC FEVER

In the 10-year period 1981–1990 approximately 1700 cases of typhoid fever were diagnosed in England and Wales; 89% were contracted abroad, mainly on the Indian subcontinent. Less than 15% were infected in the Mediterranean and Middle-East. In the same period, there were 1000 cases of paratyphoid A and B.

Pathology

Salmonella typhi causes enteric fever: *S. paratyphi* types A, B and C cause paratyphoid fever. These micro-organisms are exclusively human pathogens causing acute disease or chronic faecal carriage. Transmission is by food, milk, shellfish or water contaminated with sewage or by a single human carrier.

After ingestion and during the incubation period of 10–14 days, organisms penetrate the intestinal mucosa and spread to the regional lymphatics. Bacteraemia follows with spread of salmonellae to Peyer's patches in the small intestine.

Symptoms and signs

The onset is insidious with malaise, myalgia, anorexia, chills, headache, a dry cough, constipation and rising fever. *Typhoid fever is not usually a diarrhoeal illness*. If untreated, apathy, abdominal pain and distension are seen in the second week and deterioration with delirium in the third.

There is a stepladder rise in temperature. Rose spots, which are pink macules seen over the chest and abdomen, cropping over 1–2 weeks and lasting 3–4 days, occur in about 50% of cases. They are caused by septic emboli. Splenomegaly is present in 40%. There may also be confusion and psychiatric symptoms such as catatonia or psychosis.

Investigations

Blood, urine and stool cultures are obtained, and a full blood count shows leucopenia and lymphocytosis.

Differential diagnosis

This includes malaria, brucellosis, occult bacterial abscess, amoebic liver abscess, infective endocarditis and viral haemorrhagic fever.

Treatment

Based on the sensitivity of the organism, ciprofloxacin, co-trimoxazole or amoxycillin/ampicillin can be used for 14 days. Intravenous dexamethasone is added in severe typhoid fever.

Prognosis

The prognosis is excellent with prompt recognition and appropriate therapy but complications include relapse in 5–10% of patients within 2 weeks of completing therapy, gastrointestinal haemorrhage and perforation in a small percentage, pneumonia, thrombophlebitis, and myocarditis and pericarditis. Metastatic sepsis in the meninges, bones and joints may develop, as may toxic psychosis. Some go on to become chronic faecal carriers.

BRUCELLOSIS

Brucellosis is a zoonosis, endemic in Mediterranean countries and the tropics; 20–30 cases are diagnosed annually in Britain, mostly in returning travellers. It used to be an occupational hazard in vets, abattoir workers and farmers.

Pathology

Brucellae are Gram-negative coccobacilli. The four important species are: *B. abortus* (cattle), *B. melitensis* (sheep, goats, camels), *B. suis* (pigs) and *B. canis* (dogs).

Brucellae are spread by direct contact with animal products of conception, inhalation of infected droplets and ingestion of unpasteurised milk and cheeses. Brucellosis is a disseminated infection, and organisms multiply within the cells of the reticuloendothelial system. Granulomata form in the liver and spleen, and abscess formation occurs in the lymph nodes and the vertebrae.

Symptoms and signs

In acute brucellosis, the incubation period is usually 2–4 weeks but can be several months. The onset may be acute or insidious with fever, chills, night sweats, myalgia, arthralgia and severe fatigue. Splenomegaly occurs in 10–20%, lymphadenopathy in 10%; there is minimal hepatomegaly and variable fever.

Chronic brucellosis causes malaise, lethargy and depression. Splenomegaly is occasionally seen.

Investigations

Prolonged culture of blood, bone marrow, liver and lymph nodes is useful. Serology includes an agglutination test to measure IgM antibodies and a 2-mer-captoethanol test to measure IgG antibodies. An anti-human globulin test is useful in chronic *Brucella* infection (Table 22.3).

Differential diagnosis

Epstein–Barr virus (EBV), cytomegalovirus (CMV), enteric fever, Q fever, tuberculosis, histoplasmosis, malaria, trypanosomiasis, kala-azar, connective tissue disorders, lymphoma and sarcoidosis all need to be considered.

Treatment

Treatment, lasting 4–6 weeks, is with doxycycline 200 mg daily plus strepto-mycin i.m. 0.75–1.0 g per 24 hours. For chronic cases oxytetracycline or doxycycline plus rifampicin, or co-trimoxazole plus doxycycline or rifampicin or streptomycin is given for 6–12 weeks.

Prognosis

Unrecognised brucellosis may become chronic. Acute brucellosis may be complicated by granulomatous hepatitis, meningitis, arthritis, spondylitis of lumbar, thoracic and cervical vertebrae, paravertebral and psoas abscesses, endocarditis and epididymo-orchitis.

Table 22.3. Serological investigations of brucellosis

	Acute brucellosis	Chronic brucellosis	Past brucellosis
Agglutination test (IgM)	>1/320	Low titre (<1/80)	Variable 1/10–1/640
2-Mercaptoethanol (IgG)	>1/320	Low titre (<1/80)	Low titre (<1/40)
Anti-human globulin test	Negative	>1/160	Low titre (<1/80)

Cross reactions occur with antibodies to *Yersinia enterocolitica* 09 and Cholera vaccination.

AMOEBIASIS

Amoebiasis is a widespread human and primate infection of the gastro-intestinal (GI) tract by the protozoan *Entamoeba histolytica*. Most common in the tropics and subtropics, the infection is acquired by ingestion of cysts and is associated with poor sanitation, inadequate food hygiene and male homosexual practices.

Pathology

Amoebic dysentery affects the caecum and colon. Mucosal ulcers extend into the submucosa as 'collar stud' abscesses and infection may spread to the liver and occasionally to the lungs and brain. A granulomatous mass may rarely develop in the caecum (amoeboma).

Symptoms and signs

Many patients are asymptomatic or symptomless cyst excretors (carriers). Amoebic dysentery has an insidious onset with mild to severe bloody diarrhoea. Abdominal pain is mild and there is rectal tenesmus but no fever and little systemic toxicity. It can become fulminant, e.g. in pregnant women, the immunocompromised, or with steroid therapy.

Liver abscess affects 20–60-year-olds, M > F. Usually it is a single abscess in the right lobe of the liver. Concurrent amoebic dysentery is absent. There is sudden onset of pain over the liver, referred to the shoulder tip or scapula. Fever, anorexia and weight loss occur. Tenderness over the liver and right basal pleural effusion develops.

Investigations

In amoebic dysentery, proctoscopy is needed for a rectal smear and microscopy reveals motile, haematophagous trophozoites which contain red blood cells. The serology is IFAT-positive in 75% of cases.

For liver abscess, scanning (ultrasound or CT) shows a fluid-containing cavity. The serology is IFAT-positive in 95%. The cellulose acetate precipitation (CAP) test is positive after 10–14 days and negative after treatment.

Differential diagnosis

Amoebic dysentery
Inflammatory bowel disease (ulcerative colitis, Crohn's colitis), pseudomembranous colitis, ischaemic colitis, bacillary dysentery and bacterial colitis have similar clinical features.

Amoebic liver abscess
Pyogenic abscess, hydatid cyst of the liver and hepatoma must be considered.

Treatment

Amoebic dysentery, liver abscess and amoeboma are treated with oral metronidazole or tinidazole for 5–10 days. Percutaneous aspiration may be needed if the abscess fails to resolve, or if rupture is imminent. A colectomy is required for fulminating amoebiasis. Cyst excretors should be treated with diloxanide furoate for 10 days.

Prognosis

Most patients with amoebic dysentery respond to therapy, and haemorrhage, perforation, peritonitis and amoeboma are uncommon. Metastatic amoebiasis of the liver, lung and brain can occur. Amoebic infection can extend from the anal canal to the skin, vulva, vagina, cervix, penis or give rise to chronic post-operative sinuses.

TRYPANOSOMIASIS

Trypanosomes are flagellated protozoan parasites. *Trypanosoma brucei rhodesiense* and *T. brucei gambiense* are subspecies and cause East African and West African trypanosomiasis respectively, collectively known as 'sleeping sickness'.
T. cruzi causes American trypanosomiasis, Chagas' disease.

AFRICAN TRYPANOSOMIASIS

Approximately 20 000 cases are reported annually to the World Health Organization. Transmission is by various species of tsetse fly (*Glossina*). West African trypanosomiasis occurs in forests and riparian woodland and affects local populations, while East African trypanosomiasis is associated with savanna and mammals—antelope, bush buck, hartebeest. Tourists and game wardens are at risk.

Pathology

A trypanosomal chancre develops at the site of inoculation and causes blood and lymphatic dissemination, and eventual meningo-encephalitis. West African trypanosomiasis is a chronic protracted disease lasting for years. East African trypanosomiasis is of rapid onset, with death in < 6 months due to myocarditis or early meningo-encephalitis.

Symptoms and signs

There is variable fever, headache, malaise, myalgia and arthralgia.
A trypanosomal chancre, seen at the site of tsetse fly bite, is painful, indurated and up to several centimetres in diameter. There is a transient erythematous rash called circinate erythema.

Splenomegaly, hepatomegaly and lymphadenopathy occur, as does peripheral oedema. A variety of neurological signs including tremors, chorea, cranial neuropathy, ataxia, psychosis, somnolence and coma are present.

Investigations

Giemsa-stained blood film and tissue fluid show trypanosomes. Serology: IFAT (immuno-fluorescent antibody test); ELISA (enzyme-linked immuno-sorbent assay).

CSF examination will show raised pressure, lymphocytic pleocytosis, morular cells of Mott (foamy plasma cells), a raised protein and the presence of trypanosomes.

Differential diagnosis

Rabies and viral encephalitis must be excluded.

Treatment

Suramin is used for both types. Pentamidine is suitable for West African trypanosomiasis and if the CNS is involved, melarsoprol, an arsenical, is used. Recently, eflornithine has been advocated for West African trypanosomiasis.

Prognosis

Trypanosomiasis is fatal if untreated, usually from myocarditis or encephalitis. Intercurrent infection leading to bronchopneumonia is common. Death can be the result of drug toxicity—melarsoprol has a 5% fatality rate.

AMERICAN TRYPANOSOMIASIS—CHAGAS' DISEASE

Infection with *T. cruzi*, a widespread zoonosis of Central and South America affecting 10–12 million people, is transmitted via the faeces of triatomine bugs of the Reduviidae family. Parasites enter the body via bite sites, mucosal surfaces or conjunctivae. Transmission by blood transfusion, laboratory accident and via the placenta has been described.

Pathology

There is inflammation and subsequent fibrosis of the heart and GI tract. The cardiac conduction system and the myenteric plexus of the GI tract are affected.

Symptoms and signs

Acute disease is mostly asymptomatic. Others experience malaise, headaches, irritability and myalgia. Entry via the eye causes palpebral oedema, conjunctivitis and local lymphadenopathy (Romaña's sign). A chagoma, an inflamed ulcer at the point of entry, may be seen. Fever, subcutaneous oedema and splenomegaly all occur.

Cardiac involvement ranges from asymptomatic ECG abnormalities (first degree heart block, right bundle branch block, ST-T wave abnormalities) to symptomatic heart block and ventricular arrhythmias (causing dizziness and syncope) and myocardial failure (causing symptoms of congestive cardiac failure). GI involvement results in impaired smooth muscle function causing megaoesophagus, dilatation of the stomach and small intestine, and mega-colon, resulting in dysphagia, regurgitation, flatulence, abdominal distension and constipation. Pulmonary infarction is sometimes seen.

Investigations

These include microscopy of a blood film for trypanosomes, Giemsa stains of blood films, haemoculture and serology.

Differential diagnosis

This is very wide and includes glandular fever, toxoplasmosis, myocarditis, acute glomerulonephritis, acute schistosomiasis, tuberculosis, brucellosis, meningo-encephalitis, etc.

Treatment

Treatment is with nifurtimox or benzonidazole for acute Chagas' disease.

Prognosis

In acute Chagas' disease there is a 10% mortality from myocarditis and meningo-encephalitis. In chronic disease, between 20 and 50% of patients develop heart failure with a high risk also of sudden death.

Megaoesophagus leads to aspiration pneumonia and malnutrition while megacolon can lead to sigmoid torsion.

LEISHMANIASIS

Visceral, cutaneous and mucocutaneous syndromes are caused by organisms of the genus *Leishmania*. Disease manifestations depend on the species of parasite, geographical location and immune status of the patient. Approxi-mately 10 million people are infected annually, of whom 400 000 have visceral leishmaniasis. *Leishmania* are transmitted by biting sandflies (Table 22.4). The zoonotic reservoir includes dogs, foxes, rodents and man.

In cutaneous leishmaniasis, single or multiple painless papular-ulcerative lesions may last up to a year. They heal spontaneously, leaving atrophic, depigmented scars.

In diffuse cutaneous leishmaniasis, large numbers of parasites spread throughout the skin.

Table 22.4. Clinical types of Leishmaniasis

Form of disease	New world parasite	Old world parasite
Cutaneous		
Simple	*L. braziliensis guyanensis*	*L. major*—Mediterranean
	L. braziliensis panamensis	*L. tropica*—Mediterranean
	L. mexicana mexicana	India, Greece
Diffuse	*L. mexicana amazonensis*	*L. Aethiopica*—Africa
Mucocutaneous	*L. braziliensis braziliensis*	
Visceral	*L. Donovani chagasi*	*L. Donovani donovani*—India, China, East Africa
		L. donovani infantum—Middle-East, China, Africa, Mediterranean

Mucocutaneous leishmaniasis occurs only in Latin America, months to years after recovery from a cutaneous ulcer caused by *L. braziliensis braziliensis*. There are destructive lesions of nasal and oropharyngeal mucosa.

Visceral leishmaniasis (VL or kala-azar) is caused by the *L. donovani* complex. Parasites disseminate to the reticuloendothelial system. VL is characterised by progressive splenomegaly, hepatomegaly, pancytopenia, fever, weight loss and a tendency to secondary bacterial and mycobacterial infections.

Investigations

These include biopsy of cutaneous lesions to demonstrate intracellular amastigotes (Leishman-Donovan bodies). Serology (IFAT or ELISA) and splenic, liver and bone marrow histology are needed.

Treatment

This is with pentavalent antimonial drugs, e.g. sodium stibogluconate, meglumine antimonate and oral or topical paromomycin.

Prognosis

Ninety-five per cent will be cured by antimonial drug therapy but with VL there may be intercurrent infection, especially of the respiratory and GI tracts. Intestinal and vaginal haemorrhage occurs, as does tuberculosis with post kala-azar or dermal leishmaniasis. Reactivation may occur in immuno-compromised and HIV-infected patients.

LASSA FEVER

This is a serious acute febrile illness caused by an arenavirus which is excreted by the rat *Mastomys natalensis* in its urine, thereby contaminating food, abrasions, etc. Person-to-person spread occurs via all body fluids. It is found in West Africa.

Symptoms and signs

After an incubation period of 2–3 weeks, fever, headache, prostration and severe pharyngitis accompany lymphadenopathy, vomiting, diarrhoea and chest pain. A maculopapular rash develops on the trunk after 10–14 days and mucosal bleeding occurs. Oliguria and hypotension with renal failure and coma are extremely bad signs.

Investigations

Although largely a clinical diagnosis, leucopenia, impaired platelet function and isolation of the virus are, together with antibody studies, the important investigations.

Treatment

This is symptomatic, but special care is required to preserve hydration. Ribavarin reduces mortality. Secure isolation facilities to protect medical and nursing staff should be available.

HELMINTH INFESTATION: WORMS AND FLUKES

See Tables 22.5 and 22.6.

Table 22.5. Nematodes (round worms)

Name	Life cycle
Ascaris lumbricoides	Common in tropics from faecal contamination (eggs) of food and water Larvae traverse lungs, pharynx and then gut
Ancylostoma duodenale *Necator americanus* (hook worm)	Worms about 1 cm long Larvae from gut enter skin, travel to lung and develop in small bowel Common in tropics
Strongyloides stercoralis (strongyloidiasis)	Worms approx 2 mm long Inhabit gut Transmitted as per hook worm Pulmonary larval phase occurs Found in tropics and in AIDS
Enterobius vermicularis (threadworms)	Usually in children Threadlike worms cause intense perianal pruritus Auto infection maintains the infestation
Trichinella spiralis (trichinosis)	Worms are the result of consuming undercooked meat, the meat containing larvae which penetrate lumen of gut and disseminate widely
Toxocara canis or cati (toxocariasis)	Humans infected from dog and cat faeces Larvae then disseminate 15% of soil samples in England show larvae Visceral larva migrans causes fever with eosinophilia There may be hepatosplenomegaly

Effects/diagnosis	Treatment
Occasional pulmonary infiltrates (pulmonary eosinophilia) and fever Can obstruct gut or bile ducts or be vomited *Diagnosis*: Eggs ++ in faeces	Mebendazole 100 mg b.d. for 3 days Prevented by not using human faeces on crops
Anaemia due to gut blood loss Hb may be 5 g or less Congestive heart failure may occur *Diagnosis*: Eggs ++ in faeces	Mebendazole 100 mg b.d. for 3 days Encourage wearing of shoes and safe disposal of faeces
Usually none May be diarrhoea and malabsorption Occasional urticaria Massive infestation in patients who are immunosuppressed Causes an often fatal septicaemic disorder *Diagnosis*: Larvae in duodenal aspirate Eosinophilia	Thiabendazole 25 mg/kg (max. 1.5 g) b.d. for 3 days *or* albendazole 400 mg b.d. for 3 days *or* ivermectin 200 µg/kg o.d. for 2 days Prevention: as for hook worm Consider prophylactic thiabendazole for immunosuppressed patients
Pruritus ani Sometimes vulvo-vaginitis *Diagnosis*: Scotch tape swab from perineal skin for eggs or recognition of egg-laying female worms	Mebendazole 100 mg as a single dose repeated after 2–3 weeks: not in children under 2 Prevent finger sucking, nail biting and encourage hand washing after use of toilet
Fever, orbital oedema, muscle pains and eosinophilia May be CNS and heart involvement *Diagnosis*: Muscle biopsy for encysted larvae	Thiabendazole 25 mg/kg up to 1.5 g twice daily for 5 days
Ocular form: Causes loss of vision due to retinal or lens lesions Visceral larva migrans *Diagnosis*: ELISA toxocara antibody test	Diethylcarbamazine in a 21-day course. *Note*: ocular disease may not respond as the causative worm is dead Prophylaxis: regular de-worming of dogs Collection of dog faeces

Table 22.6. Trematodes (flukes) and cestodes (tape worms)

Name	Life cycle
Schistosomiasis	see p. 516
Fasciola hepatica (fascioliasis) (Sheep liver fluke)	Fluke (3 cm × 1.5 cm) invades biliary tree Miracidia from faecal larvae—penetrates a freshwater snail and then encysts on watercress and other aquatic flora before being eaten by sheep or man
Taenia saginata (beef tape worm)	Worm (bisexual) inhibits small gut; segments passed in faeces From undercooked beef Common in Africa, South America and Middle-East
Taenia solium★ (pig tape worm)	Uncooked pork
Diphyllobothrium latum (fish tape worm)	Uncooked fish
Echinococcus granulosus (hydatid disease)	The dog tape worm, usual intermediate host sheep—thus direct contact with dogs or contaminated pasture and sheep causative Common in sheep-rearing areas

★Cysticercosis—human infection with an intermediate stage of *T. solium*—can occur by ingestion of worm eggs. Encystation occurs in the tissues, and in the muscles they may calcify. Occasionally epilepsy, hydrocephalus and visual disturbances can occur. CNS involvement is diagnosed by CT scanning and positive serological tests. Praziquantel in a 14-day course is effective.

Effects/diagnosis	Treatment
Upper abdominal pain Fever, chills, hepatomegaly and occasionally jaundice *Diagnosis*: Eggs + in stools Eosinophilia	Bithionol 40 mg/kg given as a twice daily dose for 15 days Isolation of sheep from watercress beds
Usually none Sometimes patient notices segments or larger pieces of worm *Diagnosis*: stool segments	Praziquantel 10 mg/kg as single dose If no segments passed for 4 months, the patient is cured Prophylaxis: thorough cooking of beef
Nil *Diagnosis*: Microscopy of segments	As for *T. saginata* with purging 2 hours after treatment
General symptoms may occur with fatigue, etc. and there may be vitamin B_{12} deficiency due to consumption of B_{12} in the gut *Diagnosis*: Eggs in faeces	Praziquantel as for *T. saginata*
Large and sometimes multiple cysts in liver, lung, bone, etc. causing cystic swellings Occasional rupture into bronchus or abdomen with anaphylaxis and collapse *Diagnosis*: Complement fixation tests, CT scanning	Mebendazole and albendazole may help Surgery may be required for solitary hepatic and pulmonary cysts and secondary abscess is an important complication

Index

ON THE WARD – ON HAND

CHURCHILL'S POCKETBOOK OF

Medicine

SECOND EDITION

P. C. HAYES
T. W. MACKAY
E. H. FORREST

1996   416 pages   illustrated
plastic binding   0 443 05325 1

When you need rapid access to the essential information, **Churchill's Pocketbook of Medicine** provides a concise and convenient source of clinical data.

The intelligent layout and clear presentation highlights definitions, practical advice, clinical features and management strategies, giving you what you want when you want it.

Churchill's Pocketbook of Medicine

 contains the essential details for confident clinical practice

 gives invaluable data on drug usage, adverse reactions and interactions

 provides practical advice with a disease-oriented approach

ON THE WARD – ON HAND

CHURCHILL'S POCKETBOOK OF

Surgery

A. T. RAFTERY

1996   472 pages   illustrated
plastic binding   0 443 05057 0

This pocketbook provides a concise and didactic account of the essential features of all common surgical disorders at a size and a price to suit the pocket. It is an essential on-the-ward reference for every medical student and junior doctor. Covering all the surgical specialties in one volume, the text outlines basic principles, aetiology, management and pre- and post-operative care.

CHURCHILL'S POCKETBOOK OF

Surgery

A. T. RAFTERY

Churchill's Pocketbook of Surgery

 covers all the surgical specialties in one pocket-sized volume

 effectively communicates important clinical points with charts, tables, lists and diagrams

 quick and easy reference to practical treatment descriptions and emergency procedures.